HEALTH POLICY AND THE NHS
TOWARDS 2000

LONGMAN SOCIAL POLICY IN BRITAIN SERIES

Health Policy and the NHS Towards 2000

Judith Allsop

2nd Edition

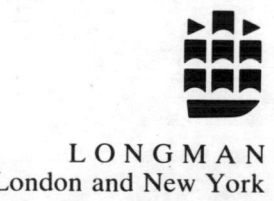

LONGMAN
London and New York

Longman Group Limited,
Longman House, Burnt Mill,
Harlow, Essex CM20 2JE, England
and Associated Companies throughout the world.

Published in the United States of America
by Longman Publishing, New York

First published 1984
Second edition 1995

ISBN 0 582 042798 PPR

British Library Cataloguing-in-Publication Data

A catalogue record for this book is
available from the British Library

Library of Congress Cataloging-in-Publication Data

Allsop, Judy, 1938–
Health policy and the NHS / Judith Allsop. — 2nd ed.
p. cm. — (Longman social policy in Britain series)
Includes bibliographical references and index.
ISBN 0–582–04279–8
1. Medical policy—Great Britain. 2. National Health Service (Great Britain) I. Title. II. Series.
RA395.G6A654 1995
362.1′0941—dc20 94–28346
CIP

Set by 5 in 10 on 11pt Times Roman
Printed in Malaysia

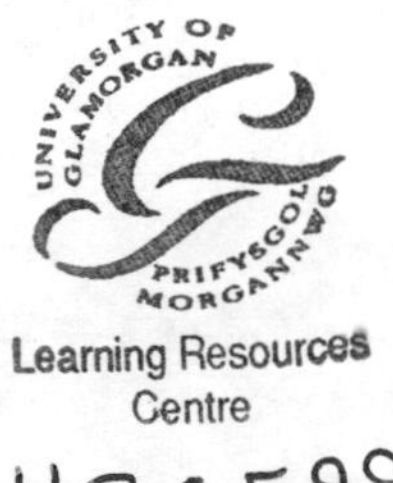

CONTENTS

LIST OF FIGURES AND TABLES

PREFACE

The first edition of this book was written in the early 1980s. Since then, there have been significant changes in the direction of health policy and the mode of delivery of health services. There has been a policy shift from an almost total focus on illness services towards a greater emphasis on the prevention of ill-health, primary care and greater responsiveness to the needs of the health service user. On the supply side, the 1990 reforms brought significant changes by introducing an internal market into the NHS.

This second edition of *Health Policy and the NHS* broadly follows the same structure as the first. The early chapters have been revised to take account of new work and the last section deals with NHS changes since the first edition of the book was written. Like the previous edition, this edition has a documents section which provides excerpts from key texts; new excerpts have been added to take account of the decade of change between the early 1980s and the present.

In various sections of the book, I draw on work I have published elsewhere – in particular, on general practice; on NHS managers (with Annabelle May) and on policies for preventing ill-health (with Richard Freeman).

Since the first edition, I have been a member of a Family Practitioner Committee, a District Health Authority and a Special Health Authority. This has provided a view of health policy from the inside from which I have benefited greatly. It was a particular fascination to listen to the language of those concerned with health policy change. Whether by conscious choice or not, the use of different words and concepts marked a shift in attitudes and were used to persuade or cajole others to accept changes in the way in which health care was provided.

I have also worked with colleagues at the King's Fund College and what was then the King's Fund Centre, on a number of projects. And I much enjoyed their company as well as learning a great deal from their collective expertise.

I am enormously grateful to a number of people who supported the production of the final draft. Claire Shirley helped to assemble the background material and always responded with promptness and good humour to a variety of requests. She took on responsibility for producing the graphics. Marie Selwood read the document through and gave invaluable editorial comments.

Oye Oduwaiye valiantly maintained the management of files in successive drafts. Jo Campling initiated the proposal for the first edition and provided helpful chivying to work on the second. I have been fortunate too, to be able to draw on the knowledge of Annabelle May, and the forbearance and practical help of Peter and Ellinor.

Judith Allsop
March 1994

INTRODUCTION

Health services and policies to promote health have developed as part of modern welfare states. The form they have taken has been shaped by the social structure and institutions in different countries as well as by socio-demographic and economic factors. The policies of particular governments have reflected both political ideology and the effect of structured interests within the health policy arena. The main focus of this book is on health policy and the provision of health services in the UK.[1] It aims to give an account of the interplay of the various factors in relation to particular policy themes. While the major part of the book relates to the period from the 1940s to the late 1980s, the development of state involvement in health policy from the second half of the nineteenth century and the period since the 1990 health service reforms is also discussed in some detail. Indeed, this historical sweep is important to identify the major shifts which have occurred in the focus of health policy and the role of government in these changes.

The book has four parts and is arranged broadly along historical lines. Part one deals with the period prior to, and including, the establishment of the NHS. Part two gives an account of the policy themes which have dominated the government's policy agenda until the late 1980s. Part three gives an account of the critiques of health policy which developed in the late 1970s and 1980s. Part four covers the health service reforms and associated policy shifts.

Part one, Chapter 1 introduces the main argument of the book. It is suggested that health policy has two main strands. The first relates to issues concerned with the protection of health in populations and the second involves the provision of illness services to individuals. Initially, the role of governments was limited to the former. However, with the development of modern medicine, the emphasis switched. Government intervention focused on mediating the effect of market forces in relation to personal illness services. Different models of intervention were possible. With the establishment of the NHS, health services in the UK were provided through what has been termed a 'command and control' economy. Not only was policy mainly determined by government but the institutions which provided health services were also dominated by Westminster.

During the latter half of the 1970s and the early 1980s, a range of critiques of health care and the NHS developed. These eventually led to a number of shifts in health policy. There was more emphasis on a wider approach which incorporated policies to prevent ill-health, and the care of those who were chronically ill or in need of support services. In 1990, competition between agencies supplying health care was introduced. This has brought a more diverse pattern of services and greater volatility in the interaction of interest groups within the health care arena. Chapter 2 examines the institutionalisation of medicine and governments' approach to health policy prior to the 1946 NHS Act. The alignment of various interest groups and the accommodations reached are described.

Part two, 'Policy Issues in the NHS', is an examination of a number of issues which have been of concern to government throughout the history of the NHS. Chapter 3 analyses the factors which led to the recurrent reorganisations as various Ministers of Health strove to increase the effectiveness through restructuring management, introducing planning systems and by top-down exhortation. Chapter 4 considers issues of funding the NHS, how Britain compares with other countries, resource allocation within the service and questions of efficiency and the measurement of outcomes. Chapter 5 looks at the dilemmas over policies for the care of dependent groups, including the proposals put forward in the 1990 Community Care Act.

Part three, 'Health and Society', considers the criticisms of health policy made during the 1970s. It is suggested that these, together with perceptions of past policy failure, helped to bring about the policy shift which culminated in the 1990 NHS and Community Care Act. Chapter 6 looks at the rediscovery of the links between poverty, social strata and ill-health. Chapter 7 examines the various critiques of health care which developed in the 1970s. These, together with other factors, led to greater questioning of health policy despite rising expenditures, and there was a sense of crisis. The American policy analyst Aaron Wildavsky (1980) referred to a sense of 'doing better and feeling worse' which was common across countries. There was a greater scepticism about the benefits of health care and a movement towards the more diffuse and difficult goal of improving the general health of the population.

Part four, 'New Directions for Health Policy', examines aspects of health policy in the 1990s. Chapter 8 describes the changes make by the 1980s Conservative governments. Chapter 9 outlines the 1990 health care reforms and the criticisms of them. Chapter 10 looks at policies in the context of general practice and Chapter 11 examines policies for prevention. Chapter 12 assesses policies aimed to empower the users of health services. Finally, Chapter 13 summarises the dilemmas within each policy area, highlights the issues which have not been included in the government's policy agenda and examines the effect of recent policy on the configuration of interests in health care.

Reference

Wildavsky, A. (1980) *The Art and Craft of Policy Analysis*, Macmillan, London.

Note

1 In the United Kingdom (England, Wales, Scotland and Northern Ireland), there are differences in the organisation of health services. These are not a focus of attention in this book. By and large, health policies, as opposed to the form of delivery, apply to the UK as a whole.

PART ONE

Foundations and Framework

CHAPTER 1

Health policy and the politics of the NHS: an overview

This chapter aims to define some of the key terms used in this book. It goes on to examine a number of alternative theoretical models for providing health services. There then follows a general account of the characteristics of the NHS from 1948 to 1990, which has been referred to as a 'command and control' economy. The policies of health care within the NHS are then described. The chapter concludes with a summary of the social and economic changes which form a background to policy shifts within the NHS.

Key concepts and models of health care intervention

The key concepts used in the book are health, health policy, health services and health care, policy paradigms, the politics of the NHS and politics within the NHS. The models discussed are the market model, the professional model and the bureaucratic model of health care provision.

Health, health policy, health services and health care

Health can be defined in two ways. The focus can be on individual ill-health. Le Grand (1982) implicitly puts emphasis on the absence of illness in the following quotation:

> Health affects every aspect of life. Our ability to work, to play, to enjoy our families and to socialise with friends, all depend crucially upon our physical well-being. Serious illnesses create enormous pain and suffering, even minor transient ailments can be depressing psychologically as well as debilitating physically. And ill health which leads to death makes all other services of satisfaction irrelevant.
>
> (Le Grand 1982: 23)

Alternatively, emphasis may be placed on protecting the health of populations. This is summed up in a quotation from the 1974 report on The Health of Canadians (the Lalonde Report) which declares:

> Good health is the bedrock on which social progress is built. A nation of healthy people can do those things which make life worthwhile and as the level of health increases so does the potential for happiness.
> (Ministry of National Health and Welfare (Canada), 1974: preface)

Both these quotations suggest why governments may develop policies for health: whether these are to protect individuals – from the devastating effects of loss of income through illness and the high cost of health care; or, whether these focus on social and health policies which allow the maintenance of health and protection from the hazards and threats which might damage it. Indeed, governments may be voted into office to take actions in these respects.

The term 'health policy' has been limited mainly to the policies of governments. That is, to the authoritative statements of intent about action which relate to the maintenance of good health in individuals and populations; the cure of disease and illness; and the care of the vulnerable and frail. Other institutions in society also make statements about health. Although these are referred to, the assumption is that as government has the ultimate authority to act, it is their policies which become a focus for debate and action.

An alternative view is that policy, far from being encapsulated in statements of intent, is the consequence of the actions taken by individuals in the process of implementation (see Barrett and Fudge 1981). In other words, in the process of implementation, policy becomes translated into something quite different from what was intended; what policy is can only be seen in terms of outcomes. The view taken here is that the policy process is cyclical. Government statements of intent have been taken as the main starting point. In being implemented, policies may be, and indeed often are, distorted by the interpretations, actions or inertia of lower-level actors. Such distortions reflect the relative power of individuals or groups. This aspect of policy is discussed later in this chapter. It is therefore particularly difficult to determine policy outcomes; research or evaluation is often required of government policies boldly stated in official documents.

The term 'health services' refers to the type and range of facilities provided by health professionals and agencies. This can be sub-divided further – thus, there are mental health services, primary care services or acute hospital services and so on. And 'health care' is taken to be the result of activities undertaken by individual health workers within various organisations.

Policy paradigms

Rein (1976) suggests that a policy paradigm is based on a particular view of the essential problem to be solved.

It is a working model of why things are as they are, a problem-solving framework, which supplies values and benefits, but also procedures, habits of thought, and a view of how society functions. It often provides a guiding metaphor of how the world works which implies a general direction for intervention, it *is* more specific than an ideology or a system of beliefs, but broader than a principle of intervention.

(Rein 1976: 103)

Rein goes on to suggest that policy paradigms are a 'curious mixture of psychological assumptions, scientific concepts, value commitments, social aspirations, personal beliefs and administrative constraints'. In order to shift, they must be challenged by an alternative view of the world which appears to fit current problems better.

Within health policy, there can be any number of policy paradigms. One which reflects different conceptions of health has already been referred to above. Government policies may focus on the care or treatment of illness in individuals and on personal illness services and/or on the maintenance and promotion of health in individuals or populations. This will have a profound effect on what problems are identified, on the way services are provided, who are considered to be the authoritative providers and who is deemed to be the main object of policy. Figure 1.1 illustrates the implications of a paradigm shift from an illness-based to a preventive model.

Illness	Health
Treatment	Prevention
Cure	Care
Disease	Behaviour producing disease
Individual	Population as unit of treatment
Illness as concern of medical profession	Health as business of everybody, biocrats, social services
Right to treatment	Duty to remain healthy

Figure 1.1 ***Shift in emphasis in the conceptualisation of health and illness***

Source: Illsley, R. (1977) Health and Health Policy.

A further paradigm shift can be illustrated in relation to the care of people with special needs. For example there has been a shift in relation to ideas about delivery – from institutional care to community care or, more recently, from a monopoly supplier to a number of competitors. Within medical care there are three theoretical options for supplying a service.

Models for the supply of medical services

Models are simply constructs of possibilities which rarely exist in any pure form. If it is assumed that all individuals will need medical care during their lifetime and there is no such thing as perfect health, access to the best possible care for those who are ill is of fundamental importance. This may be supplied according to a market, a professional or a bureaucratic model.

A market model assumes that health care is a product like any other. Where a demand exists, then market forces will supply the goods required for a price. Market theory suggests that suppliers, as individuals or corporations, will harness available technologies to provide health care relative to demand from users for that price. Suppliers will advertise their wares while competition will ensure a price which gives a margin of profit and that consumer preferences are met. In theory the consumer is sovereign while the 'hidden hand' of market forces ensures the most efficient use of scarce resources by matching supply and demand. In this context, the market has the authority to determine resource allocation.

However, particularly since the rise of medical science in the nineteenth century, two other models have developed – the professional and the bureaucratic models. Both these assume medical care is too important and knowledge too specialised to be treated as a market good. The professional model places authority over medical care with the expert – the doctor. Because it is based on technical and expert knowledge, those who need medical care must be protected from unqualified practitioners. This may include the authority to determine training and qualifications and to judge what is in the interest of the patient. The approach is essentially paternalistic. Although in modern states, arrangements may be made to ensure access to doctors for the whole population, the medical profession remains dominant in determining the shape of the health care system.

In the bureaucratic model, the state takes over the role of determining health policy. This tends to be encouraged by the democratic process as governments represent the interests of citizens who collectively put a high value on health care. In this model, the emphasis is on the rights of citizenship and the state becomes involved in distributional issues such as: ensuring access to services according to equity criteria; the allocation of resources; the management of services and the ordering of priorities. The benefits to the collectivity as well as to the individual are stressed.

In actual welfare or health states, governments mediate between the market and the professional providers in a variety of different ways. For example, Titmuss (1958) referred to the residual, occupational and institutional-redistributive models of welfare. In the residual model, the family and the market were the main props for welfare, the state had a minor role in supporting the poor. In the occupational model, the employer and the fiscal system provided the major share of welfare. While in the institutional-redistributive model the state intervenes to provide redistribution benefits through the tax system. Epsing Anderson (1990), although he does not refer to health as such, discusses the liberal, corporatist-statist and socio-democratic welfare state models.

In the UK until the 1980s, the dominant model has been institutional-redistributive. By democratic mandate, a bureaucractic, centrally controlled system of health care was introduced in 1948. The choices made by government on behalf of the population are legitimised by government's representative character. At the same time, because of the dominance of scientific medicine, this still results in a powerful medical profession. Elston (1991) describes the cultural (the high value given to medical knowledge) and social (medical dominance in the division of labour) authority of medicine and the high degree of professional autonomy it enjoys. This forms part of the NHS 'command and control' economy described in more detail below.

Health care politics and the politics of the NHS

It has been argued that because scientific medicine has dominated health care provision in most modern welfare states, there is a typical form of health care politics. Conflicts and struggles for ascendency in relation to both policy and provision occur between structured interests configured around the state, the medical profession and, in some countries, health care funders and commercial interests.

For example, Alford (1975) suggests that interests in health care can be classified into three major groupings: the professional monopolisers, the corporate rationalisers and the community interest. These interest groups have certain aims and objectives and their power is structured in particular ways. The dominant interest group, he argues, contains the professional monopolisers – doctors whose control of medical knowledge both explains and reinforces the dominance of the disease model of illness. Although numerically small, in contrast to for example nurses, their definitions of health and illness tend to dominate health policy and provision. Alford comments:

> Physicians have extracted an arbitrary set from an array of skills and knowledge relevant to the maintenance of health in a population and have successfully sold these as their property for a price and have managed to create legal mechanisms which enforce that monopoly and the social beliefs which mystify that population about the appropriateness and desirability of that monopoly.
>
> (Alford 1975: 197)

The second major interest group is composed of 'the corporate rationalisers'. This includes politicians, administrators at central and local level, and some professionals whose main objective is to achieve greater coordination and integration in the planning and delivery of health services. Their interests lie in improving efficiency and effectiveness and making the best use of the health resources of the collectivity.

The third interest group identified by Alford is 'the community interest'; that is, the cluster of organisations and individuals which seek to represent a different order of priorities, alternative perspectives on health policy and perhaps a broader view of health care. They attempt to influence health policy through a variety of means, from lobbying the legislature to picketing local hospitals. In most health systems, community interests tend to be suppressed. The major forces of authoritative decisions are the professionals and government Ministers and officials who make decisions behind closed doors.

The politics of the NHS

On the basis of the above or similar types of analysis, it has been argued that the politics of the NHS are essentially concerned with the relationships between the two powerful interest groups, the government and the medical profession. Indeed, it has been argued that UK health politics is corporatist in style. That is, health policy is developed by the government and the medical profession, achieved by negotiation and compromise away from public scrutiny (Cawson 1982).

Harrison, Hunter and Pollitt (1990) review approaches to policy-making in the NHS and conclude that a version of the corporatist thesis, a process of what they call 'mutual partisan adjustment', occurs. In other words, the various structured-interest groups adjust to each other in shaping policy within a framework of accepted conventions. The model is reproduced in Document 7 (page 296). It may be of course, that this particular explanation of policy-making applied specifically to mainstream policies within the NHS between 1946 and 1990. This issue is addressed in Chapter 13.

The corporatist approach tends to take an over-simple view of health care politics with little recognition that the political interplay of groups may vary. Empirical studies suggest diversity. For example, Mills (1993) in a collection of studies on preventive health policy, shows that a variety of interest groups seeks to put pressure on government and in some cases they have had a decisive effect on outcome (see Chapter 11). Day and Klein (1991) indicate that policies vary over time. However, NHS politics, at least between 1948 and 1989, tended to be predominantly corporate in character. I now examine the characteristics of the NHS in this period as it forms a backdrop to the more detailed consideration of policies in Parts two and three of this book.

A command and control economy

From the establishment of the emergency medical services in World War Two to the 1990 NHS and Community Care Act and the publication of the White Paper on *The Health of the Nation* (DOH 1992), the dominant policy paradigm within the NHS has been the provision of a range of personal illness services to individuals. During the 1980s, there was a shift towards the prevention of ill-health in populations, and the reforms of the late 1980s began to replace the command and control economy with the supply of health services through more loosely linked competing agencies, although many crucial features remain (Chapter 9 indicates the changes). In terms of the models introduced above, the dominant form was a social-democratic/bureaucratic model which gave considerable autonomy to professional providers, particularly doctors, within the system. Over most policy areas at a national level, NHS politics were corporatist. At the local level, within health authorities, funding was skewed towards illness services despite efforts made centrally to shift resources towards caring services for frail and vulnerable people.

As established under the 1946 Act, the NHS was democratic in the sense that it rested on a social and political consensus. The consensus was on issues of principle – that the whole population should have access to illness services on the basis of need, free at the point of delivery. Health services were funded from taxation. Policy was made centrally in the health department and there was a hierarchy of health authorities from a central department, through regions to local level authorities. The fact that the Health Minister was accountable to Parliament for policy, planning and the quantity and quality of services added another democratic element. In practice, this meant that Ministers were questioned in the House of Commons not only on policy and strategy but also on aspects of the day-to-day running of the service. Democratic accountability at the local level in the health service was much weaker, a matter which concerned some of the architects of the NHS. For example, Sir John Maude pushed hard for a health service organised under elected local authorities (Webster 1988). In the event, members of local-level Health Authorities have been appointed by Ministers to represent the views of professionals and lay people.

Perhaps because there was little challenge on grounds of principle, the NHS was organised along bureaucratic lines and decision-making has been centralised and corporatist in the sense that there has been prior consultation with the main interest groups to ensure acceptability. Health Authorities at regional and district level have been shadowed by civil servants within the central department as a check on the alignment of local policies with central policy concerns.

Governments have controlled key aspects of policy and administration. Most important has been the control of the total sum of resources allocated. As a result of annual negotiations between the central government spending departments and the Treasury, resources were set aside for health and thence distributed to the lower level authorities. Governments controlled capital expenditure and thus the pace and direction of hospital building. Expenditures were earmarked for particular programmes. The criterion of distribution was equity on the basis of varying criteria such as historic costs and later, needs. These different definitions are discussed further in Chapter 4. But increasingly, formulae have been developed to allocate budgets on a weighted population basis.

Governments also controlled the supply of labour to the NHS. The level of salaries and wages was negotiated nationally through a series of pay and review bodies representing different occupational groups within health care. Further, the numbers of training places available in medicine, nursing and professions ancillary to medicine and the numbers of senior posts and their distribution have been regulated. This has generally followed discussions between the training councils, professional associations and institutions. The numbers of senior medical posts and their distribution was agreed centrally as was the distribution of general medical practitioners to different parts of the country.

The NHS was a monopoly employer of skilled labour as there were limited alternative sources of employment for many groups working within it. In all, for most of the period from the 1940s to the 1990s, the NHS employed almost one million people. Managers in the NHS have been trained through national training programmes. Health administration and management tended to be a career confined to the NHS and progression depended upon a reputation within the service.

The limitations to control

Like most command and control economies, the NHS was criticised for its rigidity, its inefficiency and its parsimony. However, as Document 29 (page 345) shows, in relation to other health systems, in so far as health care outcomes can be measured through mortality rates, the NHS has done relatively well. From the perspective of government, there have been a number of problems. A major preoccupation has been devising methods to obtain value for money in health care spending. The pressures of demographic change as the population ages, the continuing and successful innovations in medical science, political pressures from the electorate and the lack of clearly defined limits to the responsibilities of the NHS have led to periodic funding crises.

However, while Governments were able to control the total resources to the NHS, they have had few means of affecting allocations within it. Whilst corporatist politics may have been the order of the day at a national level, at the local level governments lacked the means to enforce their policy priorities. And there were major problems in governments implementing change where these did not coincide with the concerns of professional medical interests.

In the 1970s, a number of research studies demonstrated the inability of the centre to ensure the implementation of its policy priorities (Kogan *et al.* 1978, Perrin *et al.* 1979, Brown 1979, Haywood and Alaszewski 1980 and Haywood and Elcock 1980). These studies demonstrated the dynamics of local level policy-making. Hospital consultants defined needs within their own specialism and were able to commit capital and revenue expenditure with little scrutiny from others. The locus for decision making frequently lay outside the management team altogether. Perrin comments that:

> . . . clinicians may be so formidable as to dominate decisions about resource use . . . the exercise of clinical autonomy should not be allowed to extend to a veto on the reallocation of resources to cope with changes in need . . . and what would be in the best interests of health in the area.
>
> (Perrin *et al.* 1978:46)

He concluded that there was often uncertainty between clinicians and managers about the boundaries between individual decisions and public policy. The decisions of clinicians had wider reverberations on resource use of which they were often unaware. Two examples of this are given in Document 14 (page 312).

Brown (1979) also found that the government's priority for community care fell by the wayside in favour of hospital building schemes. He comments:

> The same authorities which passed pious resolutions in support of services for the elderly committed themselves to other developments which in effect made it impossible to achieve their objectives.
>
> (Brown 1979)

The doctors who provided services in the surgeries and clinics made decisions which had a ripple effect up through the organisation. In a very real sense, individual medical decisions determined what health policy was. Acute medicine and hospital care took an increasing proportion of the health budget.

Administrators, or as they later became, managers, had little influence or power over the decisions of clinicians or the direction of policy. Neither did they have the means of persuasion over other groups of workers if they chose to withdraw labour or take other forms of industrial action – wages and salaries were negotiated nationally. On the whole, managers attempted to avoid conflict rather than attempt to lead in their hospitals.

A further point is that the NHS was also unresponsive to patients. It left them scant opportunity to exercise voice through democratic channels; few choices in relation to how their care was provided and little chance of exit as the NHS was virtually a monopoly.

The 1990 health service reforms

The political economy of managed competition

During the latter half of the 1980s, a number of shifts began to take place in health policy. First, managers were increasingly held to be accountable for policy implementation within their organisations; second, there was an increase in competitive tendering; third, contributions to private insurance were subsidised; fourth, patients' rights were strengthened through the publications of charters; fifth, the 1990 NHS and Community Care Act introduced an internal market so that there was competition between those supplying health services; sixth, the health reforms increased the powers of GPs in relation to hospital doctors; and seventh, targets for improving health status were established. Taken together, the reforms have increased the influence of market forces in making allocative decisions. This has altered the style and possibly the form of NHS politics. Part four of this book discusses the new NHS and the concluding chapter assesses the effect of a paradigm shift on health policy and the politics of the NHS.

Why do health policies shift?

The above description of policy shifts in health care and the mode of delivery did not dwell on why policies shift. There is no single explanation for policy change, rather a number of factors contribute but appear in different combinations. The ideology and political values of governments; the state of the economy; demographic change; the possibilities offered by technology as well as more apocalyptic factors such as war, scandals and epidemics have all been shown to play a part in policy change. At a macro level, Marxist or functionalist theories provide an account. The former theories are explored further in Chapter 7. There are also questions of policy maintenance and whether issues may be kept *off* policy agendas as a consequence of vested interests.

Subsequent chapters will explore these issues in relation to particular themes. However, one issue will be raised here as it related to public spending as a whole and is relatively neglected in the discussion of policy themes within each chapter. This is the fluctuating level of economic growth in the UK and its impact on social policy (see Judge 1982 for a discussion of the issue). It is worth pointing out here that consensus about the NHS began to break down during the economic downturn of the 1970s. The slower growth rates since the mid-1970s have broken the dominant economic assumption of the post-war period which rested on the view that public expenditure could be manipulated, usually in an upward direction, to achieve economic and social progress. High levels of inflation, the oil crisis of 1974 and the increase in the extent of government borrowing helped to change Westminster's attitudes towards welfare spending. This came to be seen as a public burden by, for example, Bacon and Eltis (1976) who argued that high levels of taxation and public borrowing had pre-empted investment in the private sector. Monetarist as opposed to Keynesian economic ideas were translated actively into public policy by the 1979 Conservative government although from the mid-1970s there had been relatively ineffectual attempts by Labour governments to reduce public spending.

Conservative Party monetarists clearly saw excessive public expenditure as lying at the heart of economic difficulties in the UK. It was argued that economic growth rates must be improved before welfare services could likewise be upgraded. In its reply to the Select Committee on Social Services in 1980, the Conservative government argued that economic policy must take priority over social policy and declared:

> In a time of low economic growth there is an absence of resources . . . it is no use having a bleeding heart if you haven't got the money to pay for it.
>
> (Social Services Select Committee 1980: 2)

Thus the attainment of economic goals was given priority over social policy goals. This was the view that underpinned the policy shifts of the last decade.

References

Alford, R. (1975) *Health Care Politics*, University of Chicago Press, Chicago.

Bacon, R. and Eltis, W. (1976) *Britain's Economic Problems*, Macmillan, London.

Barrett and Fudge (1981), *Policy and Action*, Methuen, London.

Brown, R. G. H. (1979) *Reorganising the Health Service*, Robertson, Oxford.

Cawson, A. (1982) *Corporation and Welfare: social policy and state intervention in Britain*, Heinemann, London.

Day, P. and Klein, R. (1991) 'Political Theory and Policy Practice: the case of general practice, 1911–1991', Paper presented at the Political Studies Association Conference, Lancaster, 15–17 April.

Department of Health (1992) *The Health of the Nation: a strategy for health for England*, Cmnd 1986, HMSO, London.

Elston, M. (1991) 'The Politics of Professional Power: medicine in a changing health service', in Gabe, J., Calnan, M. and Bury, M. (eds), *The Sociology of the Health Service*, Routledge, London.

Epsing Anderson, G. (1990) *The Three Worlds of Welfare Capitalism*, Polity Press, Cambridge.

Harrison, S., Hunter, D. and Pollitt, C. (1990) *The Dynamics of British Health Policy*, Unwin Hyman, London.

Haywood, S. and Alaszewski, A. (1980) *Crisis in the Health Service*, Croom Helm, London.

Haywood, S. and Elcock, H. (1980) *The Buck Stops Where? Accountability and Control in the National Health Service*, Institute of Health Studies, Hull.

Judge, K. (1982) 'The Growth and Decline of 'Public Expenditure' in *Public Expenditure and Social Policy* in Walker A. (ed.), *An Examination of Social Spending and Social Priorities*, Heinemann Educational, London.

Kogan, M. *et al.* (1978) T*he Working of the National Health Service,* Royal Commission on the NHS, Research Paper No. 1, HMSO, London.

Le Grand, J. (1982) *Strategy for Equality: Redistribution and the Social Services*, Allen and Unwin, London.

Mills, M. (ed.) (1993) *Health, Prevention and British Politics*, Avebury, Aldershot.

Ministry of National Health and Welfare (Canada) (1974) *A New Perspective on the Health of Canadians* (Chairman: M. Lalonde), Ottawa.

Perrin, J. *et al.* (1978) *Management of Financial Resources in the National Health Service*, Research Paper, No. 2, Royal Commission on the National Health Service, HMSO.

Rein, M. (1976) *Social Science and Public Policy*, Penguin, London.

Social Services Select Committee (1980) *The Government's White Papers on Public Expenditure in the Social Services*, 3rd Report, session 1979/80 HC 702, HMSO, London.

Titmuss, R. (1958) *Essays on the Welfare State*, Allen and Unwin, London.

Webster, C. (1988) *The Health Services Since the War,* vol 1, *Problems of Health Care: the NHS before 1957*, HMSO, London.

CHAPTER 2

Establishing the NHS

The National Health Service (NHS) came into operation on 5 July 1948 following the NHS Act of 1946. The event marked the end of a period of discussion and negotiation which began in 1942. Although there was general agreement in the war years on the need for a national service available to everyone funded from taxation and hierarchically organised around medical services, there was disagreement on the means for achieving this. As the end of the war came in sight, these differences grew and groups, particularly within the medical profession, pursued their vested interests. The steering of the NHS Bill through Parliament and the eventual agreement by the majority of doctors to join the service was a major political achievement for the Minister of Health of the 1945 Labour government, Aneurin Bevan. His success reflected a broad consensus of public and political opinion within the country for a national health service.

The Act was of crucial importance in establishing the pattern of health care in Britain. It rested on the principle of a collective responsibility by the state for comprehensive health services, to be provided on the basis of equal access for all citizens. This represented a radical new commitment. The central government was committed to funding from taxation a health service which rested on the principles of collectivism, comprehensiveness, equality and universality. The effect was a redistribution of resources to the less healthy and poorer sections of society – unskilled manual workers, women and their children – who stood to gain the most from the changes. Although later criticised for being insufficiently redistributive, in its effects, in terms of what had gone before, the increase in government responsibility for extending access to all was a large step (Walters 1980). Also radical was the nationalisation of the hospital system and its organisation on a regional basis. This gave the whole population access to specialist services wherever they were in the country. The Act too established a new structure through which health services were to be administered. This 'tripartite' structure remained for 26 years until the health service was reorganised in 1974.

Less obvious because it was part of the accepted wisdom of the time, but of equal importance, was the state commitment to a particular *kind* of health service. There was an emphasis on the provision of personal medical services. Under the new Act, doctors had a decisive role in determining what these medical services were. They had had important powers over the content and scope of medical care before the Act and retained these afterwards. However, in addition they now had responsibilities for treating the whole population with the security of employment and payment which this brought.

The Act did not, either, immediately produce new or different health care. As Watkin puts it, 'there were no new hospitals, no new drugs or treatment' (Watkin 1978: 13). The organisation of services was strongly influenced by the existing division of labour in health services and the history of state intervention during the nineteenth and early twentieth centuries. To understand the strength of the medical profession in establishing the form and structure of the NHS it is important to examine the development of the profession during the nineteenth century.

The rise of the medical profession and state intervention in health

Industrialisation and urbanisation in the late eighteenth and early nineteenth centuries brought changes in most areas of social life, including medicine. First of all, there was the gradual increase in the number of hospitals where medicine could be practised. By the end of the nineteenth century, hospitals and their medical schools developed the knowledge base for clinical practice. Equally important were the changes in social structure and the role of the state which led to an increased demand from various institutions and social classes for medical care. Both factors combined to enhance the position and status of the profession and to consolidate its control over medical practice.

During the course of the nineteenth century, the state became involved in what was essentially a private, market relationship in three stages. First, the 1834 Poor Law involved local-level poor law guardians and the central Board in making provision for the sick and, in so doing, employing doctors. The 1834 Poor Law required the appointment of a parish medical officer to look after the sick poor. This was in part to distinguish between the sick and the able-bodied pauper, which was necessary in order to apply the principle of deterrence and ensure that application to claim 'pauper status' was not encouraged. Under the Poor Law, special facilities were often provided for the sick and poor. This educated a generation of medical practitioners in the connection between poverty and ill-health. Much of the material collected in the Victorian Blue Books on social conditions drew on evidence from medical officers and other public medical practitioners. Partly as a consequence of the demand for 'qualified' parish medical offices and to protect the newly enfranchised classes from quackery there was demand through Parliament for legislation to define the qualified. The establishment of an agreed qualification for doctors was fraught with difficulty and the cause of disputes which continued, in the case of specialist qualifications, throughout the century.

A second and, many believe, crucial step in consolidating the professional monopoly over medical work was the 1858 Medical Act. This legislation brought self-regulation and a monopoly to practise which excluded the unqualified. The Act established the General Medical Council (GMC). The GMC had two functions – one related to qualifications, the other to conduct. The Council was licensed by statute to establish the requisite training for doctors. A basic qualification was recognised and a register of the qualified begun. Only those with a recognised qualification were entitled to use it. The Council also had the power to debar from practice those who were found guilty of breaking the code of conduct. This enabled the profession to draw boundaries around itself through the maintenance of a register of the qualified. Figures from the Census and the Medical Directories of the period give an indication of the success of the profession in reducing competition from the unqualified. The census of 1841 showed 30,000 doctors while the first directories 12 years later listed only 11,000 qualified practitioners (Gill 1971).

In the second half of the century, local authorities employed the medically qualified to deal with a range of public health matters from dealing with infectious disease to establishing hospitals in the towns and cities. By the time the 1911 National Health Insurance Act (which guaranteed the payment of expenses for medical care for manual workers) was under consideration, the profession was highly structured and mature. The British Medical Association (BMA), represented the interests of GPs in negotiations with government throughout the passage of the Bill.

Elliot (1972) refers to the transition of medical practitioners as a move from a pre-industrial status profession to a post-industrial occupation profession – from a profession which depended on patronage to one whose authority rested on the possession of a recognised body of skill and knowledge. Until the first quarter of the nineteenth century, medicine was practised by groups of doctors, each with a differing social status. The members of the Royal College of Physicians, established in the sixteenth century by Royal Charter, were at the apex of a pyramid. This thin top-layer were Oxbridge-educated in the medical classics, with little practical knowledge of medicine. They typically provided care for the rich, primarily in London. Members of the more recently formed College of Surgeons (separated from the Company of Barbers in 1745) had a more practically based training and tried to compete with the physicians in London, while in the provinces they practised where and how they could. Members of the Society of Apothecaries, whose skill lay primarily in the provision of medicines, tended to be the poor person's doctor.

On the whole these different groups derived their status from the social class of their patrons and they depended on their personal reputation with particular social groups to attract custom. Medical knowledge at this period still consisted of a variety of competing theories and ideas which had not been tested empirically. There were few predictably efficacious treatments. This too increased the dependency of the doctor on the social standing of their patients (Jewson 1976).

Waddington (1973) has traced the development of hospitals which began to function as centres for the development of a scientifically based medical knowledge in post-revolutionary France – and somewhat later in England. Following the 1832 Anatomy Act which allowed medical students to obtain bodies for dissection, this new knowledge was based on the three pillars of 'physical examination, autopsy and statistics'. The hospitals were a focal point for the training of doctors and thus provided a foundation for the acquisition of the two basic ingredients of professionalism: a degree of technical skill based upon scientific knowledge and a wisdom derived from experience. However, until the last quarter of the century, hospitals could do little by way of therapeutic benefit to the patient until the introduction of antiseptic surgery pioneered by Lister in 1865 and ten years later, the introduction of anaesthetics. Indeed, the conditions in hospitals were frequently so poor that the risk of cross-infection was high. In his history of *The Hospitals*, Abel-Smith (1964) observes that some of those who did not have fatal diseases when they entered hospital acquired them after admission. Partly for this reason, hospitals tended to treat mainly the urban poor. Those who could afford it preferred treatment in their own home from a doctor, usually a physician or surgeon, who was based at a teaching hospital.

The divisions within medicine

In the second half of the nineteenth century, the medical profession experienced collective social mobility (Parry and Parry 1976). Doctors were better qualified and there was a growing demand for medical care, particularly for those whose qualifications combined the skill and knowledge of the apothecary and the surgeon the forerunner of the general practitioner (GP). Indeed this term first began to be used in the late nineteenth century. The status differences within the profession, the divisions between different types of doctor – in hospital medicine, in general practice and in public health – persisted. Those who practised in the hospitals had a higher degree of specialisation and tended to come from a class who could afford the specialist education. General medical practitioners treated middle-class patients for a fee and those working-class patients who were covered by a weekly subscription to the sick clubs and friendly societies which developed as part of the labour movement. The income of GPs varied considerably as they often treated the poor for no payment.

In the last quarter of the nineteenth century, a division of labour was agreed between the GPs and hospital doctors. GPs would refer patients to specialists but not work in hospitals themselves. The BMA and the Royal Colleges decided that hospital doctors would only treat patients directly in accident and emergency departments. In most circumstances, they would treat patients referred to them by general practitioners. This division of labour was crucial in establishing the basic framework of medical care in Britain and was reinforced by subsequent legislation. It enabled the GP, the generalist doctor, to hang on to the patient despite the increasing specialisation of medicine and the rise of the hospital doctor. In most other countries, the generalist gave way to the specialist, bringing a different division of labour.

Both GPs and hospital doctors practised medicine differently from doctors who worked as medical officers. Local authority Medical Officers were concerned with collective rather than individual ill-health and were employees of the public authorities. The differences in outlook between the three types of doctor, their status differences and the type of medical work they practised were reinforced by the 1911 National Insurance Act and the 1946 Act with its 'tripartite' structure. They persist today and are one of the distinguishing characteristics of medical care in Britain.

From the mid-nineteenth century, there was a strong emphasis on public health. Chadwick, in his *Report on the Sanitary Condition of the Labouring Population* (1842), had propounded a theory of disease causation. The epidemics and infectious diseases among the poor were due, he argued, to atmospheric impurities generated by decomposing organic matter, itself the consequence of bad drainage, imperfect cleansing, inadequate water supply and defective ventilation. Chadwick's solution was to subordinate public health medicine to sanitary engineering. Disease and illness were seen to be caused by poverty, and conditions of work and living which were conducive to the spread of infection. Health policies were primarily concerned with maintaining health by removing public squalor. Chadwick had little but contempt for 'the bumbling-pretensions and hopeless disputes of doctors' and for 'the patheticality inadequate' curative medicine of his time. Document 1 (page 283) gives Chadwick's prescription for public health and shows how he made the connection between polluted environments and ill-health. The efforts of the health reformers led to a new role for the local state through sanitary reform and the building of hospitals.

The duties of the Medical Officers of Health appointed under the Public Health Act of 1848 were to implement sanitary reforms and they had to work closely with public health engineers. They were relatively isolated from other branches of the profession because of their very different orientation to health. Moreover, as public employees they did not receive the financial rewards of other members of the profession. In terms of an improvement of general health, however, they undoubtedly achieved more than those practising the inadequate curative medicine of the time.

The extension of medical and particularly hospital practice and, towards the end of the century, its increasing success brought a change in the doctor–patient relationship. Even the better-off might be treated in hospital. Between patient and doctor there was a widening gulf in knowledge. Jewson (1976) comments:

> the new occupational standing of the clinician was matched by the emergence of a new role for the sick man, that of patient. As such he was designated a passive and uncritical role in the consultative relationship, his main function being to endure and wait.
>
> (Jewson 1976: 235)

Foucault, in *The Birth of the Clinic* (1971), discusses the shift in power relationships when the focus of the doctor is on the internal malfunctioning of the body rather than on the ill person. Further, although there were status differences and divisions among doctors, these depended more on the professionally determined criteria of qualifications and training than on the social standing of the patient.

The 1911 National Health Insurance Act: access to personal health services

In 1911, National Health Insurance was introduced by the Liberal government to maintain the income of sick workers as well as to provide access to personal health services. It is significant as a first attempt by the state to cushion a section of the working class from the costs of illness. It provided limited access to general medical care for groups of working men earning less than £2 per week. The scheme was subsequently extended to cover other occupational categories of working men. The scheme – a contributory one by state, employer and employee – entitled beneficiaries to free treatment and care by an approved panel doctor. Hospital services were not at first included. Sickness benefit, a sum to compensate for loss of earning power during sickness, was also paid. The scheme was administered by 'Approved Societies' and insurance committees which had already been administering the sickness clubs and friendly societies' private and commercial schemes, respectively.

A number of key groups had a financial interest in personal health which they would not have had in measures for the poor or preventive health – the Approved Societies who organised working men's sick clubs, the insurance companies and the British Medical Association. Day and Klein (1991), in a study of general practitioners and the state, conclude that the BMA in particular established the system of private conferences which foreshadowed the corporatist politics of the NHS. In an interwar official history of the BMA, it was noted that the Association's discussions:

> had radically altered the detail of the 1911 Act: . . . the alterations were all of a nature which brought the system more into line with the wishes of the profession. The position thus secured by the Association has never been lost – on the contrary, each successive Government has acknowledged the Association as the representative organisation of the whole profession, a gain which itself would justify all the energy and money expended during the struggle.
>
> (Day and Klein 1991: 5)

Bentley Gilbert (1966) also argues that the medical and insurance pressure groups were also extremely influential in shaping the 1911 legislation. Lloyd George had first introduced this scheme in 1908, but his plan was changed significantly by the time it came into effect in 1911. Bentley Gilbert argues that this:

> . . . was the result of the powerful and conflicting pressure exerted by the three great social institutions most affected by health insurance – the friendly societies, the commercial insurance industry and the British medical profession.
>
> (Gilbert 1966: 290)

As a consequence of the 1911 Act, the state for the first time became involved with providing personal health services.

On the supply side, the main beneficiaries of the Act were the newly formed Insurance Committees and the GPs who could now claim fees and whose income base thus became more secure. GPs were free to practise as they wished and as panel doctors received an income from the Insurance Committees. Parry and Parry suggest that:

> the fact that doctors were well organised, prior to the major entry of the State into the field of personal health care, was a crucial factor in the success of [GPs in] the negotiations with Lloyd George over the principles and administration of the National Health Insurance Act of 1911.
>
> (Parry and Parry 1976: 254)

Fox (1988) concludes that by the end of World War One, the purpose of health insurance had been redefined. It was to become, in the interwar years, a programme for providing medical care as opposed to maintaining income. He attributes this shift to two factors in the 1914–18 war – the continuing extension of local authority hospital services to maintain the health of the civilian population and the success of the medical services at the front. He comments:

> Death rates from contagious diseases and from infection related to wounds were lower than in previous wars, as a result, many experts concluded, of both scientific knowledge and the way services were organised. Moreover, military experience increased the number of doctors who were familiar with the new technology and improved the co-ordination of the people and resources required to use it.
>
> (Fox 1988: 36)

The impact of war

War is often a time when the importance of health to national efficiency is recognised. At the turn of the century, anxiety about the state of health of recruits for the Boer War caused concern because it had an impact on recruitment to the army. Document 2 (page 285) reproduces contemporary material on this issue. During World War One, there was also concern about the health of the civilian population, particularly that of mothers and children. Infant mortality was high, and a contemporary, Lord Rhondda, wrote:

> Public opinion is now keenly aroused on the existing deficiency and inefficiency of our public medical service, especially for maternity and infant welfare. There is widespread and insistent demand for improvement.
>
> (quoted in Briggs 1978)

Public opinion was swayed, too, by the publication in 1915 of *Maternity: Letters from Working Women* edited by Margaret Llewelyn Davies (1978) from letters written to the Women's Co-operative Guild. These letters presented a picture of the perpetual overwork, illness and suffering which was the experience of working-class women. Almost half of the women writing to the Guild had had miscarriages or still-births. Llewelyn Davies attributed this to low wages; the lack of knowledge of maternity services; the absence of skilled advice and treatment; and the lack of a caring personal relationship between husband and wife. In 1918, the Maternity and Child Welfare Act was passed. In 1919, in the aftermath of war, this was established. This became the focus for developing a policy for organising medical services. Policies for income security and housing were dealt with by separate government departments.

The interwar years: the increasing focus on medical care

The 1911 Act covered 27 per cent of the population for GP services. By 1938 this had increased to 43 per cent. It did not include hospital or specialist treatment nor did it provide for families or dependants. During the 1920s and 1930s, there were a number of attempts to extend access to health insurance and more particularly to organise medical services in a planned way. The provision of medical services had grown up in a piecemeal way and was inadequate to meet the needs of the population for medical treatment, let alone health care. Fox (1988) argues that there was general support for a hierarchically organised medical service with hospitals as a priority; disagreements focused on how this should be funded and the details of organisation.

In 1920, Sir Bernard Dawson, who chaired the Council on Medical and Allied Services, recommended in his report that there should be a close coordination of preventive and curative services and spoke of 'the increasing conviction that the best means of maintaining health and curing disease should be made available to all citizens'. The report recommended a unified health service as the proper framework for the expansion of health insurance and a network of health centres in which services would be concentrated. In 1926, a Royal Commission on health insurance recommended an extension of coverage. However, governments were reluctant to fund such an extension in the context of economic crisis and rising unemployment.

During the latter half of the 1920s and early 1930s, interest in administrative reform of health care waned; however, the focus on hospital care remained and resources were directed towards the growth of this sector. In 1929, a Local Government Act permitted local authorities to convert Poor Law infirmaries into public general hospitals. Many of the larger boroughs supported hospitals and the voluntary ones provided increasing services for paying patients from all social groups. In some sectors there was a concern about the relationship between social factors and ill-health and an interest in preventive measures. For example, in the 1930s the BMA issued pamphlets stressing the importance of 'positive health' and called for the prevention of disease through better housing, physical education and health education. Nevertheless, it was in the area of medical services that there was most demand and that there was perceived to be the greater deficit.

In 1937, a highly critical *Report on the British Health Services* was published by the independent research institute, Political and Economic Planning. This showed how inadequate medical services were. It concluded that the publicly provided health services were:

> . . . enormously hampered by piecemeal and anomalous methods of organisation which have no justification upon health and administrative grounds and involve waste of resources and increased suffering or inconvenience to the consumer [see Document 3].

The report showed the inequity in the distribution of services. GPs practised where market forces guaranteed an income from private fees or where there were Insurance Committees which used the services of panel doctors. The distribution of hospitals was chaotic and fragmentary. Services were provided by municipal, charitable and voluntary institutions reflecting past philanthropy or civic pride rather than population needs.

The report also drew attention to the inequalities in health status and commented on the cost to the country in terms of lost production of 30 million working weeks a year. It argued that ill-health was more serious and widespread in low income families than in the rest of the community. Tuberculosis, for example, was twice as prevalent among the poor as the well-to-do. The infant mortality rate in Glasgow was 109 per thousand live births compared to 42 per thousand in Surrey.

The search for a national health service: the war years

While interwar governments were overwhelmed by economic problems and unable to find the political will to tackle questions of health services, a new spirit was generated by World War Two. For the purposes of the war effort, the state assumed reponsibility for health care. In 1938, as part of preparing for an emergency, the first survey of hospitals undertaken since 1863 was carried out. It found that there were 78,000 beds in voluntary hospitals, 32,000 in local authority hospitals and 35,000 in isolation hospitals and tuberculosis sanitoria. These were estimated to be inadequate to meet the requirements to treat civilian war casualties and the sick and wounded from the armed forces. It was concluded that the shortage was compounded by an uneven distribution between different areas of the country. A Report on Sheffield and the West Midlands commented:

> We have seen far too many examples of dark, over-crowded, ill-equipped infirmary blocks in which the chronic sick drag out the last days of their existence with few amenities of civilised life.
>
> (Nuffield Provincial Hospitals Trust 1946)

Paradoxically, what could not be achieved in peace was achieved with remarkable speed after the onset of war. Webster, official historian of the NHS, refers to the consensus at the time.

> the very strong and in some cases unanimous feelings that in the future, the best possible medical, surgical and hospital treatment must be available to everyone without the stigma of charity.
>
> (Webster 1988: 27)

In 1942, the Beveridge Report on Social Insurance and Allied Services proposed a radical approach to postwar reconstruction

(Beveridge 1942). It argued that 'basic' health services should be made available to the whole population. The health service would be free at the point of delivery, mostly without direct charges and mostly financed by general and local taxation. Beveridge was not entirely consistent on this point. He also suggested that there should be an element of compulsory insurance. However, he saw access to adequate medical care facilities as part of a comprehensive attack on the five giants standing in the way of social progress: Want, Disease, Ignorance, Squalor and Idleness. He declared that such an approach would prevent ill-health and rehabilitate the sick after illness and so make the nation fitter and more productive.

Following the Royal Commission on National Health Insurance in 1926, one of the stumbling blocks to the assumption of state responsibility had been the fear of the high level of public expenditure to which the central government would become committed. Beveridge changed the terms of the debate. In Assumption B [Document 6 page 294] he argued that the burden and cost of ill-health on a society was borne by the whole of that society, irrespective of state provision of health care. It was therefore an intrinsic part of the purpose of any social security system to save the nation from these costs. 'Disease and accidents must be paid for in any case in lessened power of production and in idleness,' he said. The impact of a health service would be to reduce the overall costs of social security by making people healthier. They would therefore demand less medical care and fewer doctors would be needed to provide less treatment. A state-funded health service was therefore part of a package leading to a greater rationality in public expenditure commitments and its introduction would also increase national efficiency.

In 1942, the wartime Coalition government announced acceptance of the principle of a national health service with a hierarchical regional hospital organisation. When plans were in a general form, there was a large measure of agreement, even from the British Medical Association. As discussions became more concrete so greater divisions of interest emerged. There was conflict about control over resources and the government of institutions. This began what has been referred to as 'the wartime paper chase' to find a health service structure which was acceptable to professionals, politicians and other interests such as the voluntary hospitals and the local authorities. The real arguments were now about the new relationships between the medical profession and the state. The different interest groups wanted different things. Within the profession, hospital doctors – especially those within teaching hospitals – wanted independence from bureaucratic control, particularly from local government. The GPs resisted a form of payment which implied that they were state employees. They also rejected local government control.

Other people, particularly Herbert Morrison, who was then Minister responsible for local government, wanted an integrated service, run by local government. However, the voluntary hospitals resisted this as representing a loss of autonomy. Despite these differences, in 1944, a White Paper was produced which reflected a compromise and which was generally supported. The hospital doctors had agreed to a salaried service while the GPs agreed to be paid by capitation. The White Paper described the deficiencies of the existing system and these are reproduced in Document 4 (page 289).

The passing of the 1946 Act

In 1945, the election victory for the Labour Party brought a reassessment of some of the agreements already reached. The Socialist Medical Association wanted a salaried service for GPs, supporters of local government wanted more control over hospitals and the differences between professional groups opened up again. Civil servants advised consideration of a structure which integrated hospitals, clinics and GPs. It was left to Aneurin Bevan as Minister of Health to take the decisions. To Bevan the hospitals were the key to the service. As a consequence of his negotiating skills and a tactic of divide and rule, Bevan reached compromises with the most powerful interest groups as the Bill was steered through Parliament. Parliament itself, as an extract from the debate in the House of Commons on the issue illustrates [Document 5], endorsed the NHS Bill as did the general public. A minority were critical. To a few, such collective action was reminiscent of a fascist state.

It was the medical profession who put up most opposition. The Royal Colleges led by the specialists and consultants were concerned by the prospect of a loss of autonomy. However, Bevan's negotiations with them proceeded with goodwill. By nationalising the hospitals, and moving toward a regionally structured service outside local government, Bevan won the cooperation of this section of the profession. In the interwar period, improvements in diagnostic and treatment techniques had led to an increasing demand for expensive equipment. Many hospitals, particularly in the voluntary sector, were in a perilous financial position, so it was to the advantage of the consultants to secure a steady flow of finance and a system of regional planning. Furthermore, Bevan, in order to gain the cooperation of the hospital doctors, gave them the right to continue with private practice, alongside NHS work. They also maintained a high degree of control over their conditions of employment. Appointments, promotion and a merit awards system (which awards large salary increments on the basis of individual contributions to medicine) were determined by consultants. Bevan is reported to have said that in order to gain their support he had: '. . . stuffed their mouths with gold' (quoted in Campbell 1987: 168). The teaching hospitals too had a separate status as they were to be financed directly by the Ministry. This enhanced the position of the doctors working within the hospitals and gave autonomy from regional control.

The local authorities and those who wanted an integrated service – combining curative and preventive and caring services provided under the Medical Officers of Health in the counties and county boroughs – lost out in the negotiations. This may have been due to the relative weakness of the public health doctors, as suggested by Gill (1971), or, as Pater (1981) contends, a harmony of interests between the Labour government and the consultants. The public ownership or nationalisation of hospitals satisfied Labour Party philosophy while a stable source of finance satisfied the consultants. The voluntary hospital movement was appeased by retaining some involvement in hospital management through special boards of trustees and through lay membership of the hospital management bodies. The local government lobby was insufficiently strong to overcome these combined forces.

That left only the GPs represented by the BMA to be lured into the service. There was bitter opposition to a salaried service and the organisation of general practice into health centres run by local authorities. Bevan conceded a method of payment by capitation fee for each patient and a considerable freedom to GPs to operate as independent contractors. The sale of practices was, however, to be stopped and a Medical Practices Committee was to be set up to attempt to get a fair distribution of GPs throughout the country. The Committee, like the Executive Councils responsible for administering family practitioners, was to be composed mainly of medical members. The role of local authorities was to be limited to building health centres. Doctors were left to practise from them if they wished.

Negotiations dragged on, however, long after the 1946 Act had been passed, and still, five months before the appointed day in 1948, there was doubt about whether the GPs would join the service. Then the trickle of those joining became a river and few, in the end, left the country to work abroad. Pater (1981) comments:

> There were histrionics on both sides, there were withdrawals and accusations of bad faith; but in the end, with what seemed trivial concessions the profession was persuaded to drop its intransigent attitude in what were, after all, not major questions.
>
> (Pater 1981: 173)

It was agreed to establish the service as it had been planned under the 1946 Act, based on the tripartite structure described in Figure 2.1 (page 31).

The aims and intentions of the NHS Act

The collective principle

A central aim of the NHS Act was that the state should provide health care free at the point of service for those in need. This was a radical departure and reflected the collectivist principle of state responsibility for its citizens. Bevan saw the NHS as the hallmark of a civilised society:

> Society becomes more wholesome, more serene, and spiritually healthier, if it knows that its citizens have at the back of their consciousness, the knowledge that not only themselves, but all their fellows, have access, when ill, to the best medical skills that could be provided.
>
> (Bevan 1961)

It was Bevan's view that the state should, through collective action, provide free access to medical services. He saw little difference between the NHS and the railways – in the case of both, centralised state organisation should be used to provide a service which was equally accessible to all citizens in distress and provided on an equitable basis according to need.

The comprehensive principle

The Minister of Health, furthermore, had a general duty to:

> . . . promote a *comprehensive* health service for the improvement of the physical and mental health of the people of England and Wales for the prevention, diagnosis and treatment of illness.
>
> (Ministry of Health 1944)

Two important areas of health care were, however, excluded from the NHS Act. Health care for school children remained for the most part in the hands of local education authorities and the health care of the worker, the culmination of a variety of Factory Acts, was to remain the responsibility of the Department of Employment and the Health and Safety Executive.

The universal principle

As well as being collectivist and comprehensive, this new health service was universalist in principle. It provided a range of health services for the whole population, free at the point of use. It has been argued that the NHS therefore embodied a set of illness rights. The use of the term 'rights' is, however, unhelpful. It is more accurate to say that health services were available without charge on the determination of need by professional service

The 1944 White Paper had described the universalist principle in the following way:

> . . . the availability of necessary medical services shall not depend on whether people can afford to pay for them, or any other factor irrelevant to real need . . . to bring the country's full resources to bear upon reducing ill-health in all its citizens . . . money should not be allowed to stand in the way of providing advice, early diagnosis and speedy treatment.
>
> (Ministry of Health 1944)

The principle of equality

The NHS Act was overtly equalitarian in its approach. Bevan argued that:

> we have got to achieve as nearly as possible a uniform standard of service for all – only with a national service can the state ensure that an equally good service is available everywhere.
>
> (Bevan 1946)

The tripartite structure was thus intended as an administrative structure which would ensure this uniformity throughout the country. The Regional Hospital Boards were to be concerned with the planning and coordination of the hospital and specialist services within their regions. In relation to the general practitioners, the Medical Practices Committee was to attain a more even distribution of GPs throughout the country by designating areas as restricted, intermediate and open and to prevent further movement of GPs to the 'over-doctored' areas. Moreover, a patient could in theory be referred by their practitioner anywhere in the country. Access to health care was not limited by particular boundaries.

The principle of professional autonomy

Although the NHS was explicitly based on the principles of collectivism, comprehensiveness, universality and equalitarianism, the principle of professional autonomy was also central to the structure and decision making in the NHS. Bevan fully endorsed and supported the importance of the professions in both the decision making and the running of the service and this meant a recognition of the centrality of the medical profession to health care. He argued:

> As I conceive it, the function of the Ministry of Health is to pr the medical profession with the best and most modern appar medicine, and to enable them freely to use it, in accordar their training for the benefit of the people of this country. Eve

must be free to use that apparatus without interference from secular organisations.

(Bevan 1946)

This clinical autonomy meant that decisions about expenditure and therefore about resource allocation within the hospitals were made by consultants within their specialisms and by GPs in primary health care. GPs were free to prescribe and refer for further specialist care at their own discretion with few limitations. The result of that arrangement was that general practice was retained in Britain while in other countries it retreated in the face of increasing specialisation.

The Medical Officers of Health in the local authorities were not concerned with the diagnosis and treatment of individual ill-health but operated within the financial constraints of local government where decisions frequently had to be made in competition with other services. They had less scope for the operation of clinical autonomy as they were largely concerned with public health matters or attempting to develop further the support services in the community for vulnerable groups.

The organisation of the service

The principle of state provision meant that financial responsibility for health services and for health policy rested with the central government. The Ministry of Health and its ministers were responsible for the institutions providing health services and were thus the central pivot of health policy. The more so as, unlike other social services such as education and housing, there was to be no elected tier in the NHS. Power, it seemed, was to lie at the centre – with ministers and their departments making policy decisions, allocating resources and administering the service. In terms of models of health care delivery, the structure leaned more towards the bureaucratic (central control) than the democratic (representation through elected representatives).

Figure 2.1 shows the tripartite structure. The hospital or group of hospitals was to have an appointed Hospital Management Committee (HMC) composed of professional and lay members who received their financing through the Regional Hospital Boards (RHBs). Regions were responsible to the Minister of Health. The 14 regions in England and Wales were responsible for coordinating and planning the provision of hospital services within their regions, also through a board composed of professional and lay members. Teaching hospitals had a separate status with Boards of Governors and direct financing from the Ministry. This was to protect special responsibilities for teaching. To Bevan, hospitals were the vertebrae of the health system. The best hospitals were those which were

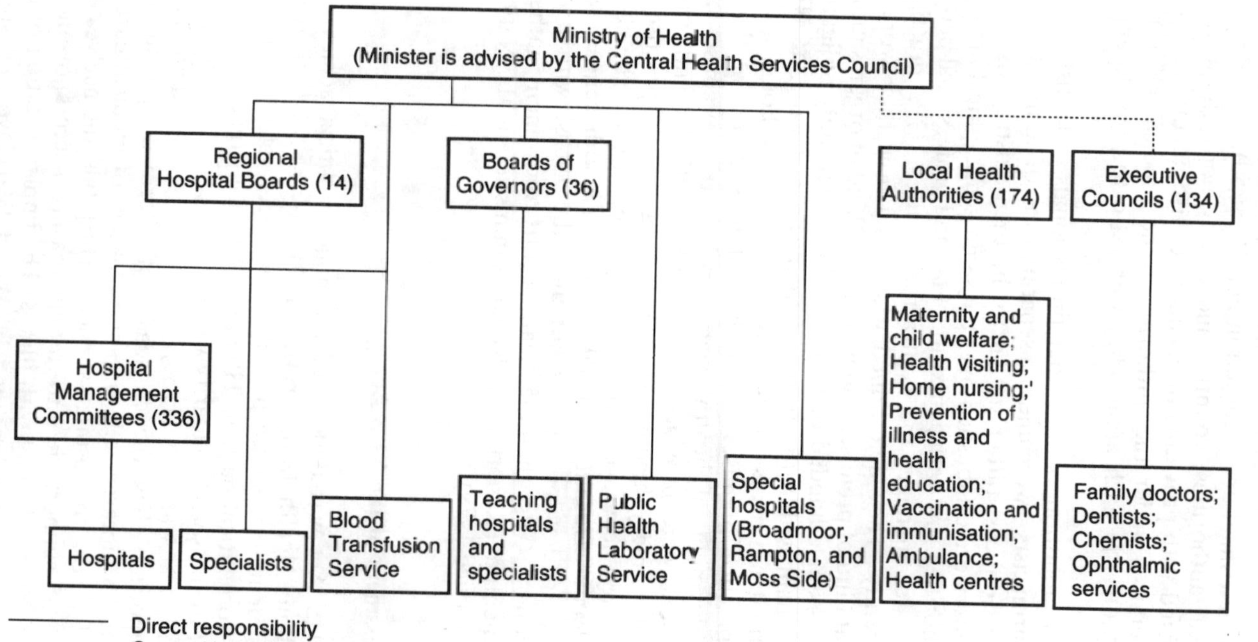

Figure 2.1 ***Organisation of the National Health Service in England and Wales 1948–1974***

large and operated according to the principles of modern science: 'I would rather be kept alive in the efficient but cold altruism of a large hospital', Bevan declared, 'than to expire in a gush of warm sympathy in a small one' (quoted in Fox 1988: 50).

The local authorities, counties and county boroughs were to be concerned with providing domiciliary, environmental and preventive services under the authority of the Medical Officer of Health (MOH) in each area. They were also to provide ambulances.

General practitioners and other professionals – dentists, opticians, pharmacists – were under a separate form of administration. Executive Councils, rather similar to the then existing insurance committees, were established over the same geographical areas as local authorities, and with a mixture of lay and professional people appointed to 'manage' the contractor services. GPs practised independently. They determined where and how they worked, from what kind of premises and within what kind of organisational structure – single-handed or with partners. Their only obligation was to remain within the terms of their contract with the NHS which stipulated access to the GP or deputy, 24 hours a day, at the practice premises or in the patient's home. Although the development of health centres, where the premises and management were provided by the local authority and where groups of primary health care professionals could practise together, were encouraged, joining a health centre was the choice of the doctor. Despite financial incentives, health centres were very slow to develop. It was not until the 1960s, with a new generation of GPs, that the health centre movement gathered any momentum (Report of the Royal Commission on the National Health Service 1979).

An assessment of the NHS Act

The NHS Act was undoubtedly a major political achievement for Labour Health Minister Bevan. However, a health service along similar lines would probably have been introduced by the other two political parties. Titmuss (1950) has argued that it was a result of the social solidarity which developed as a consequence of a nation at war. Fox (1988), however, contends that war was less important than the consensus of informed opinion which supported a hierarchically organised system of medical care that ensured access to hospital services. Hospitals themselves were assured of support due to the increasing success of medical interventions in dealing with illness. The implementation of these changes was simply hastened by World War Two and support came particularly from the middle classes for whom hospital care was a growing expense.

However, the cooperation of the medical profession had costs. The compromises reached to introduce the 1946 Act carried the seeds of future problems. First, the hospitals were split from local government, the GPs were cut off from practising any hospital medicine and they themselves were divided from the local authority nursing services. Second, hospitals were dependent on central financing and had no access to local funding. This was to prove a brake on expansion. Third, the GP services were essentially unreformed: an integrated and salaried service for GPs was impossible to achieve because of its symbolic place in the GPs' notion of their professional identity. Fourth, the compromises reached with the hospital doctors gave them a dominant position in shaping the new service. Governments were to find it difficult to impose their own priorities.

Although the NHS embodied radical ideas of universality, comprehensiveness, equality and collectivism it did so within a structure in which the functional autonomy of the medical profession was paramount. A DHSS Memorandum of 1970 put it in the following way:

> The health and personal social services have always operated on the basis that doctors and other professional providers of services have individual professional freedom to do what they consider to be right for their patients. Thus in each individual doctor-patient situation it is the doctor who decides on the appropriate objective and the appropriate priority. That is not to say that the department cannot impose overall constraints or influence behaviour, e.g. by the imposition of charges, but it is important to note that the existence of clinical freedom substantially reduces the ability of the central authority to determine objectives and priorities and to control individual facets of expenditure.
>
> (Report of the Royal Commission on the NHS 1979)

Quite apart from the ability to make clinical decisions within very elastic financial limits, the profession was also well represented on the management and decision-making bodies in the NHS – the Hospital Management Committees (HMCs), the Regional Hospital Boards (RHBs) and the Executive Councils. As Bevan had argued in the House of Commons in 1946, while steering the Act through Parliament, 'I believe it is a wise thing to give the doctors full participation in the administration of their own profession' (Bevan 1946).

Health services as they developed after 1948 were to be primarily about the delivery of appropriate medical care, with the lion's share of resources going to the hospitals. This was a consequence of both how health policy was generally perceived and of the centrality of the medical profession to decision-making. From the 1911 Act to the 1946 Act, the primary goal of health policy had changed. In 1911, the aim had been to prevent poverty for the working man and his family by replacing income and relieving minor illness by access to general medical care. This had been replaced by access for the whole population to a range of specialist hospitals via the referral system. The emphasis in preventive health had also changed, from an emphasis on environmental regulation in the nineteenth century, and nutrition, income and housing in the early part of the twentieth century, to the prevention of ill-health in individuals. Vaccination and immunisation have been actively promoted, while factors *causing* ill-health such as poor nutrition and bad housing were regarded as the responsibility of other government departments and separated from health.

If the form of the NHS in Britain was a consequence of the past provision of health care and the organisation and power of the groups who provided it, its future problems as well as its achievements also derive from the structure set up in 1948. The subsequent chapters pursue these issues.

References

Abel-Smith, B. (1964) *The Hospitals 1800–1948*, Heinemann, London.

Bevan, A. (1946) *Hansard* (House of Commons), 30 April 1946, col. 45 and 52

Bevan, A. (1961) *In Place of Fear*, MacGibbon and Kee, London.

Beveridge, W. (1942) *Social Insurance & Allied Services*, Cmnd 6404, HMSO, London.

Briggs, A. (1978) 'Making Health Every Citizen's Birthright: the road to 1946', *New Society*, 16 Nov.

Campbell, J. (1987) *Nye Bevan and the Mirage of British Socialism*, Weidenfeld & Nicolson, London, ch. 12.

Consultative Council of Medical and Allied Services (1920) (Chairman: Sir Bernard Dawson) *Interim Report*.

Day, P. and Klein, R. (1991) 'Political Theory and Policy Practice: a case of general practice, 1911–1991', Paper presented at the Political Studies Association Conference, Lancaster.

Elliot, P. (1972) *The Sociology of the Professions*, Macmillan, London.

Flinn, M. (ed.) (1965) *Edwin Chadwick, Report of the Sanitary Conditions of the Labouring Population of Great Britain*, Edinburgh University Press, Edinburgh.

Foucault, M. (1971) *The Birth of the Clinic*, Tavistock, London.

Fox, D. (1988) 'The National Health Service and the Second World War: the elaboration of consensus' in H. L. Smith (ed.) *War and Social Change*, Manchester University Press, Manchester.

Gilbert, B. (1966) *The Evolution of National Insurance in Great Britain*, Michael Joseph, London.

Gill, D. G. (1971) 'The British National Health Service: professional determinants of administrative structure', *International Journal of Health Services*, 1(4), pp. 341–53.

Jewson, N. D. (1976) 'The Disappearance of the Sick Man from Medical Cosmology 1770–1870', *Sociology*, 90, pp. 225–44.

Llewelyn Davies, M. (1978) *Maternity: letters from working women* (1915), republished by Virago, London.

Ministry of Health (1944) *A National Health Service*, Cmnd 6502, HMSO, London.

Nuffield Provincial Hospitals Trust (1946) *The Hospital Surveys: The Domesday Book of the Hospital Service*, Oxford University Press, London.

Parry, N. and Parry, J. (1976) *The Rise of the Medical Profession*, Croom Helm, London.

Pater, J. E. (1981) *The Making of the NHS*, King Edward's Hospital Fund for London, London, ch. 2.

Political and Economic Planning (1937) *Report on the British Health Services*, PEP, London.

Report of the Royal Commission on the National Health Service (1979) (Chairman: Sir Alec Merrison), Cmnd 7615, HMSO, London.

Titmuss, R. (1950) *Problems of Social Policy*, London.

Waddington, I. (1973) 'The Role of the Hospital in the Development of Modern Medicine: a sociological analysis', *Sociology*, 7, pp. 211–24.

Walters, V. (1980) *Class, Inequality and Health Care: the origins and impact of the National Health Service*, Croom Helm, London.

Watkin, B. (1978) *The National Health Service: the first phase 1948–1974 and after*, Allen & Unwin, London, ch. 1, p. 13.

Webster, C. (1988) *The Health Services Since the War*, vol. 1 *Problems of Health Care before 1957*, HMSO, London.

PART TWO

Policy Issues in the NHS

CHAPTER 3

The search for control: the NHS and its organisation from 1948 to 1982

This chapter is concerned with the 'governance' of the NHS; that is, with policies dealing with the relationship between central government and the lower-level health authorities. Until the reforms of the late 1980s, the NHS was highly centralised. In theory, the policy decisions were made by government, that is, by the Minister and the health departments, and implemented by the lower level. The Minister was accountable to Parliament for policy, planning and the quantity and quality of services. This chapter examines the changes in the management of the NHS until the early 1980s, and why they were then believed to have failed.

Within the parameters of the tensions between 'centre' and 'periphery' were resolved by different methods during this period. In general, after an initial phase of *laissez-faire*, the tendency was towards increasing central control. The reasons for this were consistent with the aims of Aneurin Bevan. The concern was to achieve national standards of provision, more effective health services, and make more efficient use of resources.

The unification of the tripartite structure

In 1948, England was divided into 13 regions with Wales as a region in its own right; Webster (1988) comments that the unification of the hospitals under Regional Hospital Boards (RHBs) was the most striking innovation of the NHS. The regions were of different population sizes although most ranged between three and four million. Oxford and East Anglia were smaller at 1.5 million. The aim was that each region should contain a university with a medical school. London was cut into four, extending outwards from central London to the coast and the Midlands. The main responsibility of RHBs was to plan for the hospital and specialist services in their area. The teaching hospitals stepped outside the regional framework. They were separately administered by 36 Boards of Governors which acted as 'agents' of the Minister. The teaching hospitals were seen as a privileged elite.

When viewed from the neglected recesses of the regions, teaching hospitals seemed like a selected club of mandarins, imbued with privilege without responsibility.

(Webster 1988: 272).

Hospitals within the regions were run by Hospital Management Committees (HMCs) either singly, or as a group. The Boards were composed of professional and lay people from very different administrative backgrounds and experience, often drawn from the membership of the province's voluntary or local authority hospital boards. They had to learn to work together to run the new service. Bevan remarked that:

. . . it is precisely by the selection of the right men and women to serve on these bodies that I hope to give them substantial executive powers, subject to broad financial control, and so prevent rigidity. Admittedly this is a field in which there is room for development in the technique of government, but the problems that will arise should not be incapable of solution.

(Klein 1980: 420)

Over the next 40 years, the greatest changes took place in the hospital service. Each hospital was eager to acquire its own share of specialist consultants and take advantage of expanding medical technology. In the 1950s, there was little or no attempt by central government to plan or rationalise these developments. The Minister and his civil servants allocated funds to the regions on the basis of expenditure in the previous year. The regions planned the service and allocated funds according to the dictates of local medical politics, a process which Ham has described for the Leeds region (Ham 1981). Teaching hospitals received separate funding and thus retained a privileged status. The share of NHS expenditure taken by the hospital sector rose consistently from the 1950s onwards.

However, there was almost no capital investment in the new hospitals or major rebuilding. So the marked inequalities in the distribution of hospitals and beds which had been a feature of the pre-war service remained. Forty-five per cent of the hospitals had in fact been built before 1891 and were deteriorating rapidly. This led an American commentator on the English health services, Eckstein, to argue:

it is high time to let the health service go on a spending spree, instead of continuing to subject it to the miserly penny-pinching necessary in the immediate post-war period.

(Eckstein 1958: 62–3)

There were less dramatic changes for local authorities who ran health and welfare services before the war and these subsequently continued to develop with funding from the rates and central government. GPs also continued to work much as they had done before the 1946 Act.

A major problem was perceived to be the lack of linkage between the three arms of the service which were administered according to entirely different criteria and policies. The boundaries of the HMCs bore no relationship to those of the local authorities in counties and county boroughs. This made for difficulties in maintaining operational continuities in patient care. GPs found it difficult to maintain linkages between the hospital and the local authority domiciliary nursing, home help and social work services. Continuity rested almost entirely on personal efforts of the professionals involved.

In 1956, the weaknesses of the tripartite structure were discussed in the Guillebaud Report (Ministry of Health 1956). A committee had been set up in 1953 to enquire into the costs of the NHS, and published their report three years later. Although some deficiencies were acknowledged, the committee felt it was not practicable to make changes in the organisation of the service at that stage. One member of the committee, however, Sir John Maude, expressed reservations. In the past he had been a strong advocate of an integrated service under local government. He now attacked the tripartite division of responsibility, believing that the administrative structure had a clear impact on the quality of service provision. He declared:

> The mischiefs to which the division of the service gives rise fall broadly under two heads (a) the administrative divorce of curative from preventive medicine and of general medical practice from hospital practice and the overlaps, gaps and confusion caused thereby and (b) the predominant position of the hospital service and the consequent danger of general practice and preventive and social medicine falling into the background.
>
> (Ministry of Health 1956)

Maude's solution was to transfer administrative responsibilities to local government – a view out of tune with the political thinking of his time and quite unrealistic given professional prejudices and the difficulties of financing the health service out of local rates.

However, the argument that the health service should have a more unified structure persisted. In 1959, the Cranbrook Report on the Maternity Services (Ministry of Health 1959) was highly critical of the split between hospital maternity services and local authority midwives. It saw the twin dangers of wasteful overlap as GPs, hospitals and local authorities duplicated procedures and failed to provide ante- and post-natal care jointly. This report was one of a number which placed great emphasis on improving access to services and continuity in care as a way of improving their effectiveness. The Committee recommended an improvement in coordination of policies and greater cooperation between the three branches of the service.

Also in 1959, the Mental Health Act made more urgent a structure which encouraged hospitals and local authorities to work together. The Act followed the Report of the Royal Commission on the Law relating to Mental Health and Mental Deficiency (1957). This had recommended care in the community for the mentally ill as offering a more humane, and cheaper, alternative to care in a mental hospital. Changes in methods of treatment had already altered dramatically the average length of stay in hospital for mentally ill patients. If community-based services were to be successful, it argued that hospitals, local authorities and general practitioners needed to cooperate closely. The Mental Health Act paved the way to community care by introducing more informal admission procedures to mental hospitals.

A change in the structure of services rested on the willingness of the medical profession to contemplate change, and in 1962, the Porritt Report (Medical Services Review Committee 1962) indicated that at least the leaders of the profession were sufficiently concerned about the problems of the tripartite structure to contemplate reforming it. The report was the work of a committee composed of representatives of the medical profession and conducted independently of the Ministry of Health. It suggested a form of unified administration of the three branches of the service under Area Health Boards. Although not worked out in detail, the report indicated that the profession accepted in principle the need for greater integration. However, it was to take another decade and another 'paper chase' to reach a compromise which was both feasible and acceptable to bring about the reorganisation of 1974.

Reform and managerialism

Meanwhile reform was in the air. The 1960s was a period of rapid economic growth and there was an optimism about the possibilities for the future. There were several major commissions and committees of enquiry which recommended radical changes in the structure of institutions. In 1968, the Redcliffe-Maude Commission made recommendations for the restructuring of local government in England as a whole. Also in 1968, the Seebohm Committee on the Personal Social Services reported and was followed by the Social Services Act of 1970. This established the social service departments and centred social work (including medical social work) in local government. In 1968, there was a regrouping of departments and functions in central government to create a social service ministry, the Department of Health and Social Security, under Richard Crossman. The department was responsible for personal social services, health and social security. In the same year, the Fulton Committee recommended a radical overhaul of the civil service and the establishing of the Civil Service College.

Major constitutional change through the devolution of power to regions was also on the agenda. The reform of the NHS was considered alongside local government. It was planned to dovetail the reorganisation of social services and health services within the reform of local government structure. Both took place on 1 April 1974. A common theme running through the reforms was support for larger units of administration and the more active management of lower-level authorities from above. While it was a period of economic growth there was the perception of rising demand particularly for health and social services as the numbers of elderly people in the population increased. The Ministry of Health was therefore concerned to control and rationalise expansion.

Haywood and Alaszewski in *Crisis in the Health Service* (1980) outline the ideas which characterised the new 'managerialism'.

1 There was a belief that organisational change could be used as a strategy for 'improving' service provision. Changes in structure would bring about improved access to better quality services because they would be better managed. Coordination of policies between different aspects of the service in hospital and community would facilitate cooperation between the different professions involved in care. The increase in specialisation in health care had exacerbated problems of coordination.
2 There was an assumption that larger units of organisation would bring economies of scale and thus be more efficient. Efficiency was more important than easy access to services by patients or families.
3 It was believed that the problems of managing public services were similar to those faced by any large organisation. Previously health care organisations had been seen as unique. The absolute value given to the preservation of life, the presence of pain and death; the care rather than the cash relationship; and the vocational aspect of employment; all these factors had precluded managerial models. A team from Brunel University, in a study on NHS management, specifically ignored the human aspects of organisation and concentrated on the mechanics. They declared: 'For our purposes the patient is not part of the organisation' (quoted in Draper and Smart 1974).
4 It was believed that a rational division of tasks between types and levels of employee could be used to structure the organisation and bring benefits in resource use. The principle was applicable to both managerial and professional hierarchies.
5 Planning was seen as a neutral tool. Targets could be set and progress made towards them. Commenting on the approach, Parston (1980) suggests that planning was seen:

> . . . basically as a methodology, a set of procedures applicable to a variety of activities aimed at achieving selected goals by a systematic

application of resources in programmed quantities and time sequences designed to alter the projected trends and redirect them towards established objectives.

(Parston 1980: 95–6)

The approach to organisational change was mechanistic and planned from the top downwards. The methods were first applied to the planning of hospitals, many of which still suffered from their piecemeal development prior to the setting up of the NHS and the lack of capital investment since 1948.

Managerialism and the professions

During the 1960s and early 1970s, the size of the NHS workforce increased and so did the complexity of the division of labour. To illustrate, in 1949 the total number of staff employed in the NHS in England was approximately 400,000, but by 1980 there had been an increase to over 800,000 employees (Office of Health Economics 1982). If Scotland and Wales are included then the NHS employed almost one million workers or 4 per cent of the working population. It was, and is, the largest civilian employer in the country. Nurses were by far the largest group of staff employed by the NHS; their numbers doubled between 1949 and 1979 and by 1980 they comprised 37 per cent of the NHS labour force.

In the 1960s, governments looked to the principles of scientific management to provide a basis for the organisation of professional work. In 1966, following the Report on Senior Nursing Staff Structure chaired by Brian Salmon, a businessman from Lyons, the food distributors, nursing was reorganised. The Salmon Committee recommended a division between nurse managers and nurse practitioners. Nurse matrons who combined professional and managerial leadership were to be replaced by a hierarchy of nurse managers.

Under the changes brought about as a result of the report, management became a specialist function in its own right. There were three levels of nursing management. The top-level managers were concerned with the making of policy while the middle and first-line managers were responsible for its execution. There was also to be a division between nurse managers and nurse teachers with the higher-ranking posts going to the former. Carpenter summarises the effect of the change. He argues that:

A nursing discipline and nursing knowledge are becoming less important compared with abstract managerial abilities that transcend local peculiarities and idiosyncrasies. It is increasingly the case that nursing background is required less for its utility than to legitimise the position of managers over a workforce, many of whom may have frustrated professional aspirations. . . . The Salmon reform over-emphasised the

> importance of managerial changes in job content to the detriment of clinical changes. It created formal structures in which power, prestige and remuneration increased with distance from the point of patient contact.
>
> (Carpenter 1977: 183–5)

Carpenter also suggests that the emphasis on managerial values in nursing lay behind the increasing growth of union membership among nurses during the 1970s and the pursuit of higher wages and improved conditions of work. On the other hand, had the changes following the Salmon Report not occurred, there would have been little preparation for the increased role in decision making for nurse managers brought about by the reorganisation of the health service in 1974.

In 1967, a similar attempt to promote a managerial consciousness in the medical profession was made through the setting up of the Cogwheel Working Party which made its first report in 1967 (Ministry of Health 1967). Unlike the Salmon Committee, Cogwheel had substantial representation of medical interests and was not chaired by a businessman. The strategy for change was one of persuasion rather than the imposition of an entirely new structure.

The first Cogwheel Report aimed to address the problem of medical management and the uncoordinated activies of clinicians across specialisms. It rightly declared:

> The hospital sector is the most complex, sophisticated and costly sector of the medical care services; problems of management proliferate in an organisation with many branches, many functions and many specialities: we believe that many clinicians fail to appreciate fully the importance of their role in management problems.
>
> (Ministry of Health 1967)

The report recommended the grouping of clinicians into Firms and Divisions, with a representative Medical Executive Committee to make coordinative decisions in relation to the allocation of medical resources over the hospital as a whole. There were two further Cogwheel Reports monitoring the changes. However, by 1972, less than half of the large hospitals had introduced changes along Cogwheel lines (Watkin 1978). Consultants were reluctant to become managers of resources, and studies of decision making in hospitals carried out for the Royal Commission on the NHS (1979) indicated that individual consultants continued to make the key decisions on the use of resources with little reference to their colleagues.

Hospital and health and welfare planning

The 1962 hospital plan

The Hospital Plan aimed to apply rational planning principles to the provision of hospital beds. It laid down bed norms, that is, a standard for the number of beds per population in the different sectors. The Minister of Health, then Enoch Powell, was concerned with the rising costs of hospital care. Britain's hospitals were old and in a poor condition. Investment had been low, and limited to additions to existing hospitals and the expansion of outpatient facilities. The belief was that beds could be used more efficiently by reducing the average length of stay and new buildings would ensure a better distribution of beds. The Plan was based on a region-by-region review of the country's hospitals and on a series of estimates of the appropriate ratio of beds to the population in the main specialisms. The Plan envisaged a reduction in beds in most specialisms: acute medicine from 3.9 to 3.3 per thousand; mental illness 3.3 to 1.8 per thousand. The numbers of beds for 'mental subnormality' patient were to remain constant. However, reflecting a belief that most births would take place in hospital, the numbers of maternity beds was planned to increase to provide for 80 per cent of all births by 1970. The Plan proposed massive new investment. Ninety new hospitals were to be built and others modernised.

The Hospital Plan signalled the beginning of a hospital building programme which continued into the 1970s. However, new hospital building proved to be more expensive, and slower, than had been envisaged. In 1976, David Owen was to write:

> . . . the hospital building programme in 1972/73, like so much expenditure in this country, was completely out of control. Even if Britain had been able to sustain the rate of economic expansion, the forward planning of hospitals was completely unrealistic.
>
> (Owen 1976: 113)

These problems were partly due to inflation and partly due to the rigid and inflexible control which the Ministry of Health, and later the DHSS, kept over standards and costs in the building programme. However, the Hospital Plan provided a 'rational basis' for the development of the hospital service. It also reinforced the dominance of the hospital sector and therefore acute medicine in the NHS. The Plan affected, too, the funding of the new health authorities after 1974. The revenue consequences of the new building made it more difficult to shift resources to community care. Once built there are political costs of not opening and using new hospitals. And running costs of the new hospitals were often high. For example, it is more expensive to clean and heat a modern open-plan hospital than the traditional oblong ward.

The development of the district general hospital

The concept of the District General Hospital (DGH) was also part of the move towards greater efficiency through larger units of operation. The Hospital Plan promoted a movement towards DGHs with 600–800 beds serving a population of 100,000 to 150,000 providing treatment and diagnostic facilities for both inpatients and outpatients in all the more common specialisms including geriatics and mental illness. It was believed that there should be a greater integration of the mentally ill into the mainstream of hospital provision as this would improve standards of care and help reduce the length of stay. However, most weight was given to the importance of bringing a wide range of facilities together for the purposes of efficient management and economies of scale.

In 1969, the Bonham-Carter Report on the functions of the DGH (DHSS 1969a) recommended building large specialist hospitals. The assumption was that no consultant in a specialism should have to work on his own and that for each speciality there ought to be at least two consultants with appropriate supporting staff. This meant even larger hospitals than envisaged by the Hospital Plan. Hospitals with 1000 beds and serving populations of about 250,000 people were proposed. The view was that people in each hospital catchment area should have access to a range of specialisms. This benefit was said to outweigh the disadvantages of longer travel for some patients and their visitors. As a result of the Hospital Plan and the Bonham-Carter Report, many small hospitals were to close over the next decade despite considerable local opposition.

During the 1970s, in the face of escalating costs, the DGH policy was modified. The disadvantages of overcentralisation and inconvenience to patients was now recognised. The idea of community hospitals, small local hospitals combining the facilities of a primary health care centre with accommodation for a selection of inpatients, outpatients and day patients, was developed and implemented. Community hospitals were thought to be particularly appropriate to rural areas. In 1976 David Owen, as junior Minister of Health, expressed the hope that they would be organised in old inner-city hospitals as well. He introduced the concept of the 'nucleus' hospital. This was based on the principle of developing hospitals in blocks or phases around a basic core. In the 1980s, restrictions on capital spending and uncertain future growth brought a more pragmatic approach to hospital building. Overall, bed numbers continued to decline.

The health and welfare plans

A 10-year plan for the health and welfare services was also published in the early 1960s (Ministry of Health 1963). There was an opportunity for joint planning as health and welfare services were provided by both health and local authorities. In the event, the plans were simply an aggregation by the Ministry of Health and the local authorities' guesstimates of what they thought they would achieve within the period. There was no attempt to ensure any compatibility of plans. This had implications particularly for the mental illness services where the reduction in beds was not compensated for by the local authority plans for community-based care. Conversely, local authority plans showed a projected increase in the numbers of community midwives at a time when hospitals were increasing bed provision for maternity cases.

In 1970, another opportunity for joint planning was presented following the establishment of the Social Services Departments. Local authorities were asked to prepare plans covering their personal social service capital and revenue programmes for the period from 1973 to 1983. A DHSS circular asked the health authorities and social service departments to make joint arrangements for forward planning. These plans would be reviewed at regular intervals, as an aid to service development and to make the best use of resources (Webb and Falk 1975). For the first time, the DHSS produced guidelines on appropriate *levels* of provision. The guidelines acted as norms and were a combination of existing service levels and ideas about good practice. Webb and Falk comment that it was virtually impossible to produce coordinated plans in the time available. Most authorities produced a set of 'feverishly concocted trend plans'.

The efforts invested in service development during the 1960s and 1970s led to a gradual improvement in planning techniques and needs forecasting. While this was hardly a 'rational' exercise it promoted a dialogue between those providing health services on the one hand and social services on the other.

The reorganisation of the NHS in 1974

The 1974 reorganisation aimed to transform the NHS into a unified, managed service with a strong planning system designed to implement government priorities. The restructuring process itself was lengthy and spanned the terms of three different Health Ministers and what Watkin (1978) called 'a sea of words'. Two Labour Ministers, Kenneth Robinson and Richard Crossman, produced Green Papers in 1968 and 1970, while a Conservative Minister, Keith Joseph, published a Consultative Document in

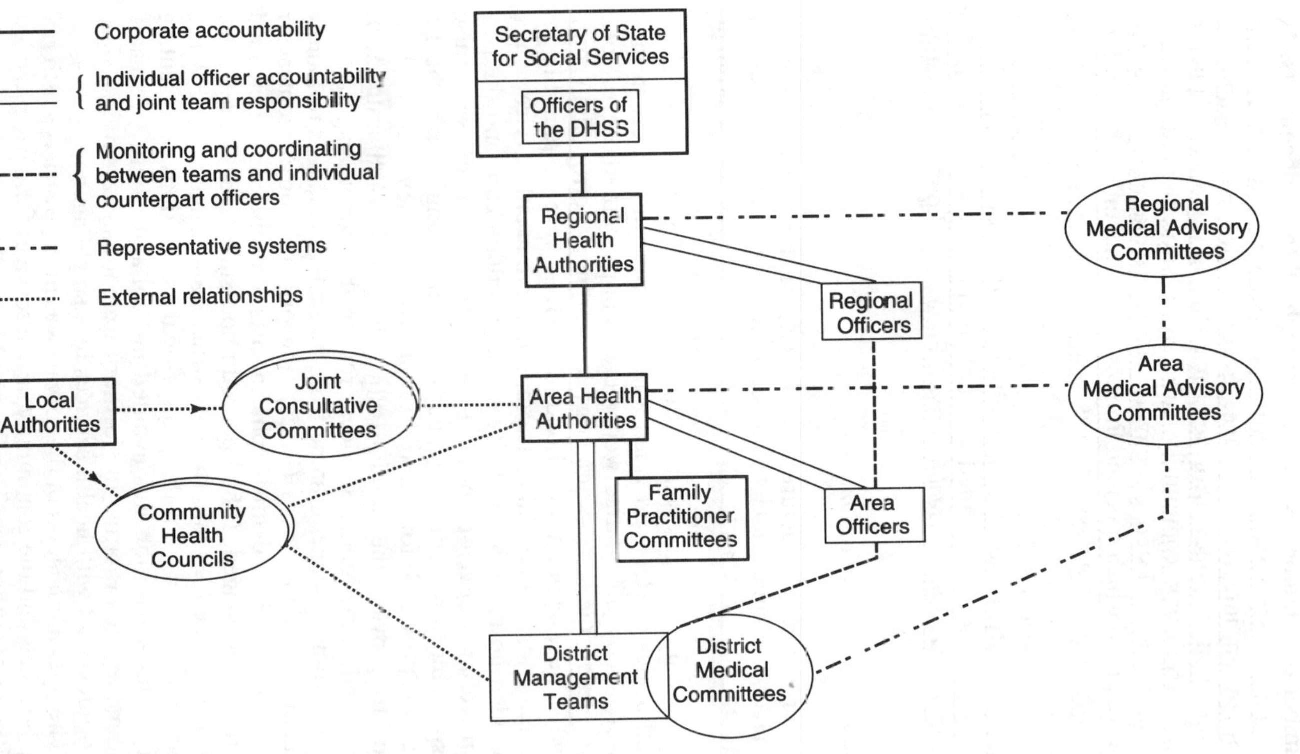

Figure 3.1 ***The organisation of the National Health Service 1974–1982***

1971, and a White Paper in 1972 (DHSS 1971, DHSS 1972). A number of common themes run through all these documents.

First, the tripartite structure was perceived to stand in the way of an integrated service. Second, the centre wanted to ensure that its policy priorities for reducing regional inequalities and introducing community care were implemented and that resources were listed effectively. Third, a management system was required which specified lines of command and accountability. Fourth, a planning system was necessary to ensure coordinated service development between hospitals and community. Fifth, the health service needed a more democratic structure to increase the influence of local communities on decision making. Levitt (1977) provides a detailed account of the new structure in *The Reorganised National Health Service*. Figure 3.1 shows the structure.

Administrative unification

Under the new structure, the 14 Regional Health Authorities (RHAs) remained intact although their powers and responsibilities were changed. They were to take charge of strategic planning of community health service provision as well as of the hospital services within the region. The 90 Area Health Authorities (AHAs) provided a new administrative tier. In most cases, AHA boundaries were coterminous with those of local authorities (the metropolitan districts and non-metropolitan counties). The exception was London. AHAs were responsible for planning for and providing a comprehensive health service, which included hospitals, community and domiciliary care and the preventive and developmental health services. They were also responsible for identifying needs and managing within the resources provided for them by the RHA. They had a duty, too, to provide the administration for, and collaborate with, the family practitioner services, responsible for managing GPs. Apart from a change of name from Executive Councils to Family Practitioner Committees (FPCs), the organisation of contractor services (the GPs, dentists, pharmacists and opticians) remained virtually unchanged. It had proved impossible to devise a way of integrating the GPs into the new structure in England and Wales due to opposition from the professional associations representing GPs. This separation was avoided in Scotland where GPs came under the Area Boards. In Northern Ireland, social services were also integrated with health services in a single agency.

The operational level of the service was in the districts which ran the hospitals and the community health services formerly provided by the local authorities. The District Management Teams (DMTs) were responsible to the AHA Management Team who in turn were accountable to the RHA. At AHA and RHA level, there was an appointed board of members who, like the previous boards, represented local and professional interests.

In England and Wales, the new structure aimed to foster links between health and social services departments by making providing and planning for service provision mandatory. Joint Consultative Committees (JCCs) with members from each authority were established to ensure collaboration. Overall, the assumption of the reorganisation was that the AHAs with their broader span of responsibility would remove barriers to a 'comprehensive' view of health care.

Management

The new management and planning structure was to be the vehicle for change. Management teams in each authority, both region and area, were responsible for running the service. The Grey Book *Management Arrangements for the Reorganised NHS* (DHSS 1974) declared that management should be achieved through consensus decisions. The management team was drawn from the major professional groupings in the service. The team consisted of the administrator; the treasurer; the nursing officer; the community physician; two doctors elected by their colleagues, a consultant from the Medical Executive Committee and a GP. There was to be no hierarchy in the management team. All members were to have equal status. At area level, the Area Management Team (AMT) was responsible to an appointed body of members, who were the formal executive body of the authority. It was intended that the members and the Chair should concentrate on general policy making and monitoring performance, while the AMT had an executive and servicing role and was responsible for producing an area plan covering the separate districts.

At district level, the point at which services were actually provided through hospitals, clinics and the like, the role of the DMT was ambiguous. It was collectively responsible for keeping district services under review, implementing area policies, and its members were also individually responsible for their own sectors of work. For those at operational level, this division of responsibility between area and district was to prove muddled and confusing.

Planning

According to the White Paper (DHSS 1972) explaining the changes, the new planning system was 'the single most important influence for better resource allocation in the service'. It was to be the way of achieving a national strategy of objectives, standards and priorities.

The planning system had three key features. First, it was applied in a standard way throughout the country. Second, it included all aspects of NHS provision. And third, it involved collaboration with local authority social service departments through the JCCs and the public, via the newly created Community Health Councils (CHCs). Whereas guidelines on policy flowed down from the DHSS to the regional level and then to the area level, the actual preparation of the plans, informed by the guidelines, was carried out at district level, then agreed with the area and on to the region and the Department. This was the planning cycle to ensure monitoring and review. It also included a short- and long-term dimension, that is, strategic and operational planning.

At district level, Joint Care Planning Teams – for specific need groups – which included GPs and representatives from the social service departments were to develop joint plans for care. These were coordinated and supported by *area* level joint planning teams who worked with the JCCs at area level. These were composed of members and officers from the AHA and the local authorities and had a budget for projects.

The planning system represented, *par excellence*, a belief in rationality. It was based on the assumption that problems could be analysed, future trends predicted and a policy developed to provide for future contingencies. Planning was seen as a neutral tool, as a way of directing resources to identified priorities and needs across authorities' boundaries.

Centralisation and priority setting

The more centralised structure of the reorganised service was intended to reduce the extent of regional inequalities in the service, and to develop the 'Cinderella' services: pushing services for the elderly, mentally ill and handicapped and the physically handicapped in the direction of community care.

There were to be many difficulties in putting these priorities into practice, which are discussed in subsequent chapters. The methods for achieving a shift in priorities were not developed centrally until after reorganisation had taken place. In 1976 the Regional Allocation Working Party (RAWP) recommended an increase in expenditure to the poorer regions at the expense of richer ones. The Priorities documents, *Priorities for Health and Personal Social Services in England* (DHSS 1976), and *The Way Forward* (DHSS 1977), recommended increases in expenditure on the Cinderella services.

The reorganised health service provided a framework for policy change. Crossman, when Health Minister, saw the reorganisation as a way of achieving social reform and he was influenced by his reading of the recent past in the NHS. His diaries (Crossman 1977) indicate his alarm and concern about the difference in standards of care between different types of hospital, particularly between the teaching hospital and the local DGH and between the acute and long-stay hospitals.

Ten years earlier, Barbara Robb's *Sans Everything* (1967) had served to raise the level of awareness of the problem but a series of enquiries into particular hospitals created acute concern in the Department of Health. In 1969, the Inquiry into Ely Hospital (DHSS 1969b) revealed a horrifying story of inertia. It commented on:

> an unduly casual attitude towards death and a continued acceptance of old-fashioned, unduly rough and undesirably low standards of nursing care.

Other scandals and enquiries followed: in 1971, Farleigh (DHSS 1971a) and in 1972, Whittingham (DHSS 1972b) and later Normansfield (DHSS 1978, Klein 1978). At Whittingham, the committee of enquiry accepted that allegations that troublesome patients received the 'wet towel treatment' (a wet towel was twisted round the patient's neck until they lost consciousness, and methylated spirits poured over patients' clothing and then set alight) were substantially true. The message seemed clear; there was too little public accountability and scrutiny. Standards were poor and so was management. In 1969, the Hospital Advisory Committee had been set up to 'inspect' the long-stay hospitals and improve standards of care. It was expected that a restructured NHS would help to improve standards.

Keith Joseph, who followed Crossman as Minister of Health, also believed in the importance of good management and accountability. His view was that centralisation with a clear definition of tasks and roles at region, area and district would ensure both efficiency, improved quality of services and a shift in priorities. He, too, was concerned about the Cinderella services. He commented when Secretary of State for Health and Social Services:

> This is a very fine country to be acutely ill or injured in but take my advice and do not become old or frail or mentally ill here.
>
> (Mooney, Russell and Weir 1980: 159)

Democratic accountability in the NHS

The 1974 reorganisation increased democratic accountability in the NHS in three ways; through increasing the membership of health authorities to represent local interests better, through setting up internal management and advisory structures to involve the workforce in decision making and through the establishment of Community Health Councils (CHCs) to represent local pressure groups.

CHCs were a new innovation. There were to be 207 of them, one for each district of the NHS. Half their members were nominated by local authorities, one-third by voluntary organisations and the rest by the regional authorities. The CHC's role was to act as a watchdog for the public. It had limited powers. It had the right to information; it could visit health service facilities and had to be consulted about service changes. The role of the CHC is discussed further in Chapter 12.

Democracy of the syndicalist variety was reflected in the representation of the professions and trade unions within the management structure itself. First, a network of professional advisory committees was established so that the management teams could be kept informed of the views of the different professional groups. Second, the management teams themselves contained members of the *major* professional groupings so that decisions could be widely discussed and information disseminated.

Reorganisation and general practitioners

No discussion of the reorganisation of 1974 is complete without some reference to the role of general practitioners. FPCs and GPs remained an anachronism in the blueprint for a planned and coordinated structure. The coordination of community nursing staff and GPs was a major problem and continued to be so following reorganisation. Nursing staff and GPs operated in different social, professional and organisational worlds. Even attachment of nurses to practices did not solve the problem.

GPs had continued since 1948 to be self-employed practitioners under contract to provide services to the NHS. Although the overall coordination of the contractor services and the planning of health centres became the responsibility of the AHA in 1974, in effect this important area of primary health care remained outside the administrative control of the health authorities and operated much as before.

Health centres, which were Bevan's attempt to provide a setting in which a number of health workers could practise from the same premises, were initially slow to develop. This was despite a financial incentive. If doctors chose to form health centres, local authorities would provide premises and pay part of the management costs. By 1963, there were 18 purpose-built health centres in operation in England and Wales. By 1969, there were 139 and by 1971, 300. By March 1977 there were 731 centres, providing practice premises for 17 per cent of all GPs. Integration between local authority health services and GPs developed through nurse attachment and this has helped to blur the distinction between health centres and the larger group practice. Reedy (1977), in a survey, found that 68 per cent of practices in England had at least one attached nurse; the larger the practice the greater the likelihood of attachment.

The Royal Commission on the NHS

The 1974 reorganisation of the NHS had been an ambitious attempt to increase the efficiency, priority setting and democracy of the NHS. However, the effect of the reorganisation on those working in the NHS was traumatic and the years following were associated with industrial disputes, public dissatisfaction and loss of financial control. The planning and management systems were soon seen to have failed. The response of the government was to set up a Royal Commission in 1978. Its report contained an analysis of the 1974 reforms.

The Commission commented on the impact of reoganisation on staff. Looking back from the 1990s and a decade of almost continuous change, their comments have a certain irony. They condemn the lack of real preparation of top management for their task and were critical of the process and impact of change, declaring that this had brought:

> An immense amount of administrative work in preparation for the new machinery; disruption of ordinary work, both before, and after, reorganisation caused by the need to prepare for and implement changes; the breakdown of well-established formal and informal networks and the loss of experienced staff through early retirement and resignation; stresses and strains on some staff of having to compete for new jobs.
> (Report of the Royal Commission on the NHS 1979: 37)

The Commission Report pointed to a number of weaknesses. In 1974, the approach had been mechanistic. Reforms were imposed from above with too little attention paid to relationships and values of those working in the service. By and large, it had failed to achieve the desired integration between agencies, although in some instances, greater integration had been achieved at the cost of 'additional work, uncertainty and frustration'. The report declared that the top-heavy planning system and the emphasis on consensus management had slowed down decision making, and made priority setting more difficult. Over issues such as where to develop or cut back there were, inevitably, conflicts of interest and opinion which had resulted in no action being taken. Moreover, there was often insufficient or inadequate information on which to base decisions, and consequently there were fundamental difficulties in implementing the government's priorities.

Patients first, and the 1982 reorganisation

In 1979, *Patients First*, a consultative document published by the incoming Conservative government, introduced a focus on the patient, which persisted in government rhetoric into the 1990s. The document recommended further restructuring. It declared that the 1974 reorganisation was 'too ambitious, was in some ways ill-conceived and created a number of undesirable side-effects', a view which was widely shared. They recommended that the structure should be simplified and responsibility for making decisions be moved closer to the locality for which health services were being provided. It declared that large areas should be broken up into districts. They believed that the 'natural community', that is, the catchment area of the hospital, was an important factor in drawing boundaries for districts rather than coterminosity with the local authorities.

Patients First recommended that the district should become the key accountable body in the new structure, responsible for *providing* services as well as *planning* for them. The locus of decision-making would thus move downward. The DHA would make decisions to meet local needs with a tighter system of management and a simplified planning structure. Contrary to the Royal Commission's recommendations, FPCs, which were responsible for managing the contracts of GPs, were to retain their existing status. In the foreword to the White Paper Patrick Jenkin, then Health Secretary, opined:

> I believe it wrong to treat the NHS as though it were or could be a single giant integrated system, rather we must try to see it as a whole series of local health services serving local communities and managed by local people.
>
> (DHSS 1979: 1)

'Managed by local people' was used in two senses. The first was a representation of local interests through membership of the authorities. Despite the emphasis on the community, however, local *authority* membership was to be reduced on the grounds that members should be concerned with local needs. Research had indicated that few local authority members had sufficient time to devote to health authority work. The membership of the DHA should be about 20, instead of more than 30, and four members were to represent the local authority. There was to be a consultant, a GP, a nurse, a university nominee, a trade-union member and the remainder were to be 'generalists'. All members were to be chosen for their personal qualities and for the individual contribution they could make to the service. Paradoxically, despite emphasis given to involvement by local people, CHCs were threatened with extinction on the grounds that with more locally based membership of DHAs they would be unnecessary.

The second aspect of 'managed by local people' was the greater flexibility allowed to local managers in administering the service. The composition of the Management Team continued to include the heads of service who, much as before, were responsible for managing, coordinating and planning the service through reaching a consensus among members.

Responsibility for decision making was placed on the professionals. Collaboration with local authorities remained, with arrangements for JCCs, although this became more complex where a new health authority spanned two or more local authorities. Districts were responsible to RHAs and the Minister in broadly the same way. Regions did not alter their boundaries, nor was any major change in their functions recommended.

The 1982 reorganisation

On 1 April 1982, 192 DHAs and nine special health authorities were established in England based on existing districts or an amalgamation of districts. Figure 3.2 shows the new structure.

CHCs survived the consultation to be reconstituted on the basis of the new districts while FPCs became fully autonomous bodies based on the previous area boundaries. They were not coterminous with districts and in some cases covered a number of DHAs. Within the districts, the units of management varied to suit local needs. Some were based on institutions such as hospitals while others crossed these boundaries to cover 'care' groups such as the elderly.

The reorganisation did nothing to resolve the problems of the conflicts and state of stasis generated by conensus management. Although a management tier was abolished, the planning and control was still far from top down. This led Alaszewski, Tether and Macdonnell (1981) to describe the changes as 'another dose of managerialism'.

As soon as the changes were introduced in 1982, the health service entered into a decade of financial constraint. The responsibility for making choices about spending decisions and cutting the service were pushed to the local level. Blame for any deterioration therefore lay with the districts and not central government (Klein 1980). They faced the difficulty of managing with a shrinking resource and had to deal with criticisms from local groups.

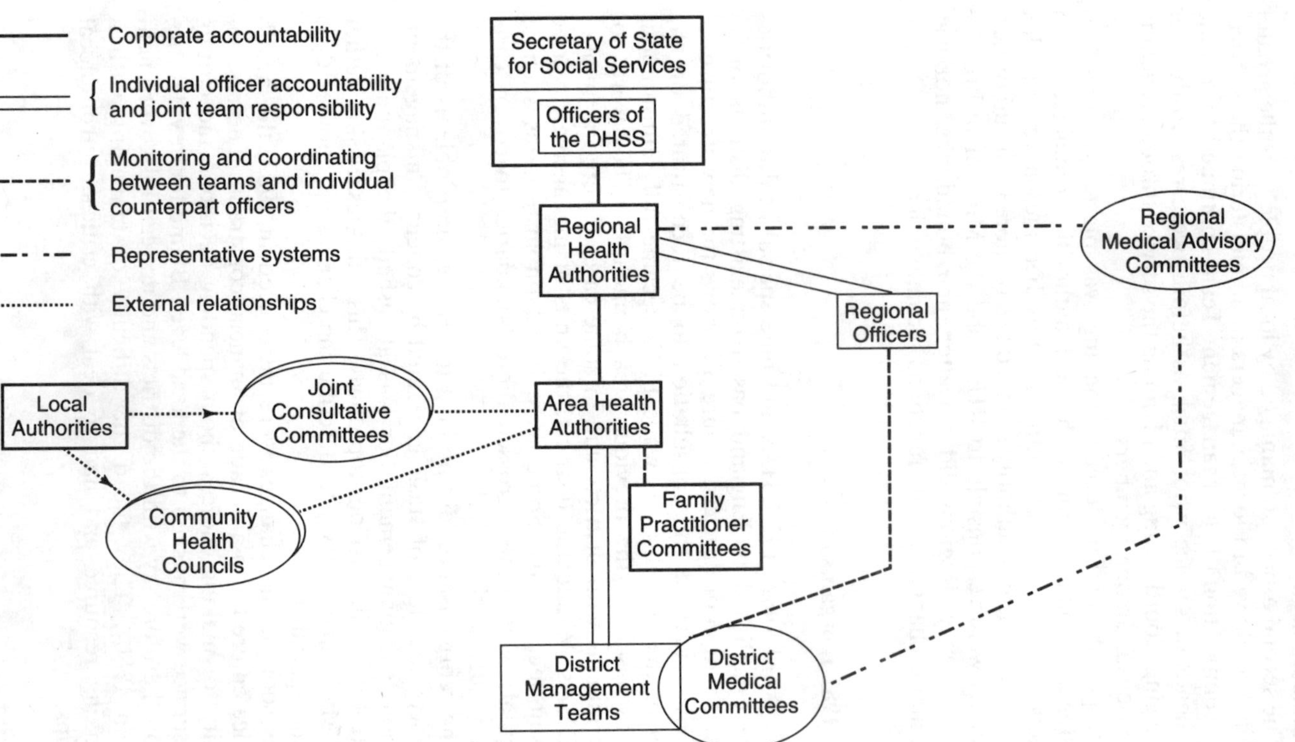

Figure 3.2 ***The organisation of the National Health Service 1982–1990***

Final comment

Looking back on the decade of reorganisation in the 1970s, it may be thought that little had been achieved in the service as one restructuring followed another. However, despite its faults, the 1974 reorganisation began the transformation of the NHS into a national service with national standards. The more *laissez-faire* period of the 1960s was replaced by a planning system which identified national priorities even though local strategies were often inadequate. Inequities in distribution had been identified and the community services were managed alongside hospitals for the first time. Perhaps most importantly, management had developed as a distinct task and a cadre of trained managers began to emerge. This was to prove crucial in the cost-cutting 1980s in achieving the increases in productivity and in handling the conflicts which resulted.

References

Alaszewski, A., Tether, P. and Macdonnell (1981) 'Another Dose of Managerialism?' Commentary 15a *Social Science and Medicine*, vol. 1, Jan. 4, pp. 5–15.

Carpenter, M. (1977) 'The New Managerialism and Professionalism in Nursing', in M. Stacey *et al., Health and the Division of Labour*, Croom Helm, London.

Crossman, R. (1977) *Diaries of a Cabinet Minister*, vol. 3, Hamish Hamilton and Jonathan Cape, London.

Department of Health and Social Security and Welsh Office (1969a) *Report of the Committee on the Functions of the District General Hospital* (Chairman: Sir Desmond Bonham-Carter), HMSO, London.

Department of Health and Social Security (1969b) *Report of the Committee of Inquiry into Allegations of Ill-treatment of Patients and other Irregularities at the Ely Hospital, Cardiff*, Cmnd 3975, HMSO, London.

Department of Health and Social Security (1970) *The Future Structure of the National Health Service*, HMSO, London.

Department of Health and Social Security (1971a) *Report of the Farleigh Hospital Committee of Enquiry*, Cmnd 4557, HMSO, London,

Department of Health and Social Security (1971b) *National Health Service Reorganisation: Consultative Document*, DHSS, London.

Department of Health and Social Security (1972a) *National Health Service Reorganisation: England*, Cmnd 5055, HMSO, London.

Department of Health and Social Security (1972b) *Report of the Committee of Enquiry into Whittingham Hospital*, Cmnd 4861, HMSO, London.

Department of Health and Social Security (1974) *Management Arrangements for the Reorganised National Health Service*, HMSO, London.

Department of Health and Social Security (1976) *Priorities for Health and Personal Social Services in England: a consultative Document*, HMSO, London.

Department of Health and Social Security (1977) *The Way Forward*, HMSO, London.

Department of Health and Social Security (1978) *The Normansfield Hospital Inquiry*, HMSO, London.

Draper, P. and Smart, T. (1974) 'Social Science and Health Policy in the United Kingdom', *International Journal of Health Services*, 4 (3) pp. 453–70.

Eckstein, H. (1958) *The English Health Service: its origins, structure and achievement*, Harvard University Press, Cambridge, Mass.

Fulton Committee (1968) *Report of the Committee on the Civil Service*, Cmnd 3638, HMSO, London.

Ham, C. (1981) *Policy-making in the National Health Service: case study of the Leeds Regional Hospital Board*, Macmillan, London.

Haywood, S. and Alaszewski, A. (1980) *Crisis in the Health Service*, Croom Helm, London.

Klein, R. (1978) 'Normansfield: vacuum of management', *British Medical Journal*, 23–30 Dec., pp. 1802–4.

Klein, R. (1980) 'Between Central Control and Local Responsiveness: striking the balance', *British Medical Journal*, 9 Feb., p. 420.

Levitt, R. (1977) *The Reorganised National Health Service* (rev. edn), Croom Helm, London.

Medical Services Review Committee (1962) *A Review of the Medical Services in Great Britain* (Chairman: Sir Arthur Porritt), Social Assay, London.

Ministry of Health (1956) *Report of the Committee of Enquiry into the Cost of the National Health Service* (Chairman: C. W. Guillebaud), Cmnd 9663, HMSO, London.

Ministry of Health (1959) *Report of the Maternity Services Committee* (Chairman: Earl of Cranbrook), HMSO, London.

Ministry of Health (1962) *National Health Service: a hospital plan for England and Wales*, Cmnd 1604, HMSO, London.

Ministry of Health (1963) *Plans for Health and Welfare Services of the Local Authorities in England and Wales*, Cmnd 1973, HMSO, London.

Ministry of Health (1967) *First Report of the 'joint Working Party on the Organisation of Medical Work in Hospitals* (Cogwheel Report), HMSO, London.

Ministry of Health (1968) *The Administrative Structure of Medical and Related Services in England and Wales*, HMSO, London.

Ministry of Health and Scottish Home and Health Department (1966) *Report of the Committee on Senior Nursing Staff Structure* (Chairman: Brian Salmon), HMSO, London.

Mooney, G. H., Russell, E. M. and Weir, R. D. (1980) *Choices for Health Care*, Macmillan, London, ch. 11.

Office of Health Economics (1982) *Compendium of Statistics 1981*, Office of Health Economics, London.

Owen, D. (1976) *In Sickness and in Health*, Quartet Books, London.

Parston, G. (1980) *Planners, Politics and Health Services*, Croom Helm, London.

Reedy, B. (1977) 'The Health Team', in *Trends in General Practice*, Royal College of General Practitioners.

Report of the Royal Commission on the Law relating to Mental Health and Mental Deficiency 1954–1957 (1957) Cmnd 169, HMSO, London.

Report of the Royal Commission on the NHS (1979) (Chairman: Sir Alec Merrison), Cmnd 7615, HMSO, London.
Robb, B. (1967) *Sans Everything: a case to answer*, Nelson, London.
Watkin, B. (1978) *The National Health Service: the first phase 1948–1974 and after* Allen & Unwin, London.
Webb, A. and Falk, N. (1975) 'Planning the Social Services: the ten year plans', *Policy and Politics*, 3 (2), pp. 33–54.
Webster, C. (1988) *The Health Services since the War,* vol. 1, *Problems of Health Care before 1957*, HMSO, London.

CHAPTER 4

Expenditure and resource allocation policies in the NHS

Funding health care, particularly in a tax-based service, is a contentious issue. Governments wish to claim how well they are doing, how many more patients are being treated, how many new developments have been introduced. Or, if they wish to inject realism into the debate, politicians may declare that potentially, demand for health care is 'infinite', and priorities must be set. Those who work in health care, those who need services and those who oppose a government in power may equally point to acute shortages, waiting lists and unmet needs. Funding health care is a matter of both politics and economics.

From the inception of the NHS, politicians have expressed concern about costs. In 1948 Aneurin Bevan, then Minister of Health, declared:

> We will never have all we need. Expectation will always exceed capacity. This service must always be changing, growing and improving, it must always appear inadequate.
>
> (Foot 1962: 209–10)

It was another conservative politician, Enoch Powell, Minister of Health between 1960 and 1963, who wrote:

> There is virtually no limit to the amount of medical care an individual is capable of absorbing . . . the appetite for medical care *vient en mangeant*,
>
> (Powell 1966: 27)

Governments in the UK have contained NHS spending at a macro level but as the service is largely free at the point of delivery, demand is likely to outrun supply. Cost containment has been achieved through a variety of informal rationing mechanisms. These mostly depend on those who provide services working within allocated budgets. Until the early 1980s, these arrangements rested on an implicit agreement between the various interest groups in health care which depended on trust. Expenditures were allowed to rise annually to allow for development and, the concordat between interest groups in health care held (Klein 1989). However, in the 1980s, governments, concerned to reduce government expenditure, looked for alternatives. In 1982, the Conservative government, having contemplated a market-orientated system, concluded that:

> . . . the principle that adequate health should be provided for all, regardless of their ability to pay, must be the foundation of any arrangements for financing health care.
>
> (Thatcher, M. Prime Minister's speech at the Conservative Party Conference, October 1982)

However, they sought to improve efficiency through inducing economy by almost nil growth, strong management and a variety of cost-cutting measures. As a consequence, the 1980s were dogged by charges of both profligacy (from the government) and parsimony (from those providing care and from opposition parties). Evidence can be found to support both positions. However, a recent study by the OECD comparing seven countries concluded that although the UK spent less of its GDP than most other countries, and less than would be expected in a country with the UK's standard of living 'it nevertheless had a better health record than might be expected from its relatively low levels of spending and activity' (OECD 1992: 119). It ranked second for perinatal mortality and third for male life expectation. Document 29 (page 345) provides further comparative figures. This chapter aims to consider the pressures on NHS expenditure, make comparisons between the NHS and other health systems, and examine the patterns of expenditure and activity over time and look at how different governments have approached issues of internal allocations and value for money.

The rising pressure of demand

In 1972, as Secretary of State for Health, Richard Crossman (1972) referred to the effects of demography, equality and technology in creating pressures for ever increasing health care spending.

Demography

In common with other post industrial societies, following World War Two, Britain experienced a transformation in the demographic structure which affected welfare spending. As far as health spending is concerned, the most significant factor is the proportion of elderly people. In 1961, just under 12 per cent of the population were aged over 65. By 1991, this had risen to 16 per cent. Trends within this age group are also important as the proportion of very elderly people is also rising. In 1961, 1.9 per cent of the population was over 80 years old. By 1991, this had almost doubled to 2.8 per cent (*Social Trends* 1994).

Elderly people are heavy users of health services. They affect demand in a number of ways: in the numbers of GP consultations; the number of prescriptions; the numbers of admissions to hospital and the length of time spent in hospital when admitted. To give just one illustration: in 1988, although those over 75 years of age were only 7 per cent of the population, they accounted for 43 per cent of the inpatient workload (OHE 1992). As a consequence of these factors, per capita spending rises rapidly with age. For example, in 1991–2, the average per capita spending for the population as a whole was £2240. For those over 85, it was almost three times as much at £7500 (Hills 1993). As numbers have risen, so has the proportion of elderly people in relation to the working population. In 1951, there were 21 people of pensionable age to every hundred of working age. By 1991, there were 30 to every hundred (*Social Trends* 1994).

Technology

Crossman referred to the pressure of 'technology'. The consequences of technological change have been a further factor with which all governments have had to wrestle. As early as 1952, Dr Ffrangcon Roberts in *The Costs of Health Care* had argued that Beveridge was wrong to assume that the demand for health care was finite and that demand for health care would fall as the health of the population improved. Medicine, he argued, was expanding and new and more expensive methods of treatment were being developed. The result of this would not be the final conquest of disease but would leave doctors more difficult problems to solve – those relating to the treatment and care of degenerative and chronic illness. These would be *more* prevalent as there was an increase in the numbers of people reaching old age. New and more sophisticated methods of diagnosis would also change ideas on the nature of disease and costs would be incurred as doctors felt obliged to use all the techniques at their disposal to establish beyond doubt what their patients were suffering from.

During the 1950 and 1960s, many new and potent drugs were being brought into use. The sulphonomides and antibiotics which began to be introduced in the 1930s were very widely used by the 1950s, when they accounted for half the ingredient costs of NHS prescriptions. Even Bevan commented:

> I shudder to think of the ceaseless cascade of medicine which is pouring down British throats at the present time. I wish I could believe that its efficiency was equal to the credulity with which it is being swallowed.
>
> (quoted in Campbell 1987: 183–4)

Tranquillising drugs and new drugs to control chronic conditions such as diabetes mellitus and high blood pressure were also part of the drug revolution. While these might be used to keep people out of hospital, other diagnostic, life support and life-saving equipment was so capital intensive that it could only be provided within a hospital setting. In the 1960s, surgical techniques were changing in relation, for example, to the treatment of cancer and, in the 1970s, transplant surgery developed to be followed by keyhole surgery in the 1980s. In the same period, chemotherapy and radiotherapy appeared to offer the hope of cure, or at least the remission of symptoms, in the treatment of cancer. Kidney dialysis had become routine treatment. New techniques were also being developed for diagnosis. In the 1980s, computerised imaging and the possibility of filmless X-rays made new claims on hospital finances. Centralised sterile supply units developed to support surgery and other activities while intensive care units and post-operative recovery units provided a battery of equipment for life support in a variety of situations, from accident cases to premature babies.

The existence of such techniques and the publicity given to medicine helped to raise public expectations. In societies with a strong emphasis on work and productivity, high levels of education and the knowledge that time spent being ill is time lost for work or leisure, has tended to make medical care into a consumer good. Payer, in a fascinating book, *Medicine and Culture* (1990), explores the differences in notions of health and sickness between Britain, France, Germany and the USA.

The increasingly technological nature of medicine is reflected in the rising numbers of professional and technical staff (shown in Table 4.1). Since the NHS was established the number of professional staff in England increased rapidly. Between 1949

Table 4.1 **NHS staff in post by main staff group (WTEs) 1981–89**

Main group of staff	*1981*	*1985*	*1987*	*1989*	*% change 1981–91*
Nursing and midwifery	47.5	49.3	50.6	50.9	3.5
Medical and dental	5.0	5.3	5.4	5.8	12.7
All prof. and Technical	7.9	9.1	9.9	10.2	24.4
Maintenance and works	3.3	3.2	3.0	2.7	–22.1
Ancillary	20.9	17.1	14.4	12.9	–40.5
Admin and clerical	13.2	13.7	14.3	15.2	11.6
Ambulance	2.2	2.2	2.4	2.4	3.5
Total	824,400	812,900	799,300	796,600	–3.4
%	100	100	100	100	

Source: Annual Report of the Chief Medical Officer for 1992, (1993) DOH, London.

and 1980 there was an increase in the numbers of doctors and nurses of 168 per cent. By 1980, the UK NHS employed over a million workers. Since this time, as competitive tendering has been introduced in the 1980s, the size of the NHS workforce has fallen and the mix of staff has changed. The proportion of skilled professional staff has increased in proportion to the less skilled. For example, between 1981 and 1991, the numbers of professional and technical staff rose from 133,300 to 173,000 (*Social Trends* 1994). However, by international standards, the NHS employs a low number of doctors. As Document 29 (page 345) indicates, the UK has the lowest ratio of doctors to population of any OECD country at 1.4 per thousand. The EC average is 2.6 (OECD 1992). The percentage of administrative staff is also low compared to countries with more complex systems of administration.

Table 4.1 shows the staff in post by main group and the percentage increases between 1981 and 1989.

Inequalities

In a national service, in which every hospital and every consultant wished to acquire the best and latest in up-to-date equipment, there were pressures to universalise the best. Indeed, from the 1970s, inequalities in the distribution of health services were high on the agenda of successive Ministers of Health. The NHS came into existence with a geographical maldistribution of resources in relation to population distribution. This was a legacy from the past, of a combination of market forces, past philanthropy and civic pride. The south was better off than the north, the towns more fortunate than the country. Areas with a larger concentration of higher socio-economic groups were better off than those with a predominantly working-class population. In 1946, specialist care for children, the treatment of venereal disease, cancer and the practice of orthopaedics were virtually unobtainable outside London and the other large cities. It was found that:

> . . . the number of residents per GP was twice as great in Kensington as in Hampstead, thrice as great as Harrow, four times as great in Bradford, five times in Wakefield, six times in West Bromwich, and seven times in South Shields.
>
> (PEP 1944, quoted in Gray 1993: 36)

In the early decades of the NHS these inequalities were reinforced by the NHS funding methods, discussed later in this chapter. As these geographical inequities became politically unacceptable, resources were reallocated, but this created an upward pressure overall. From the 1980s, when some of the most blatant inequities has been eradicated, there was increasing pressure to improve services for disadvantaged groups such as disabled people and

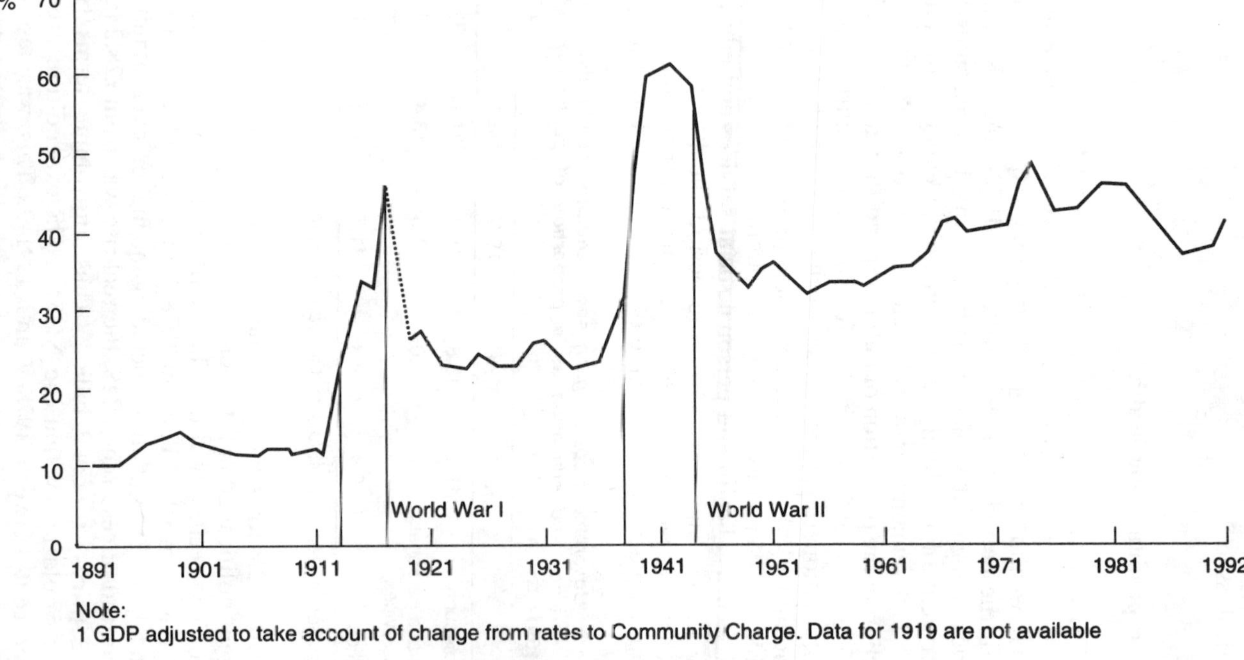

Note:
1 GDP adjusted to take account of change from rates to Community Charge. Data for 1919 are not available

Figure 4.1 ***General government expenditure as a percentage of GDP 1891–1992***
Source: Social Trends (1994) HMSO, London.

those from ethnic minorities whose special needs had been hitherto ignored. Also, as Chapter 12 indicates, there has been increasing pressure to offer greater choice as consumerism became a political issue.

Public expenditure and health

In the UK, there has been a long-term trend towards a higher proportion of Gross Domestic Product (GDP), a measure of national wealth, being devoted to public expenditure. During most of the period from 1951 to the mid 1970s, the UK enjoyed historically high rates of economic growth. This accounted for 75 per cent of the total increase in public expenditure (Judge 1982). The remainder was a result of increased taxation and a reduction in the proportion of public expenditure going to military spending. Figure 4.1 shows the trends. The downturns following the international economic crisis in the 1970s, and in the 1980s coinciding with the Thatcher governments should be noted.

Table 4.2 compares the share of public spending devoted to social security, health and personal social services and education between 1951 and 1990. Over the period, health and personal social services were subject to less fluctuation than other sectors. This may reflect a higher degree of central control over supply.

Table 4.2 ***Government spending on social security, health and personal social services and education as a proportion of public expenditure 1951–1991***

	1951	*1961*	*1971*	*1981*	*1991*
Social security	11.8	15.8	16.4	31.1	32.1
Health and personal social services	10.1	9.0	11.5	13.4	13.8
Education	6.8	9.8	11.7	14.3	12.9

Source: Social Trends, HMSO, London (various years).

Figure 4.2 shows the percentage real growth achieved under different political administrations.

Looking specifically at the Thatcher/Major years, total expenditure grew from £9.2 billion in 1978–9 to £37.3 billion in 1991–2. When adjusted for inflation, including the higher levels of inflation for pay and prices in the NHS, the real rise was from £28.2 (using 1991–2 prices) to £34.3 billion. Thus, in volume terms (what money would buy within the NHS), NHS expenditure grew by 22 per cent between 1978–9 and 1991–2. This was less than 2 per cent a year. However, in the early 1990s, in the wake of the health reforms, volume expenditure has begun to rise. From 1991 to 1992–3 the rise was 3.9 per cent.

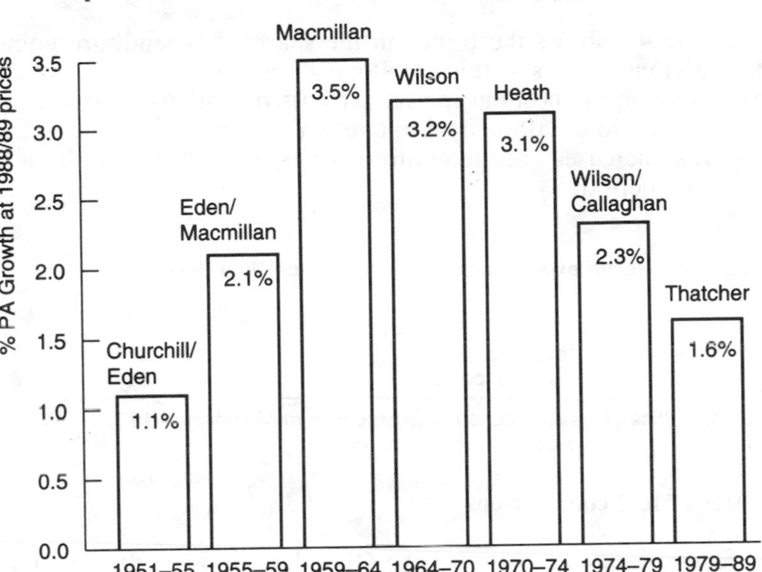

Figure 4.2 **Total NHS spending: percentage real growth per annum 1951–1989**
Source: Appleby, J. (1992) Financing the NHS, Open University Press.

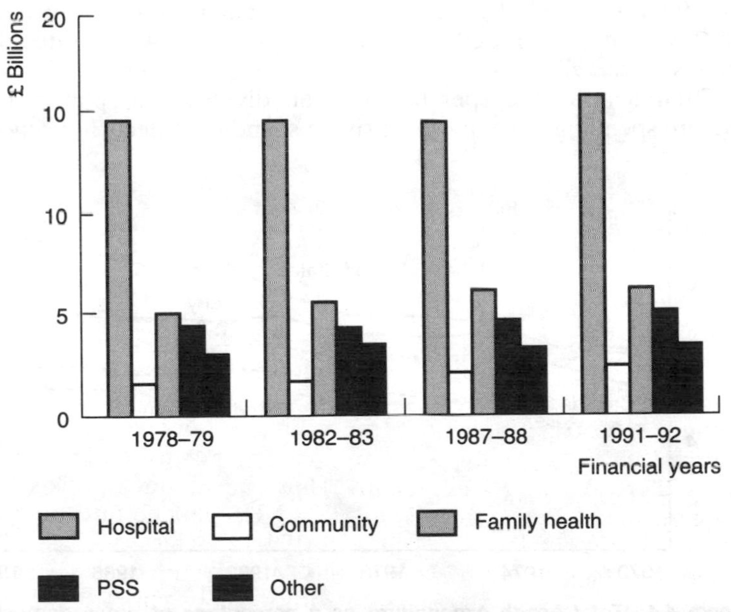

Figure 4.3 **UK NHS and PSS volume expenditure by sector 1978/9–1991/2**

Figure 4.3 shows the trends in the share of expenditure going to different sectors within health and personal social services. Spending on the hospital service far outstrips other services.

Table 4.3 looks at the data in another way and shows the actual and real increases in expenditure per person on health in the UK over the period.

Table 4.3 **Health expenditure per person in the UK 1960–90**

	1960	*1970*	*1980*	*1990*
Health expenditure per person	16	36	207	494
'Real' health expenditure per person	100	148	234	296

Source: Office of Health Economics, compendium of statistics (1993).

International comparisons

In terms of the proportion of the GDP devoted to health, the UK spends less than most other OECD countries. In 1990, it ranked 17 out of 22 developed countries. New Zealand, Ireland, Spain, Portugal and Greece spent less (OHE 1993). On this measure, therefore, the UK has relatively low health expenditures, particularly when compared to its European neighbours. The overall level of economic performance of a country tends to affect the amount of overall health spending. Thus, the USA at 12.4 per cent of GDP in 1990, is the world leader, followed by Canada at 9.0, France 8.9 and Sweden 8.7. The UK trailed at 6.1. Figure 4.4 illustrates the trends since 1970.

Total health care spending can be divided into public and private spending. The level of private spending reflects household

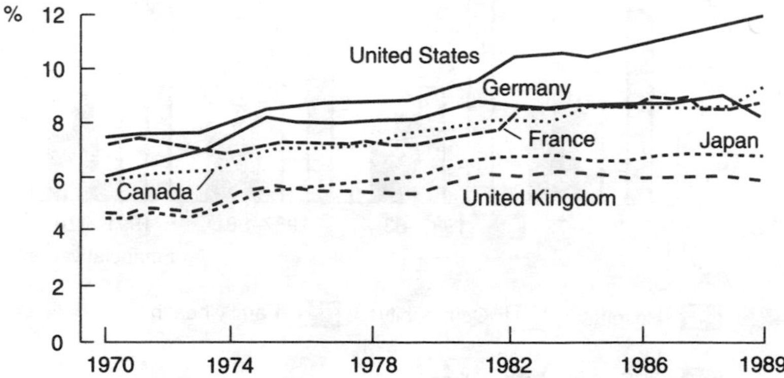

Figure 4.4 ***Total health expenditure as a percentage of gross domestic product, selected OECD countries, 1970–1989***

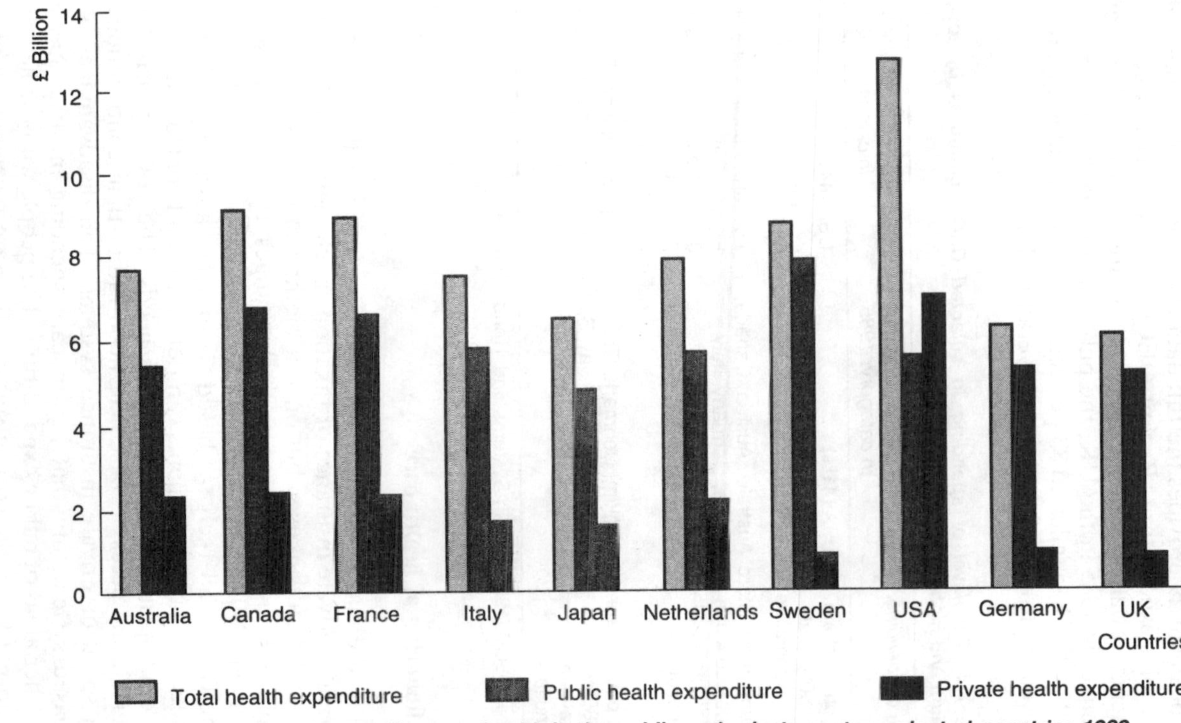

Figure 4.5 ***Comparison of expenditure on health in the public and private sector: selected countries 1989***
Source: OECD (1993) Health Systems and Trends, 1960–91.

choice. Countries vary widely in the balance between public and private spending. In the US more than one half of the total spending is private. Other leading spenders, such as the Scandinavian countries spend only a relatively small percentage privately.

Document 29 provides the full data expressed as proportions of per capita expenditure. Recent OECD figures suggest a general tendency towards reducing the public share of expenditure. For example, in 1985 in the UK, the public share was 86 per cent but by 1991, this had fallen to 83 per cent. The same trend is apparent in Sweden. Table 4.4 shows the overall ranking.

Table 4.4 **The level of spending in selected OECD countries by low, medium and high: 1985 and 1991**

Level of spending	*Selected OECD countries in category: 1985*	*Selected OECD countries in category: 1991*
Low: public share below 60% total health expenditure	USA (41%)	USA (44%)
Medium: public share between 60% and 80% of total health expenditure	Australia, Austria, Canada, France, Germany, Italy, Japan, Netherlands, Switzerland	Australia, Austria, Canada, France, Germany, Italy, Japan, Netherlands, New Zealand, Sweden, Switzerland
High: public share over 80 per cent of total health expenditure	Belgium, Denmark, Greece, New Zealand, Norway, Spain, Sweden, UK	Belgium, Denmark, Greece, Norway, Spain, UK

Source: OECD (1993) Health Systems and Trends 1960–91.

The financing of health care

Health care may be financed through three main methods: social insurance; private insurance or taxation. Each method has advantages and disadvantages, but once a method of funding has been established, it is rare for radical changes to occur (Epsing Anderson 1990).

The UK has a largely tax-based system. The advantages of such systems are that governments can determine and control the level of overall spending to meet health needs. The coverage can be universal, and access is based on need rather than contributions as in social or private insurance systems. The disadvantages of tax-based systems are that health care spending must compete with other areas of public expenditure. The people who use health care do not know the cost of services they are receiving because there is no need for pricing and costing. Market theory suggests that in this situation demand will be high, but access to health care may be provider-determined (as in the UK) or through some other form of rationing. Users may thus be unable to express demand or preferences directly. In other words, they may want to spend more on health care but this is determined by the political rather than the economic process. Taking a comparative view, the 1992 OECD report comments:

> At best, they [tax-based systems] seem to be capable of supplying good quality health care according to clinical need, financed at a reasonable cost. However, they are frequently attended by waiting lists and seem to encourage a brisk and impersonal style of service. At worst, the result is overloaded and low-quality services which are supplied by ill-motivated staff in shabby premises.
>
> (OECD 1992: 16)

The most common form of health care funding is through some form of compulsory social insurance which provides universal or partial cover based on contributions from employers, employees and the state. Schemes typically provide benefits to cover loss of earnings during sickness and access to health care services. Vulnerable or low-income groups may be covered through some form of tax subsidy. Social insurance systems are usually government controlled and regulated. The expense of such schemes may be high as they tend to be patient led. The administrative costs of social insurance also tend to be high as arrangements must be made to collect contributions, record status and reimburse payment. Medical treatments must also be priced and bills collected. The advantages are that, like tax-based systems, risks are pooled, people have greater choice over how much they consume, there is a clear relationship between contributions and costs of health care even though they are borne by contributors as a whole.

Private insurance gives the greatest choice to individuals to consume health care once they are accepted as subscribers. However, the take-up of insurance depends on the willingness and the ability to pay. The risk of ill-health is unpredictable and may be underestimated or ignored. Those with the least ability to pay premiums are often at the highest risk. Conversely, from the insurers' point of view, there are incentives to 'cream skimming'. Insurers may exclude those who are most vulnerable. Schemes also tend to vary and many are shallow in their coverage. Once insured, individuals have a tendency to over-consume as medical care becomes a free good. The administrative costs of private insurance tend to be high. Countries which rely on private insurance, such as the US, may have a combination of high medical costs and low population cover. In actual health systems there may be elements of the three methods.

Financing health care in the UK

In the UK, health care spending is dominated by the NHS. In 1991, around 89 per cent of health expenditure was attributable to the NHS and 11 per cent to the private sector. As Figure 4.5 above showed, private funding is a much lower proportion than other countries. Within the NHS, most funding is derived from taxation. In 1992, 79 per cent came from taxes, 16 per cent from national insurance contributions and the remainder, 6 per cent, came from charges to patients and other payments. In recent years, contributions from national insurance have tended to rise, with a slight fall in the proportion of the tax contribution.

The public sector NHS

The contributions coming from the different sources of revenue for the NHS have varied little over the years. This has ensured that health spending was, and is, a major issue in each expenditure round. A settlement is agreed each year in Cabinet for England, Scotland, Wales and Northern Ireland and allocated to the Health Departments. Expenditure per head on health care has historically been higher in Scotland, Northern Ireland and Wales and still remains so. For example, in 1982–3, expenditure per head in England was £243 per capita, in Wales £262 and in Scotland £308 (*Regional Trends* 1985). In England, separate allocations are made for community and hospital services, about two-thirds, and the remaining third goes to the family practitioner services. While hospital services have historically taken a major and rising share of NHS expenditure, in more recent years (from 1992), there has been a shift towards community and family practitioner services, which is discussed further in Chapter 10.

Resource allocation policies between health authorities

Within the NHS, resources are allocated to regions and from there to districts. Until the 1970s, budgets were allocated from the central department downwards on the basis of their spending in the previous year through a cyclical process. A budget was prepared by the local Hospital Management Committee (HMC) which related its planned *future* expenditure to recent *past* expenditure. Each October the HMCs were required to submit forecasts of the revenues they required to maintain services and meet 'urgent developments and improvements'. These were passed upward and the Minister decided on the growth rate. The total budget was then divided among the regions broadly in proportion to their expenditure in the last year for which figures were available. The process was imprecise and was based on the principle of 'What you got last year, and an allowance for growth, and an allowance for scandals'. As a consequence, inequalities in distribution persisted.

In the 1960s and 1970s a number of studies highlighted the regional inequalities in the distribution of resources. Writing in 1972, Cooper and Culyer (1972) examined thirty-one health care inputs such as GPs, hospital specialists, beds to population served, specialisms and outpatient facilities and found an uneven distribution. Sheffield did particularly badly. Compared to Oxford, it was less well endowed on all indicators. Newcastle had twice as many gynaecologists per adult female as Sheffield and Birmingham and twice as many consultants.

As Labour Minister of Health, Richard Crossman was determined to tackle this issue, although he described it as one of the most difficult he had to face. In 1971–2, the best endowed region had 42 per cent more resources than the average in terms of expenditure per head of population, while the worst region had 23 per cent less. In 1975 a resource allocation working party (RAWP) was set up to develop a formula for reallocating resources to regions on a more equitable basis. In 1976, RAWP (DHSS 1976) recommended a formula based on weighted capitation which reflected healthy needs; measured by age, sex, mortality rates, fertility, marital status. The formula was then adjusted for additional patients treated across regional boundaries and an additional Special Increment for Teaching (SIFT) was added. The components of the formula were then aggregated and the resources available nationally were divided to produce a revenue target for each region in England with separate allocations for other parts of the UK. The London regions lost under the RAWP formula while the northern regions gained. RAWP did not affect the total size of the NHS budget, but provided a principle for its equitable distribution. The intention was that regions would apply the RAWP formula to areas and districts within their boundaries to achieve an equity within districts.

In 1977/8, when it was first applied, RAWP was widely criticised, mainly by the losers. Some criticisms were technical; others political. It was argued that the data were poor and the measures inadequate. Mortality rates did not give an indication of the amount of sickness. Nor was sufficient account taken of deprivation or the supply of related services such as primary care and personal social services. Strong opposition came from the Oxford and Thames regions, and the London teaching hospitals. They argued that the NHS was a national rather than regional service and rather than replicating services locally people should come to the centres of excellence. They claimed that these institutions and internationally renowned research centres would be put at risk through lack of funds. It was also argued that extra resources would not necessarily be quickly transformed into facilities and services, and that centres of excellence, once lost, could not be quickly replaced. In the 1990s, precisely the same kind of arguments are being put forward by the great teaching hospitals in London which are being closed, or threatened with closure, to reduce the numbers of 'unnecessary beds' in the capital (Tomlinson 1992).

Implementation of RAWP

Despite the criticisms, the formula was applied to regional budgets from 1977–8; and Figure 4.6 below shows the progress towards meeting the targets of equity in resource allocation by 1989 when the exercise was deemed to have achieved its goal. The policy has created most difficulty for regions which lost out financially particularly as NHS resources during the 1980s were shrinking in relation to demands. At this time, cuts were not always made rationally but in the areas where they were easiest or least painful. Studies of the Oxford region have indicated that community hospitals and 'social beds' were reduced rather than acute medical services which affected the health authorities' capacity to keep people in the community and realise policies for increasing resources for dependent groups (Maynard and Ludbrook 1980). Politically, RAWP was resisted, most publicly by Lambeth, Southwark and Lewisham Area Health Authority, which refused to reduce services in its three teaching hospitals. Members of the authority were suspended in 1979 but this was later ruled illegal by the courts. The Commissioners put in to run the service were also subsequently replaced. However, by

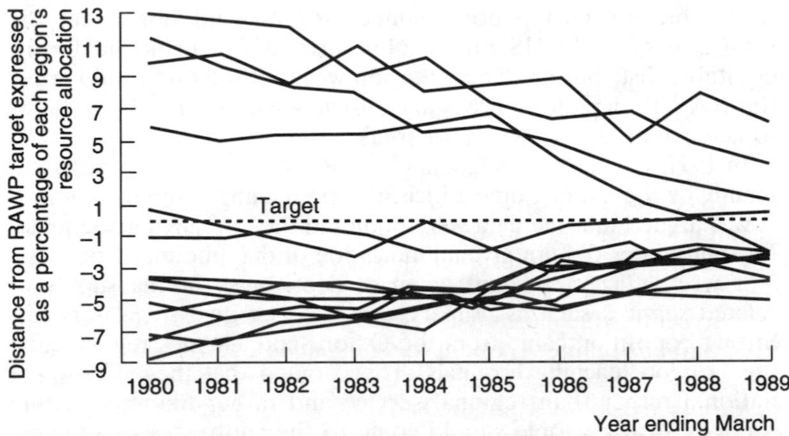

Figure 4.6 **Distances from the RAWP revenue target of the 14 RHAs in England 1980–89**

Source: DHSS (1988) Review of the RAWP formula, London.

the mid-1980s, RAWP achieved its objectives. Health service facilities have been developed in the shires and in those regions with the greater needs. Figure 4.6 shows that regions now receive funding broadly in line with budget targets.

Initially, it was intended that the RAWP principle should be applied within regions to the areas and districts. However, there were barriers to implementation which were a combination of local politics and the problems of reversing existing plans. Elcock and Haywood argue in *The Buck Stops Where?* (1980) that the revenue consequences of capital projects already started kept resources in districts where new hospital facilities were being constructed or planned. On the basis of their research, they conclude that:

> Our health authorities frequently adopted budgetary policies which were intended to dilute, evade or even reject the reallocation policy set out by RAWP.
>
> (Elcock and Haywood 1980: 48)

In the 1990s, capitation funding brought a new dimension to resource allocation (see Chapter 9).

The search for economy, efficiency and effectiveness

Because health care is funded centrally in the UK, considerable emphasis has been placed on obtaining value for money. The 1944 White Paper stated that the government wanted to ensure that:

> . . . in future every man, woman and child can rely on getting all the advice and treatment and care they may need in matters of personal health; that what they get shall be the best medical and other facilities available; that their getting these shall not depend on whether they can pay for them, or any other factor irrelevant to real need.
>
> (Ministry of Health 1944)

This open-ended commitment was contained in a number of ways in different periods. Most demands for health care have been generated by service providers. Demand is professionally led. There are two points of entry to the NHS where the consumer can voice a demand; to the GP, who acts as a gatekeeper to the hospital service, and to the hospital casualty department. Klein (1975) argued that consumer demand fell in the early years of the NHS. Contacts between patients and GPs fell by an estimated 25 per cent, which meant a reduction of 20 million or more in the number of annual patient 'demands'. In contrast, the number of patient visits to hospital accident and emergency departments rose only by about a million. All this has happened in a period when the total population of potential consumers rose by over 20 per cent. What increased dramatically was doctor-determined demand. Referrals from GPs for hospital services, and both outpatient and inpatient numbers have increased. In 1991, for the first time since its inception, the average number of visits per person per year to the GP rose from four to five (General Household Survey 1991).

Funding the NHS: the 1950s to the 1970s

As suggested above, in the early decades of the NHS, funding for the hospital and community services was based on historic costs. In the first years of operation, allocations were insufficient and supplementary estimates were raised in 1948–9 and 1949–50. Charges were introduced in 1951 on teeth and spectacles as part of Hugh Gaitskell's budget. This led to Bevan's resignation as Minister of Health. In 1952–3, expenditure on the health service was £383 million rather than the £170 million estimated by Beveridge (Watkin 1978).

The primary concern of policy-makers was to contain the size of the NHS budget. In 1953, the Guillebaud Committee was set up with the following terms of reference:

> to review the present and prospective cost of the NHS, to suggest means, whether by modifications, reorganisation or otherwise, of insuring the most effective control and efficient use of such Exchequer funds as may be made available; to advise how, in view of the burdens on the Exchequer, a rising charge upon it can be avoided while providing for the maintenance of an adequate service, and to make recommendations.
>
> (Ministry of Health 1956)

In 1956, the Committee reported and on the basis of work carried out by Abel-Smith and Titmuss, found that far from being extravagantly high the cost of the NHS had fallen from 3.8 per cent of GNP to 3.3 per cent between 1949–50 and 1953–4 in real terms. Actual costs had risen but this was largely due to increases in the levels of salary paid to the NHS employees (Abel-Smith and Titmuss 1956).On the basis of these findings, there was no change in the organisation of the NHS, and in the 1960s, expenditure rose along with economic growth. Salary rises outside expected estimates were met by government.

From the early 1970s, when the growth of the economy slowed down, allocations were cash limited but with an allowance for inflation. If the inflation was higher than predicted, there were additions to allow the planned volume of service to be provided. From 1976–7, no allowances were made for inflation and if it was higher than predicted, savings had to be found from the service.

The 1980s: economy, efficiency and effectiveness

In the 1980s, there was increasing emphasis on economy (cost savings), efficiency (providing a service of a given standard for a lower cost or of an improved standard at the same cost) and effectiveness (ensuring that for a given input of resource there was a positive gain in outcome). A major problem for policy-makers was the lack of adequate data by which value for money could be measured. Despite the mass of activity data on health care – the number of patients being admitted and discharged, for example, are routinely recorded – there was little analysis of data on which to assess performance either in terms of inputs related to outputs or the evaluation of outcomes.

Economy – cutting costs and rationing access: By the 1980s, when the reduction of public expenditure became a policy priority for the Thatcher governments, allocations to the NHS were less than the 2 per cent required to match inflation and demographic change and most areas of health care were cash-limited. As Figure 4.3 above indicates, compared with the 1970s, the annual rates of growth were lower. This produced a sense of crisis. In 1986, the Social Service Select Committee drew attention to the relative shortfall thus:

> Taking into account efficiency savings, on the most favourable interpretation of the Government's own data for the last five years, the Government has done no more than half what, by its own admission, it should have done: resources for the hospital and community service ought to have grown by 2 per cent in volume terms, but they have actually grown by only 1 per cent since 1980 81. The most telling way of representing the shortfall is to say that between 1980–81 and 1985–86 the cumulative total under-funding on the Hospital and Community Health Services current account was £1325 billion at 1985–86 prices, after taking full account of the cash-releasing cost improvements.
>
> (Social Services Select Committee 1986: xiii)

It can be concluded that in the 1980s, rates of growth did not keep pace with demand and there was relative resource starvation due to cumulative underfunding (Robinson and Judge 1988). However, in the early 1990s, health services in the wake of the NHS reforms have begun to grow more rapidly.

Rationing: One highly visible way of rationing health care is by delaying treatment through the queue or waiting list. Waiting lists grew during the 1980s and early 1990s. In 1993, there were almost one million people waiting for treatment. Eighteen per cent had been waiting for more than 12 months. The average waiting time was five weeks but one in five people had to wait more than six months. Although the number of people waiting for more than a year has now fallen, those waiting for less time has increased. Queues tend to be longer in certain areas such as, for example, elective surgery and fertility treatment. Waiting lists, however, are not an accurate measure of demand. They are a construct resulting from GPs' referral behaviour, the working practices of consultants, and the need to maintain a queue in order to use expensive facilities such as operating theatres to full capacity (Yates 1987).

Doctors are important decision-making agents in the health service in another sense, too. As well as determining the quantity demand, they also make rationing decisions about which consumer demand will be satisfied and in what way. Very little is known about the process or effects of this decision-making but an illustrative example can be given. A study on the choice of patients for renal dialysis and transplantation found that recipients were likely to be between the ages of 15 and 45, without other health problems, married with children, rather than single. Others were likely to be refused treatment (*British Medical Journal*, editorial, 1978). Weale discusses these issues in *Cost and Choice in Health Care* (1988).

Another way of rationing is simply not to provide a service. In the UK, the availability of some treatments such as fertility treatment and intensive care cots for very premature babies has been very limited. Aaron and Schwartz (1984) compare provision between the US and the UK in relation to ten types of hospital treatment. In six of these, provision in the US was much higher. There were major differences in the numbers of diagnostic tests, intensive care beds and the availability of renal dialysis and the rate of operations for a wide number of common conditions such as tonsillectomies, hysterectomies and hernias. This is attributed to medical economy, medical scepticism and the stoicism of the British patient (see also Payer 1990).

Efficiency in the NHS: Performance indicators, cost improvements and throughout

Performance indicators: The 1980s saw a number of measures to increase efficiency. Following the recommendations of the Korner Committee (DHSS 1980) on information systems, there were instructions to health authorities to develop routine methods for collecting standardised financial and activity data using information technology. These is a plethora of figures on activity in the NHS; patients treated in different specialisms, as patients and outpatients; waiting times for admission; numbers of beds and their use and the length of stay in hospital; hospital equipment; numbers of staff employed. The aim of the Korner Committee was to recommend a system of data collection which would bring benefits in managing the service. Subsequently the introduction of IT systems for financial management, personal functions and patient records has been rapid. Ironically, it has been in this area that the sharpest criticisms have been made about a waste of large amounts of public money. Wessex RHA and the West Midlands

RHA have been criticised for purchases of ineffective IT systems. In 1993, a Public Accounts Committee report listed a catalogue of issues involving such mismanagement.

Another attempt to improve the basis for analysing NHS activity is through the use of Performance indicators (PIs). Developed in 1980, PIs were designed to make comparisons between districts and to draw attention to districts where performance was 10 per cent above or below the performance for all districts. While PIs have the advantage of drawing attention to performance which is out of line, the information gained is difficult to interpret. Further investigation may be necessary to find the reasons for differences. Currently, a standard set of PIs are collected so that hospitals, departments and procedures can be compared. But they remain crude and they generate more questions than answers. The collection of reliable data on costs, quality and outcomes can allow comparisons to be made between treatments, clinicians and hospitals. Such information is valuable to patients or their agents so that they can make informed choices. Although such data have been published on educational institutions, it is not yet available for hospitals. Howard Davies, former Director of the Audit Commission comments:

> Unfortunately, it is not clear that the government are quite as enthusiastic about publishing information about services for which they are directly responsible, such as the NHS. In my view, it is vital that performance data should be independently collected and verified by an external agency, and not seen simply as useful management information. It is equally essential to ensure that information is presented in a form which individuals can understand.
>
> (Davies, *Times Health Supplement*, April 1993: 9)

There are dangers in using PIs as measures of outcome. For example, Fitzpatrick and Dunnell (1992), report a US study of cancer mortality in seven California hospitals. No allowance was made for the variation in severity and complexity of health problems in interpreting results which revealed considerable differences in the death rates between the 'worst' and the 'best' hospital. However, work is currently taking place to develop quality indicators for a number of common conditions.

Cost improvements: In 1984, the DHSS introduced a programme of cost improvement. RHAs and DHAs had to find cost savings without cutting patient services. There was also a number of special scrutiny exercises carried out under the leadership of Lord Raynor. These included an examination of NHS residential accommodation and the non-emergency ambulance service. A National Audit Office report concluded that the exercises had led to 'significant achievements' (NAO 1986), saving enough money to match the development money for the year. However, there was considerable variation between authorities and in some places the report suggested that health authorities had cut services and passed these off as savings.

In 1990, the Audit Commission, which carries out an external audit of local authorities for government, extended its functions to cover the health service. It has carried out a number of specific value for money audits of areas of NHS activity such as day surgery (Audit Commission 1991) and children's services (Audit Commission 1993) in order to highlight good practice. A general finding was that considerable gains could be made if best practice was universalised. There were considerable variations in performance in terms of both cost and quality.

Increasing throughput: These various policies have been aimed to increase efficiency. If this is measured by throughput, there have been clear productivity gains. The numbers of inpatients and outpatients treated has grown steadily. This is despite a decrease in the numbers of hospital beds. On the eve of the NHS, there were 544,000 beds available in the UK. The number fell so that by 1971, there were 526,000. By 1989, this had fallen again to 373,000. In 1959, there were over a thousand hospitals, and by 1979, 543 hospitals (OHE 1993).

Despite the decline in the numbers of beds, the numbers of inpatients and outpatients treated has risen steadily. This is due to the substantial reductions in the lengths of stay and, in recent years, the increase of outpatient and day patient activity. Between 1981 and 1991, the number of inpatient cases increased by 17 per cent. The average number of staffed beds available fell by almost 25 per cent yet the number of patients treated per available bed per year increased by 25 per cent. The average length of stay fell from 18 days for all specialisms in 1982, to 11 days in 1991. And for acute specialisms, the fall was from 8.6 days in 1982 to 6.1 in 1991 (OHE 1993). Of particular note is the increase in day surgery. This rose from 24 per cent of all surgery in 1982, to 34 per cent in 1990. The Royal College of Surgeons suggests a feasible target for the end of the century would be 50 per cent of surgery cases undertaken as day cases (Day Surgery Task Force 1993). This is an example of an area where new technologies have led to cost reductions (see Document 30, page 347).

In 1992, the DHSS claimed that cost improvements had generated total savings of £973 million between 1984–5 and 1989–90. Savings in labour costs were estimated at 25 per cent; rationalisation of patient services at 25 per cent; competitive tendering at 14 per cent; and supplies and energy at 12 per cent. Although more patients have been treated in fewer beds this has not led to a fall in the costs of treatment per head. These have risen. The figures above suggest one reason why this may be so – there are more highly paid staff. A further reason is that while people are in hospital they tend to be treated most intensively in the few days after admission. Daily costs fall with the length of stay.

The closer investigation of activity in the NHS has shown marked differences between the way beds are used by different consultants, in different hospitals. A number of studies draw attention to this. For example, in 1976, Abel-Smith reported a study of the duration of stay for the surgical treatment of septic ulcers in Scotland. The median length of stay of patients under different surgeons varied between 6 and 2 days. In 1981, a study of the acute hospital sector related the numbers of patients treated in particular specialisms to the input of medical manpower (DHSS 1981). It made comparisons between the 'productivity' of clinicians in different specialisms. Such studies often raise more questions than they answer. Feldstein (1967), in a study of hospital use in the 1960s, suggested that available beds tend to be filled and people who were admitted to hospital for a particular condition in one area were not in another according to bed availability. Length of stay may also reflect social conditions. A procedure which can be carried out on an outpatient basis in one area may be inappropriate in another with very deprived social conditions. A procedure which can be carried out on an outpatient basis in one area may be inappropriate in another with very deprived social conditions. Despite the problems of interpretation, it is important to continue to find ways of assessing value for money. As a consequence, this means unpacking the process of medical work. Decision-making becomes subject to scrutiny rather than remaining concealed under the cloak of clinical judgement.

Effective services cost benefit analyses, random controlled trials and medical audit

Cost benefit analysis has been used to assess the costs and benefits of different treatments. The benefits are assessed in terms of the effectiveness of treatment measured by a number of possible outcomes over time. For example, the benefits could be measured in terms of objective or subjective criteria, in terms of the relief of symptoms, quality of life or survival for a stated length of time. This method has been used to develop measures termed QALYs, Quality Adjusted Life Years. It may lead on to assessing which forms of intervention are the 'best buy' in terms of health care (Document 30).

This method has been applied at different levels within health care. For example it can be used to assess two alternative methods of caring for patients having renal dialysis. They may have the dialysis at home, which means bringing equipment to them, as a day patient or as an inpatient staying in hospital overnight. Cost benefit analysis can also be used to help determine priorities for health programmes. The costs of a programme may be set against the benefits in terms of decreases in morbidity and mortality.

The US state of Oregon has conducted the best-known experiment in assessing priorities for administering the Medicaid public insurance programme. It had insufficient funds to give the full range of available medical treatments to everyone in the state and wished to find a method of rationing health care which involved the public in the debate. The Health Commission in charge of the programme developed a set of measures which ranked interventions in terms of the calculation of benefits over costs. These procedures were then ranked and a public consultation exercise was undertaken before decisions were made. The rationing of health care by these overt methods has been the subject of controversy and debate. The issues are discussed in Honigsbaum, *Who Shall Live and Who Shall Die?* (1992).

The World Bank's 1993 report on health uses a similar approach but a different measure – DALYs (Disability Adjusted Life Years) as a measure to assess the extent of 'health' in terms of a reduction in disabilities incurred through illness and added years of life through particular interventions. The concept of 'health gain' has also been developed to evaluate benefits. These issues are discussed further in both Chapter 6 and 11.

These economic approaches to assessing health care interventions may have profound effects for relationships in health care at the level of doctor/patient as well as between interest groups. On the individual level, there is a conflict of ethical principles involved. Principles based on individual rights suggest that each person is entitled to medical treatment irrespective of the cost or the benefit. The individual must be the final arbiter of choice about which course of action to pursue. Utilitarian principles focus on the costs and benefits to the social group and on collective methods for solving these problems. So far, technical problems of measurement, and unease about the moral issues has limited the used of QALYs as the basis of rationing decisions but, as will be indicated in Chapter 9, in the new NHS when health authorities make decisions to purchase care, implicitly or explicitly they make choices between priorities.

Random controlled trials: Professional providers have also been concerned to promote value for money in terms of good quality medical practice. In a path-breaking book in 1972, *Effectiveness and Efficiency, Random Reflections on Health Services*, Cochrane argued that few procedures in health care had been rigorously evaluated and many practices rested on habit, custom, tradition and privilege rather than on rationality. Cochrane called a procedure effective when the result of a particular medical action altered the natural history of a disease for the better. He called for the greater use of Random Controlled Trials (RCTs) in the prevention, diagnosis and treatment of illness. RCTs are used to test the efficacy of treatments. People are allocated to two groups at random with one group receiving the new treatment and the other, control, group receiving no treatment or a placebo or an old treatment. The groups should be similar so that differences can be attributed to the treatment rather than to the characteristics of those involved in the trial. Because of the possibility of the placebo effect (the psychological effect of knowing that a treatment is being given may produce an improvement in the patient), double-blind trials may be carried out where neither the patient nor the investigator knows what treatment is being taken.

Randomisation is an important method for establishing the efficacy of new treatments scientifically. However, it raises ethical issues. It can be argued that it is unethical to withhold treatment which may be effective. This, however, begs the question. How do we know that a treatment is effective unless it is shown to be so? It could equally well be argued that it is unethical to give treatments where the effects are unknown. Currently, most new drug treatments are subject to RCTs. An example is a large clinical trial of the use of Tamoxifen as a preventive agent for women at high risk of breast cancer.

Medical audit: Another method of assessing professional practice is through medical audit. This has been defined as:

> . . . the systematic, critical analysis of the quality of medical care, including the procedures used for diagnosis and treatment, the use of resources, and the resulting outcome and quality of life for the patient.
>
> (Secretary of State for Health 1989: 30)

Working for Patients declared that doctors were required to take part in an audit (Secretary of State for Health 1989). Arrangements for this should be agreed locally between managers and professsionals. Audit might take the form of case note review where notes are examined to follow through particular treatments and their consequences. Process or treatment protocols may be developed as a result of medical review where treatments are assessed against each other. Such exercises can provide the guidance for clinicians, including more junior staff, and may be used in training. In a recent study Kerrison, Packwood and Buxton (1993) consider the extent and pitfalls of audit.

An example of national medical audit is the National Confidential Enquiry into Perioperative Deaths (NCEPOD). Perioperative deaths are those which occur within thirty days of a surgical procedure. This enquiry was carried out by surgeons and anaesthetists to establish the cause of death on the basis of a completed questionnaire. Cases are then selected to audit practice both in the clinical and practical management of cases, and to make recommendations about how patient care could be improved. The most recent report highlights areas where clinical management could be improved and where there is a shortage of resources (NCEPOD 1993).

There are a number of problems with medical audit. First, it runs counter to the principle of clinical autonomy and so its implementation may be resisted by clinicians. Second, in many areas of medical practice, there are differences in practice which offer valid alternatives for particular patients. If approached too rigidly, protocols can inhibit innovation. Lastly, evaluations of treatments have tended to rely heavily on clinical criteria which have emphasised 'hard' data (for example, blood pressure, breathing tests, scanning readings). There is less acceptance of patient evaluations of health status or on the aspects of medical care which patients deem important. Further examples of audit methods may be found in Davey and Popay (1993) and the Audit Commission's report *What Seems to be the Matter?* (1993).

Conclusion

This chapter has described the main flows of resource distribution in the NHS and the variety of methods through which politicians and providers have sought to achieve greater value for money. As the resources allocated to health care have risen, so the methods of assessment and evaluation has become more technical and sophisticated. However, many problems of implementation remain. At the same time, issues of access and equity have remained important. Over the period, it is apparent that the centre has increased its control over the authorities at the periphery and, through the evaluation of particular protocols, has entered into the detail of medical work. The introduction of the internal market has added another dimension to the search for value for money as the purchasers use the criteria of cost and quality to evaluate where they will place their contracts. This is discussed in Chapter 9.

References

Aaron, H. and Schwartz, W. (1984) *The Painful Prescription*, Brookings Institute, Washington, DC.

Abel-Smith, B. (1976) *Value for Money in Health Services*, Heinemann, London, Ch. 7.

Abel-Smith, B. and Titmuss, R. M. (1956) *The Costs of the National Health Service*, Cambridge University Press, Cambridge.

Appleby, J. (1992) *Financing Health Care in the 1990s*, Open University Press, Milton Keynes.

Audit Commission (1991) *A Short Cut to Better Services: day surgery in England and Wales*, HMSO, London.

Audit Commission (1993) *Children First: a study of hospital services*, Audit Commission, London.

British Medical Journal (1978) Editorial, 'Selection of patients for dialysis and transplantation', 2, pp. 1449–50.

Campbell, J. (1987) *Nye Bevan and the Mirage of British Socialism*, Weidenfeld & Nicolson, London.

Cochrane, A. L. (1972) *Effectiveness and Efficiency. Random Reflections on the Health Services*, The Nuffield Provincial Hospitals Trust, Oxford.

Cooper, M. H. and Culyer, A. J. (1972) 'Equality in the National Health Service: intentions, performance and problems in evaluation', in Hauser, M. M. (ed.), *The Economics of Medical Care*, Allen & Unwin, London.

Crossman, R. (1972) *The Politician's View of Health Service Planning*: 13th Maurice Bloch lecture, University of Glasgow.

Davey, B. and Popay, J. (1993) *Dilemmas in Health Care*, Open University Press, Milton Keynes.

Davies, H. (1993) 'Making the Social Market Work', *Times Health Supplement*, April, pp. 7–10.

Day, P. and Klein, R. (1991) 'Britain's Health Care Experiment', *Health Affairs* (fall), pp. 39–59.

Department of Health and Social Security (1976) *Sharing Resources for Health in England*. Report of the Resource Allocation Working Party, HMSO, London.

DHSS (1980) Steering Group on Health Service Information (Chairman: Edith Korner), established 1980.

Department of Health and Social Security (1981) *Report of a Study of the Acute Hospital Sector*, DHSS.

Department of Health and Social Security (1983) *Health Care and its Cost*, HMSO, London.

Elcock, H. and Haywood, S. (1980) *The Buck Stops Where? Accountability and Control in the National Health Service*, Institute for Health Studies, University of Hull.

Epsing Anderson, S. (1990) *Three Worlds of Welfare Capitalization*, Polity Press, Cambridge.

Feldstein, M. S. (1967) *Economic Analysis of Health Service Efficiency*, North Holland, Amsterdam.

Fitzpatrick, R. and Dunnell, K. (1992) 'Measuring outcomes of Health care' in E. Beck, S. Lonsdale, S. Newman and D. Patterson (ed.) *In the Best of Health? The Status and Future of Health Care in the UK*, Chapman and Hall, London.

Foot, M. (1962) *Aneurin Bevan – a biography*, vol. 1, *1897–1945*, MacGibbon and Kee, London.

Gray, R. (1993) 'Rationing and Choice' in B. Davey and J. Popay *Dilemmas in Health Care*, Open University Press, Milton Keynes.

Hills, J. (1993) *The Future of Welfare: a guide to the debate*, Joseph Rowntree Foundation, York.

Honigsbaum, F. (1992) *Who Shall Live and Who Shall Die?* King's Fund College, London.

Judge, K. (1982) 'The Growth and Decline of Public Expenditure', in Walker, A. (ed.), *Public Expenditure and Social Policy*, Heinemann Educational, London.

Kerrison, Packwood and Buxton, M. (1993), *Medical Audit: Taking Stock*, King's Fund Centre, London.

Klein, R. (1975) 'The National Health Service' in Klein, R. (ed.), *Inflation and Priorities: Social Policy and Public Expenditure*, Policy Studies Institute, London.

Klein, R. (1989) *The Politics of Health Care,* Longman, London.

Maynard, A. (1977) 'Avarice, Inefficiency and Inequality: an international health care tale', *International Journal of Health Services*, 7 (2).

Maynard, A. and Ludbrook, A. (1980) 'Budget Allocation in the National Health Service', *Journal of Social Policy*, 9 (3) July.

Ministry of Health (1956) *The Cost of the NHS*, Cmnd 9663, HMSO, London.

Mooney, G., Russell, E. and Weir, R. (1980) *Choices for Health Care*, Macmillan, London.

National Audit Office (1986) *Value for Money Developments in the NHS*, Report by the Controller and Auditor General, HMSO, London.

NCEPOD (1993) Report of the National Confidential Enquiry into Perioperative Deaths, NCEPOD, London.

OECD (1992) *The Reform of Health Care: a corporative analysis of 7 OECD countries*, OECD, Paris.

OHE (Office of Health Economics) (1992 and 1993) *Compendium of Statistics*, Office of Health Economics, London.

OPCS (1991–2) Social Survey Division, *General Household Survey*, No. 22, HMSO, London.

Payer, L. (1990) *Medicine and Culture: notions of health and sickness in Britain, the US, France and West Germany*, Gollancz, London.

Powell, E. (1966) *Medicine and Politics*, Pitman, London.

Public Accounts Committee (1994) *8th Report of the PAC*, HMSO, London.

Regional Trends 20 (1985) Central Statistical Office, HMSO, London.

Roberts, F. (1952) *The Costs of Health Care*, Turnstile Press, London.

Robinson, R. and Judge, K. (1988) *Public Expenditure and the NHS: trends and prospects*, King's Fund Institute, London.

Schieber, G. and Pouillier, J.-P. (1991) 'Recent Trends in International Health Care Spending', *Health Affairs*, 1.

Secretary of State for Health (1989) *Working for Patients*, HMSO, London.

Social Service Select Committee (1986) *Public Expenditure on the Social Services, 4th Report*, I, HMSO, London.

Social Trends 24 (1994) Central Statistical Office HMSO, London.

Tomlinson (1992) *Inquiry into London Health Services, Medical Education and Research*, HMSO, London.

Tudor Hart J. (1968) 'The inverse care law' in Cox, C. and Mead, A. (eds), *The Sociology of Medical Practice*, Collier-Macmillan, London.

Watkin, B. (1978) *The National Health Service: the first phase 1948–1974 and after*, Allen & Unwin, London.

Weale, A. (1988) *Cost and Choice in Health Care*, King's Fund Institute, London.

World Bank (1993) *Investing in Health*, World Bank.

Yates, J. (1987) *Why are we Waiting? An analysis of hospital counting lists*, Oxford University Press, Oxford.

CHAPTER 5

Policies for care in the community

Policies in relation to the care and treatment of very dependent people has been a dominant theme within the 'service' stream of policy in the NHS. By the early 1960s, it had become apparent that the care and treatment of the elderly, those with special needs (termed physically and mentally handicapped until the mid-1980s) and mentally ill people, whose requirements were for care rather than cure, posed special problems for an 'illness-based' NHS. In the 1970s, strategies were developed for each 'client' group through the preparation of reports, White Papers, and consultative documents. The policy documents had two common themes. First, that services should be provided in the community rather than in institutions, and second, that there should be cooperation between health authorities and local authority social service departments. The problems of achieving change form the theme of this chapter.

A problem of dependency or a right to services?

It is not the membership of a particular group, as such, which creates a need for care, but the degree of dependency. Illsley (1981) has used the term 'dependency groups' to refer to 'individuals with impaired abilities to function independently'. A common characteristic is that their condition is not amenable to curative treatment; there is a potential cost of long-term use of medical and social services and needs are multiple and not the responsibility of a single profession. This definition covers those with chronic illness, with disabilities, elderly frail people and those with challenging behaviour. People suffering from mental illness may or may not have long-term needs for treatment.

Caring for dependent people has been seen as a social problem, but as MacIntyre argues:

> Social problems are what people think they are, and if conditions are not defined as social problems by the people involved in them, they are not problems to those people although they may be to outsiders or social scientists.
>
> (MacIntyre 1977: 41)

The social care of dependent people poses particular difficulties for advanced industrial societies due to the value system of possessive individualism and the shrinking family unit. Those who are not 'owners of themselves', who are unable to produce, may have a marginal status and care must be provided by others. Although health and welfare services have developed to meet various contingencies, care for very dependent people remains very much the responsibility of families and neighbours. Who should provide what services raises fundamental questions of roles and responsibilities in society. As Abrams (1977) points out, there is a conflict of interest between the collectivity and the group. From a public point of view the provision of caring services is very costly and family or neighbourly care very cheap. But from the point of view of the individual, the situation is reversed. The costs of caring for others can be exorbitant while contributions to state welfare provision are relatively low – or at least unavoidable and relatively low, if they are spread through the tax system.

The 'problem' of the care of the dependent has become more apparent for a number of reasons. The demographic changes described in the last chapter have led to increases in the number of very old people. This group is more likely to have acute episodes requiring inpatient care and to need more support from a variety of services to remain at home. Older people are also more likely to suffer from mental illness. The elderly mentally infirm fall between two stools, often requiring the opportunity to move between hospital and community. It is estimated that between 5 and 7 per cent of people over 65 have moderate to severe dementing illnesses and the prevalence rises steadily with age to about 18 per cent of people aged 80 and over. Estimates of people suffering from dementia in the UK range from 100,000 to 500,000 (Taylor and Taylor 1989). Demographic trends mean that this will increase by 25 per cent over the next 15 years.

The prevalence of mental illness, or mental distress – there are a number of distinct forms of mental illness – is widespread. Four to five million people consult their GP for conditions such as depression or anxiety every year. There are nearly two million psychiatric outpatient attendances and some 200,000 admissions to hospital in England for a mental illness each year. The numbers of admissions to hospital have increased, rising from 160,000 in the early 1960s, but admissions now tend to be for shorter periods. Of the 60,000 patients in hospital at any one time, about half have been inpatients for a year or more and 30 per cent for five years or more (Taylor and Taylor 1989).

The increase in the population has also brought a rise in the numbers of people with mental and physical disability and in addition, more children born with special needs are surviving into adulthood due to the developments in medical science and rising living standards. The Economist Intelligence Unit (1973) estimated that there has been an annual increase of 0.9 per cent in the numbers of those who are severely disabled, an increase of

5,000 per year. As well as demographic changes in the incidence of disabling illness, there have also been social changes which have brought a greater awareness of incidence of disability and chronic illness. The Chronically Sick and Disabled Persons Act of 1970, for example, increased the extent of registration of disabled people, while studies carried out for the DHSS in the 1970s collected accurate data on disability for the first time. An estimate of the numbers of people in different age groups and with different degrees of disability is given in Table 5.1. With knowledge of the extent of the problem comes political pressure to increase provision.

In 1988, just over six million adults in Britain were estimated to be disabled. Having a disability does not mean that someone will have regular or frequent contact with health or social care agencies. For many people there is a need for employment, housing or income support or personal assistance. The need for health care depends on the severity of the disability which is likely to be influenced by age. There has been a steady increase in the numbers of people claiming state disability and invalidity benefits. This may be due to the numbers of older people or increasing knowledge of entitlement. Medical factors are not thought to have played a part in the increase (Lonsdale 1992).

Not all elderly, mentally ill people and individuals with special

Table 5.1 ***Estimated and projected numbers of people with disabilities living in private households, by age: Great Britain 1968–2001***

Age group	*Degree of disability*	*1968–69*	*1981*	*2001*
16–64	Very severe	42	42	44
	Severe	120	123	131
	Appreciable	215	220	233
	Total disabled	377	385	408
65–74	Very severe	35	42	37
	Severe	99	123	108
	Appreciable	206	257	224
	Total disabled	340	422	369
75 and over	Very severe	80	109	126
	Severe	123	170	197
	Appreciable	172	240	278
	Total disabled	375	519	601
16 and over	Very severe	157	193	207
	Severe	342	416	436
	Appreciable	593	717	735
	Total disabled	1092	1326	1378

Source: Adapted from Harris, A. (1971) HMSO, London and 'Populations projections 1978–2018', (1980) HMSO, London.

needs are dependent, or if they are, this may not be for extended periods. Among the elderly, for example, more than 95 per cent live in their own homes, either alone or with a spouse, while less than 4 per cent live in institutions (Equal Opportunities Commission 1982). However, the number of single elderly is likely to increase in the future, particularly women in this group. Traditionally, women have tended to provide care; however, changes in family structure and in attitudes may have reduced this pool of labour. Moroney (1976) and others have argued that there will be fewer carers available in the community as a consequence of social changes. The higher incidence of marriage has reduced the numbers of single women who were traditionally the carers while the smaller family sizes from the 1930s onwards has reduced the numbers of children in families to share the caring task. The fact that more women are in employment – including married women and those with children – has also increased the social and financial costs for this group of potential carers. Participation rates in employment have increased for women at all ages. A Department of Employment forecast is that women's participation rate will reach around 80 per cent in some regions by the year 2000 (*Employment Gazette* 1990).

Although very few women now do not marry, family patterns are changing and family formation is not necessarily stable. The increasing rates of divorce and the growth of cohabitation also has implications for who will care for whom. By 1989, 4 per cent of couples were cohabiting but not married. Between 1970 and 1991, the proportion of births outside marriage in England and Wales rose from 8 per cent to 30 per cent and between 1951 and 1987, the annual divorce rate rose from 2.6 to 12.7 per cent (Hills 1993). The number of families with a single parent continues to increase, rising from 8 per cent of all families in 1971 to 18 per cent in 1991. At the same time as the rising demand for care, the changing family structure and the declining number of potential informal care-givers, social and economic policies in the 1980s have created inceasing poverty – particularly among families with children. It is not possible to predict how these changes will affect the caring capacity of families but it is likely to alter current patterns of family obligation. An additional factor is increasing longevity. Will 70-year-old offspring be willing to or capable of caring for their 90-year-old parent or a dependent adult son or daughter?

In evidence to the Social Services Select Committee one witness, from the British Association of Social Workers, commented:

> There are elderly people, people over the age of 65, who are still caring. In my borough, we have 60 people over the age of 65 caring for sons and daughters who have mental handicaps. That is something which is not going to go away.
>
> (Select Committee on Social Services 1990: viii)

Most care for dependent people currently comes from informal care-givers. In 1990, 16 per cent of all adults were caring informally for someone who was elderly, sick or disabled. This has risen by 2 per cent since 1985. For 4 per cent of adults the care was for someone who lived in the family home (Evandrou 1987).

Governments have recognised that the informal network provides the most important form of care. In 1989, in *Caring for People*, the government stated:

> . . . the reality is that most care is provided by family, friends and neighbours. The majority of carers take on these responsibilities willingly, but the government recognises that many need help to be able to manage what can be a heavy burden. Their lives can be made much easier if the right support is there at the right time, and the key responsibility of statutory service proprietors should be to do all they can to assist and support carers. Helping carers maintain their valuable contribution to the spectrum of care is both right and a sound investment. Help may take the form of providing advice and support as well as practical services such as day, domiciliary, and respite care.
>
> (Department of Health and Social Security 1989: 9)

It is providing support for carers that has become the focus of policy even though socio-demographic trends suggest changing patterns in the future. In 1984, the General Household Survey identified around six million carers/helpers in Great Britain of whom 3.7 million carried the main care responsibility and 1.4 million devoted at least 20 hours a week to caring (Select Committee on Social Services 1990).

The right to services

Dependency may be perceived as a burden to public authorities and possibly families, but 'dependent' people themselves increasingly stress their rights to enjoy opportunities like everyone else. Over the past decade, there has been a variety of articulate pressure groups run by, or on behalf of, elderly, disabled and mentally ill people. Those with disabilities have been particularly articulate. The concept of 'normalisation' was developed (Wolfensberger 1992) and this has come to represent the right of disadvantaged people to an ordinary life. The concept stressed the right of each individual to participate in activities which are valued by everyone – such as independent living and access to employment. Many groups have thus stressed entitlement and criticised the over-reliance on medical and other professional judgement in relation to the care of people with disabilities (Oliver 1984). They stress instead the practical, social and emotional needs to which the condition of disability gives rise.

The Director of the British Council of Organisations of Disabled People told the Social Services Select Committee:

It worries me . . . when I hear this word 'care'. The fact that the government paper *Caring for People*, has 'caring' in the title worried me intensely, because many, many disabled people do not need caring for, but there are people who are entitled to benefits and there are people who need basic services in order to lead full and independent lives.

(Select Committee on the Social Services 1990: vi)

Just as those with disabilities have expressed their rights, so have women who have been the traditional carers stressed their need for support in the caring task. For example, Nissel and Bonerjea (1982) suggest that women who give up work altogether to care lose on average £4,500 a year while those who reduce their hours of work lose on average £1,900 a year. Carers all bear considerable indirect costs in loss of employment-related benefits, while the emotional costs of carers have also been shown to be high. Although a Disability Living Allowance may be claimed by someone needing care for more than 35 hours a week and an Invalid Care Allowance is available for those looking after that person, Hills (1993) concludes that these benefits are much smaller than the typical forgone earnings.

In relation to government expenditure on the community services, an Equal Opportunities Commission study, *Who Cares for the Carers?*, comments:

The expectation that a woman will provide the necessary care within the family whatever the cost to herself, still underpins the reality of community care. Cuts in health and social services and cash benefits intensify the demands placed on carers, they mean there are less physical resources to aid them, less alternatives to relieve them, and less money to support them. Savings in public expenditure increase the cost to carers in terms of her social life, her employment prospects and ultimately her physical and mental well-being.

(Equal Opportunities Commission 1982: ch. 4)

These costs are borne individually and do not figure in any public expenditure account. The price paid is the restriction placed on women's opportunities. Perhaps more than in other areas of health policy, governments have been led, or driven, by pressures from groups in the wider community with special interests. These have been voluntary organisations, professionals and groups of users. As governments have moved to involve those who use services in the policy process, so the diversity and complexity of the policy process has grown.

Government policies for community care

During the past 30 years, governments have emphasised the need to provide community care. The framework which supports community care policies involves the development of a network of services provided by a variety of organisations. These include:

NHS inpatient, day patient and outpatient facilities; a range of community-based services involving GPs, nurses, psychologists, health visitors and other health workers; local authority housing and social services, including sheltered housing, day care and education centres, meals on wheels and home helps. Private (for profit) and voluntary (not for profit) facilities may also be available. This can include residential care, nursing homes and other forms of accommodation.

These services are complicated to organise because they are based on meeting the needs of the individuals in their own homes around their existing networks of support and particular needs. A large number of agencies may be involved simultaneously and, over time, shifts between different types of care may be necessary. Effective policy has been slow to develop. There has also been a lack of clarity over a number of key issues – the meaning of community care, the allocation of responsibility between agencies, and the costing of community care. Governments have been reluctant to resolve issues and state a clear policy because of the implications for public expenditure.

Since the 1960s, there has been an emphasis on certain themes:

1 An increasing focus on the needs of individuals rather than services
2 The importance of providing locally based rather than institutionally based care and support
3 The need to find an organisational framework for coordinating activity.

The main objective of community care has been to maintain individuals in their own homes wherever possible, rather than provide care in a long-stay institution or residential establishment. This was an objective which has been spelt out in government reports and legislation from the Philips Committee's Report on the elderly in 1954 and the 1959 Mental Health Act onwards. Governments have been attracted to community care, as it was taken for granted that it was the best option from a humanitarian and moral perspective. It was also cheaper. The Guillebaud Committee (Ministry of Health 1956) summed up the assumptions in relation to elderly people. It suggested:

> Policy should aim at making adequate provision wherever possible for the care and treatment of old people in their own homes. The development of domiciliary services for this purpose will be a genuine economy measure and also a humanitarian measure enabling people to lead the life they much prefer.

However, admission rates to large hospitals continued to rise and people discharged from mental hospitals found little support from community-based services.

Opinion turned against long-stay institutions. The view that patients in such establishments were vulnerable to mistreatment was supported by popular and scholarly writing. In 1968, Goffman in *Asylums* had argued with both wit and insight that the organisation and environment of institutions diminished the quality of life for their inmates. This message had been forcibly brought home to politicians and the public by the scandals in the long-stay hospitals during the 1960s. The Normansfield Inquiry of 1978 (Department of Health and Social Security (DHSS) 1978) was a further indication that the large mental hospital was fatally flawed in conception.

In 1975, the Government published a White Paper, *Better Services for the Mentally Ill* (DHSS 1975b). This remains a key document as it spells out a national policy for mental health. The emphasis was on normalisation – on enabling people with dependency needs to live an ordinary life. The White Paper states:

> The aim is for people to be able to use the service they need with a minimum of formality and delay without losing touch with their normal lives . . . the philosophy is integration rather than isolation and the aim for the future must be to develop a much more locally-based service.

It specified four policy objectives:

1 The expansion of local authority services to provide residential, domiciliary and day care as well as social work support,
2 The relocation of specialist services to more local settings
3 The establishment of a structure for developing links between health and social services
4 An improvement in staffing levels.

In 1985, the government, in their response to the Social Services Committee, described the ideal service. A locally based psychiatric unit was the core of the service. A local day and inpatient service would ensure ready access for those requiring treatment for acute episodes, but psychiatrists and therapeutic teams were expected to work closely with GPs and the primary care team and in the patient's home setting, away from the hospital base. There should also be an integration with social service departments. The proposals meant a reduction in the requirements for long-stay hospitals.

In 1971, objectives had also been set for people with learning disabilities. A DHSS White Paper, *Better Services for the Mentally Handicapped* (DHSS 1975a) had spelt out a policy for community care (see Document 12 (page 309)). However, change was slow. Following the Jay Report on *Mental Handicap Nursing and Care* (DHSS 1979), the aim was to provide care in the community for all those with learning disabilities. *Mental Handicap: Progress, Problems and Priorities* (DHSS 1980) defined the aims. There were to be no new long-stay facilities and existing hospitals were to be run down. In 1981, it was estimated that of the 15,000 people still in hospital, half could be discharged immediately if there were facilities available in the community (DHSS 1981a).

In the mid-1970s, the *Priorities* document (DHSS 1976) and *The Way Forward* (DHSS 1977) had provided policy guidelines so that health authorites would shift resources towards community care. The reports contained indicative figures on the necessary resource shifts. The 1974 planning system provided a basis for cooperation. It was explained at the time as follows:

> The real objective is not to achieve the joint consideration of plans which have been prepared separately by the two sides and brought together at a late stage to see how well they match up, but to achieve joint planning from the initial stages.
>
> (DHSS 1973)

Joint Consultative Committees with funding available for this type of project were to oil the wheels of service development. The budgets were to be used for a variety of projects such as hostels and schemes which supported carers. For example, a night-sitting or bathing service for the elderly could be developed through joint financing.

In 1981, joint-financing amounted to £416 million. It benefited particularly the elderly and those with learning disabilities. Forty per cent of this money went to services for elderly people, and 33 per cent for people with learning disabilities (Booth 1981). Joint collaborative machinery, Booth suggests, would have been largely redundant without the incentive of joint-financing money. He argues that the *process* of planning was particularly important. It helped to build up relationships between those working within the different organisational structures of health and social services. This was more important than the production of detailed and time-consuming plans.

A shift in priorities? The late 1970s

In 1981, a research report on community care (DHSS 1981b) suggested that there had been steady increases in staff and facilities in community-based services. The number of GPs had been rising steadily at 1.5 per cent a year. Most groups of nurses in the community had also increased. Between 1949 and 1979 the numbers of community nurses rose by 238 per cent, from 9,529 to 32,162. There was a particularly sharp rise between 1967 and 1971, that is, *before* the Priorities documents. However in 1979 there were still 10 nurses in hospitals compared to every one in the community. There were also increases in the numbers of day-centre places and in home helps. This latter service was crucial in allowing elderly people to remain in their own homes. The elderly make up 90 per cent of the home help case-load.

What is not known from these data is whether the increase in personnel had kept pace with demographic and social change. Almost twice as many pensioners lived alone in 1971 than had in 1961. It was also not known whether sources were sufficient to cover community care needs. Few guidelines were available and very little was known about how some groups of professionals spent their time or how effectively. Did an increase in GPs mean that they worked more with elderly people? And did this enable people to remain in the community when they otherwise could not have done? Like many other aspects of health and social care, it was easier to obtain measures of service input than outputs. Effectiveness was not measured at all. It was not known what benefits followed from increases in manpower and facilities. Governments in the 1970s were as unclear as anyone about the consequences of their policies. In 1979, the Royal Commission on the NHS commented that:

Even after listening to the careful explanation by representatives of the DHSS about the way in which the needs of particular priority groups are taken into account in the allocation of resources to health authorities, we

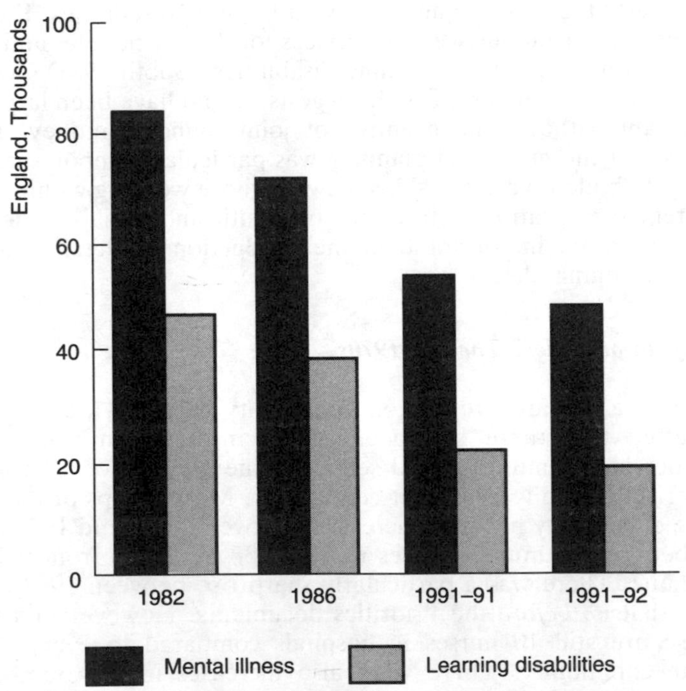

Figure 5.1 ***Mental illness and learning disability hospitals and units: average daily available beds 1982–1992***
Source: Social Trends, (1994) HMSO, London.

remain mystified. We are bold enough to think that this *is* because there is cloudiness in the department's thinking about these matters, which are as important as anything in the department's care.

In relation to mentally ill people, 88 per cent were still treated as inpatients, the remaining 12 per cent were treated as outpatients or by the local authority. This concealed a growing and changing population. Figure 5.1 shows the reduction in the average number of beds available daily between 1982 and 1992.

For those with learning disabilities, there had been an increase in community facilities. For example by 1981, it was concluded that there had been a significant shift in the way in which they were cared for. In 1969, the numbers of adults and children with learning disabilities in hostels was 7.8 per cent and 21 per cent respectively of those in public care. By 1977 these proportions had risen to 19.3 per cent and 36 per cent respectively. The DHSS Report, *Mental Handicap: Progress, Problems and Priorities* (DHSS 1980) agreed that there had been progress but that a considerable number of people in this group remained in hospital because there was no alternative provision.

The position of elderly people was less clear and services for this group were affected by cuts in public expenditure in the late 1970s. In 1982, Webb and Wistow concluded that the proportion of expenditure devoted to the elderly was declining marginally within local authority budgets, although this is contrary to national policy guidelines from the DHSS. Meals on wheels had hardly grown in volume and had failed to keep pace with the growing numbers of elderly people. Day-care places had similarly fallen in proportion to the population aged over 75 since 1979/80 and additionally, between 1976 and 1980, expenditure on aids and adaptations was reduced. The evidence suggests that numbers of frail or chronically elderly occupying acute hospital beds had not diminished and the level of frailty of the elderly occupying local authority residential homes and sheltered housing had increased. Community care it seemed had not kept pace with demand.

Care in action: a change of emphasis?

Care in Action (DHSS 1981a) outlined the 1979 Conservative government's policies and priorities for the health and social services. These remained much as before. Priority *groups* were identified as the elderly, mentally ill, and those with special needs. Priority *services* were those in the community. However, these priorities were not ranked and neither were they linked to resource allocation targets. In other respects, *Care in Action* brought a marked change of emphasis. The document drew attention to the need to reduce public expenditure. The strategy to achieve the meeting of social needs was what Klein (1981) called a 'non-strategy'. It relied on two factors, the careful husbanding of NHS resources to achieve savings and the 'innovative' use of the informal, voluntary and private sectors in care. These were seen as the primary sources of community care if not community treatment, and statutory and private sources were seen as supplementing and supporting this provision. Earlier, in 1977, the Wolfenden Report on *The Future of Voluntary Organisations* had described the notion of the 'mixed economy' of welfare. It had drawn attention to the plurality of caring agencies and the separate but complementary roles of the statutory, the commercial or private sector, the voluntary sector and the informal sector of family, friends and neighbours in caring for dependent groups.

In 1980, Patrick Jenkin, then Secretary of State for Health, outlined his approach:

> . . . we cannot operate as if the statutory services are central providers with a few volunteers here and there to back them up. Instead we should recognise that the informal sector lies at the centre with statutory services and the voluntary sector providing expertise and support.
>
> (Jenkin 1980)

In fact the Conservative government proceeded to encourage the development of the private sector. It did so in two ways. It reduced the allocations to local authorities and more importantly, in 1979 the DHSS had begun to meet the full cost of care in private residential and nursing homes for those on income support. The policy appeared to be almost accidental but it had profound effects

Table 5.2 **Residential accommodation for elderly and younger physically handicapped people in England and Wales 1977–85**

				Type of home
	Local authority	*Voluntary*	*Private*	*All homes*
Number of homes				
1977	2 799	1 065	1 920	5 784
1981	2 861	1 161	2 609	6 631
1985	2 880	1 144	5 602	9 626
% change				
1977–81	2.2	9.0	35.9	14.6
1981–85	0.7	–1.5	114.7	45.2
Number of residents				
1977	114 811	30 046	24 578	169 435
1981	115 833	33 047	34 830	183 710
1985	113 853	32 057	72 333	218 243
% change				
1971–81	0.9	10.0	41.7	8.4
1981–85	–1.7	–3.0	107.7	18.8

Source: Adapted from DHSS statistical collections.

on private sector growth. It also let local offices set limits on the board and lodging payments they considered appropriate for their area. In 1983, there was a leap in the level of allowable payments (Day and Klein 1987). As a result, the number of residential places in private rest homes for elderly and disabled people nearly doubled between 1979 and 1984. The expenditure on residential and nursing homes increased from £6 million in 1978 to £460 million in 1986 (Knapp 1992). The proportion of people in private residential homes receiving help with their fees through support payments increased from 14 per cent in 1979 to 35 per cent in 1984 and by 1987 it had reached 54 per cent (Bradshaw and Gibbs 1988). Tables 5.2 and 5.3 indicate the extent of change in the early 1980s.

Table 5.3 ***Health and Social Care Services for People with a mental illness 1980–89***

	1980	*1983*	*1986*	*1989*
Number of inpatients	77 297	69 030	60 280	56 200
Inpatient costs (£m. 1989 prices)	1 172.2	1 210.7	1 196.9	1 262.7
Cost per patient (1989 prices)	15 255	17 539	19 856	22 468
Places in local authority staffed homes	2 333	2 557	2 646	2 703
Places in local authority unstaffed homes	1 391	1 616	1 824	1 994
Places in voluntary homes	1 381	1 603	2 134	2 325
Places in private homes	761	764	1 731	3 912
Places in day centres	4 907 (1981)	5 159	5 545	6 396

Source: Social Services Select Committee (1992) HMSO, London.

Criticisms of community care in the 1980s

By the early 1980s, there was a broad-based lobby of groups expressing concern about policies for community care. This consisted of those providing care, academics and pressure groups. In 1986, an Audit Commission Report, *Making a Reality of Community Care* (Audit Commission 1986), and a Social Services Select Committee Report (1985) on community care for mentally ill and people with special needs provided a coherent critique, backed by evidence, on the shortcomings. A report from Roy Griffiths, *Community Care: an agenda for action* (DHSS 1988), documented the shortcomings and laid out an agenda for policy. The issues are now summarised.

Problems of boundaries

It was argued that definitions of community care had changed and shifted. There were with no clear boundaries between the reponsibilities of various agencies, no agreement on priorities or budgets which related to the actual costs of care. Most important, there was no philosophy of care. Griffiths also commented on the lack of coherence at the centre. He stated:

> . . . community care has been talked of for thirty years and in few areas can the gap between political rhetoric and policy on the one hand, and between policy and reality in the field on the other hand, have been so great.
>
> (DHSS 1988: iv)

Deinstitutionalisation

By the 1980s, there was profound concern that the rundown of long-stay mental hospitals and the discharge of patients was made without adequate services to provide care. The numbers of resident inpatients fell from 150,000 in the 1950s to 50,000 at the end of the 1980s. There has been no adequate mechanism introduced to ensure that community care is in place before a hospital closes. The Audit Commission (1986) concluded that, particularly in relation to mental illness, community care had not kept pace. In 1985, the Social Services Select Committee commented:

> Any fool can close a long stay hospital: it takes more time and trouble to do it properly and compassionately.
>
> (Select Committee on Social Services 1985: xxii)

In fact, few long-stay hospitals closed completely as there were patients who were too dependent to move. As a consequence, unit costs rose. In a critical report, the National Audit Office (NAO 1987) commented that there had been undue emphasis on the rundown of mental hospitals rather than the build-up of community services. Pressure groups alleged that the increase in homeless people and the increase of the prison population was due in part to the closure of long-stay institutions.

Conflicting interests and the problems of collaboration

The Griffiths Report commented on divided responsibilities at the centre and at local level. This led to:

> . . . a feeling that community care is a poor relation; everybody's distant relative but nobody's baby.
>
> (DHSS 1988: iv)

Collaboration between agencies with different organisational structures has always proved difficult. In relation to the care of dependent groups this has been exacerbated by the number of agencies involved and the complexity of needs. Document 23 (page 330) gives a graphic representation of the issues. In addition, there is a range of professionals involved in care with distinctly different approaches to the definition of need. While there is a major distinction between the social and the medical models of care, within these categories there are other specialisms, each with a distinctive knowledge base. Conflicts have existed at all levels and been manifested in overt and covert ways. In the mid-1970s, for example, the medical profession was overtly antagonistic to priorities for community care and non-treatment models of care. In a phrase which tellingly revealed underlying attitudes, an editorial in the *British Medical Journal* (1976) thundered the hostility of the medical profession:

> By putting people before buildings and by giving practical expression to the public sympathy for the old and the handicapped, Mrs Castle [the then Minister of Health] has, perhaps, allowed sentiment to overrule intellect. (1976: 787)

At the local level, cooperation between service-providers had been as difficult as collaboration between agencies. On the basis of research, Booth (1981) and Wistow (1982) concluded that planning had not developed in the joint way that was intended. They spell out the policy dynamics. Local authorities and Area Health Authorities (AHAs) tended to plan separately. Each operated within a micro-political system with its own organisational imperative, system of financing and professional and political perceptions of priorities. Changes occurred only at the margins as most expenditure in health and social services was already committed. The balance of influence in the local political system also had a stronger effect than directives from the centre. While joint financing had aided collaboration, the use of monies had tended to be *ad hoc* and incremental rather than part of a larger scheme of planned growth and development.

Community care tended to mean different things to the local authority and the health authority. To the former it meant a reduction in the amount of residential accommodation, while to the latter, it could refer to alternatives to hospitals such as residential accommodation, nursing homes or sheltered housing (which increased the opportunity to discharge patients from hospital and release 'blocked beds'). Booth's studies found that social service departments frequently perceived the AHA as trying to off-load their problems on to social services, leaving little room for bargaining and reciprocity. For example, hospital consultants could reduce the length of stay, or discharge patients, without reference to social services or their ability to cope with very dependent people.

Within health authorities, decisions tended to be made by clinicians rather than managers or planners. The former were frequently more concerned with protecting their own specialisms than working with others. Moreover, mechanisms for enforcing government priorities simply did not exist. Studies by Haywood and Alaszewski (1980), Brown (1979) and Hunter (1979) on decision-making suggested that policy-making in health authorities had tended to revolve around the influence of clinical interests and commitments to existing projects and expenditure. Authorities on the whole were not willing or able to make changes in allocations unless additional monies were made specifically available. Moreover, there was what Hunter calls a high 'puzzlement' factor. Managers were often uncertain about how to change. In addition, there were no sanctions on those who did not support community care policies. Central government directives were treated as rhetoric and ignored unless there was a particular local commitment. Hunter and Judge (1988) describe some notable exceptions in areas such as Exeter, which developed integrated community-based services; but these were the exception rather than the norm. In sum, the activities of the health authorities at the periphery have been of crucial importance in affecting the implementation or non-implementation of government policy.

Variations in provision

These difficulties were compounded by local variations in need, differences in levels of provision and a scarcity of data on the subject. For example, although there were data on demographic trends in relation to the numbers of single-elderly nationally, these were often not available at a local level. Similarly, there was little information about the extent to which needs were being met by local services, particularly by the voluntary and informal sector. Again, although such data have been collected in national surveys – by, for example, Audrey Hunt in the 1978 OPCS Survey on *The Elderly at Home* or through Nissel and Bonerjea's 1982 small-scale survey *Family Care of the Handicapped Elderly: Who Pays?* – these did not give any picture to local or health authorities of patterns of need, or the shortfall of services for dependent groups in their own areas.

The availability of social care also varied considerably from area to area depending on a number of factors; local employment markets, local housing policies, the extent and organisation of voluntary agencies. The pattern of provision of health and personal social services has developed in a variety of ways as legislation has tended to be permissive. The structure of families and social and neighbourhood networks, too, are crucial in determining the level of demand and need for publicly provided care. There were little data of this kind available unless local studies were undertaken.

Conservative policies for community care

Under Conservative governments, there was a marked lack of strategy. The decision to provide subsidy through social security had led to unplanned growth of the private sector while local level authorities were left to devise their own strategies for community care. However, no special funds were earmarked. The Select Committee on Social Services in its report on the public expenditure White Paper in 1980 stressed this point when it commented:

> We are struck by the apparent lack of strategic policy-making at the DHSS and the failure to examine the overall impact of changes in expenditure levels and changes in the social environment across the various services and programmes for which the department is responsible . . . Community care of the elderly and disabled demands financial commitment . . . there is strong evidence to suggest that the need to make short term savings in Personal Social Services budgets may be obstructing the shift to community care.

The 1986 Audit Commission Report found that arrangements for community care were in disarray and there were a number of organisational and financial disincentives to efficient provision. And there were particularly perverse incentives to increase residential care through social security payments. The result was poor value for money. Too many people were in care settings costing more than £200 a week when they could be receiving more appropriate care in the community at a lower cost of £100 to £130 a week to public funds. They had also found that the amount local authorities spent varied considerably. In well over half the local authorities, spending was less than £1 per head. In addition, provision was uneven, with a clustering of private accommodation in coastal towns in Southern England. The Commission's general conclusion was that:

> At best there seems to have been a shift from one pattern of residential care based on hospitals to an alternative supported in many cases by supplementary benefits payments – missing out on more flexible and cost-effective forms of community care altogether. At worst, the shortfall in services will grow, with many vulnerable and disabled people left without care and at serious risk.
>
> (Audit Commission 1986: 2)

Roy Griffiths (DHSS 1988) accepted the findings of previous inquiries and was concerned to focus his recommendations on the needs of people rather than on what particular agencies provided. He was convinced that the local authority social service departments were well placed to provide community care which was based on a social model. His formula was similar to that proposed for NHS mangement in 1983; he wanted to change the way in which managers approached their task and to obtain greater value for money. Griffiths recommended that social service managers should not provide community care directly but design programmes for its implementation and organise the necessary purchases from other groups. The meeting of individual needs should be organised by care managers who would buy services as appropriate either from groups of their own staff, or from the voluntary or private sector. Here was a mixed economy of care which would 'widen consumer choice, stimulate innovation, and encourage efficiency'. With 'care management', those in need of care could choose their own form of 'normalisation'. Griffiths also recommended that funding for community care should be 'ring-fenced' so that it would be used for this, and not other purposes.

This prescription conflicted with government policy which aimed to reduce public spending. It also increased the role of local government – the powers of which the Thatcher administrations had consistently aimed to curb.

The government waited 18 months before publishing its response – *Caring for People* (DHSS 1989). This White Paper followed Griffiths' recommendations that local authorities should purchase care and increase choice and independence of clients through individual case assessments and care management. A 'care manager' would be appointed for each client who would purchase a package of care on the client's behalf. The changes are designed to increase competition between a range of potential suppliers. *Caring for People* also put a particular emphasis on supporting care-givers in *practical* ways to enable people to stay at home. It also encouraged the use of the private and voluntary sectors while clarifying their responsibilities so that they could be held accountable for price and quality.

In 1990 the NHS and Community Care Act implemented these proposals. They were to be phased in over a period of three years from 1991. The funds which were previously used to support elderly people and those with special needs in residential homes were now transferred to local authorities. However, this funding was capped. Commenting on this transfer, the Select Committee on Health suggested:

> . . . this represents a fundamental shift from a demand-led system, based on individual entitlement at given income levels, to one based on the assessment of need, within a fixed budget. The transfer of funds to local authorities will provide a budget within a single agency to cover the costs

> of different packages of social care, whether in a residential or nursing home, a person's own home, or another community-based setting.
>
> (1993: 3rd Report)

In 1993–4, £400 million was transferred from the Department of Social Security to local government. In 1994–5, this will rise to £105 billion and in 1995–6, to £157 billion. Additional sums may be spent from the local authorities' budget. These sums are intended as transitional payments to enable local authorities to discharge their new responsibilities. Thereafter, the sums will be absorbed into the general local government support grant. It has been suggested that this transfer of funds is 'a poisoned chalice' for local government. It is insufficient to meet their new responsibilities and will deflect blame from central government for the care of a growing group of vulnerable people.

It is also argued that the policies may create a new set of perverse incentives, that is incentives to act in ways which are contrary to policy aims. For example, *Caring for People* draws a clear distinction between social and medical care. Yet, for elderly and mentally ill people in particular, the line between the two cannot be drawn precisely, because needs fluctuate. As both health and social services will be attempting to minimise costs there may be temptations for each agency to push responsibility on to the other. Hills comments:

> . . . one reaction appears to be like passing the parcel as the NHS saves costs by closing down long-stay geriatric wards, shifting to social security funding of residential care, which has been passed in turn to local authorities.
>
> (Hills 1993: 75)

A further complication is that in many areas a split has developed between the hospital and community trusts. This in effect creates a new tripartite system and, if GPs are included in the equation, a four-way split, between statutory agencies which contribute to care. Joint planning is more necessary than ever. Yet past evidence suggests that there are professional and organisational disincentives. The onus now falls on managers of clients to sort out a care package. This means cooperation between individuals from different professions. Just as General Practice Fundholders (GPFHs) contract for hospital services, from 1993 they will also contract for community services, and in the future this may extend to social services. They will need a new batch of skills to carry out the task (Morris 1993).

It has also been suggested that the potential for switching resources from their present configuration is limited. One estimate is that, at most, 17 per cent of residents are currently inappropriately placed. Furthermore, choice could be said to have been reduced as the care manager will make choices on the client's behalf. Previously, clients had the freedom to make their own decisions about residential care as it was subsidised from the social security budget. The changes may therefore actually *reduce* choice. One of the Audit Commission's criticisms was that there were considerable variations in the quality of community services in different parts of the country. The potential for disparity under the new arrangements is even greater. Furthermore, unlike the NHS with the NHS Management Executive (NHSME) to monitor standards, there is no central authority. The Social Services Inspectorate is much smaller and has few powers or resources to affect change when they find inadequacies.

Conclusion

The health and community care reforms (the former are discussed in Chapter 9) have begun a process of shifting responsibilities which are likely to continue through the decade. The changes in the organisational structures and in the mechanisms for providing services make assessment at this time impossible. There are some certainties. Demand is likely to increase – due to continuing reductions in the length of hospital stay and the increase in the dependent population indicated by demographic trends. In relation to supporting this group, there has been a fundamental shift in the value system. Instead of a focus on meeting needs, packages of care will rely on income assessments. In 1992, another report from the Audit Commission suggested:

> . . . if community care is to have any chance of success, the change process itself will need to be managed with considerable skill.
>
> (1992: 36)

The gap between rhetoric and reality is far from being closed and community care has entered a period of greater uncertainty and instability than hitherto.

References

Abrams, P. (1977) 'Community Care: some research problems and priorities', *Policy and Politics*, 6 (2), pp. 125–52.

Audit Commission (1986) *Making a Reality of Community Care*, HMSO, London.

Audit Commission (1992) *Community Care: managing the cascade of change*, HMSO, London.

Booth, T. A. (1981) *Collaboration between the Health and Social Services, Part I: a case study of joint care planning, Part I and II, Policy and Politics, 9, 1*, pp. 23–50 and 9, 2, pp. 205–226.

Bradshaw, V. and Gibbs, E. (1988) *Public Support for Private Medical Care*, Avebury, Aldershot.

British Medical Journal (1976) Editorial, 3 April, pp. 787–88.

Brown, R. G. H., (1979) *Reorganising the Health Service*, Robertson, Oxford.

Day, P. and Klein, R. (1987) 'Residential Care for the Elderly: a Billion Pound Experiment in Policy Making', *Public Money*, 6, 4, pp. 19–24.

Department of Health and Social Security (1973) *Report from a Working Party on Collaboration between the NHS and Local Government on its activities to the end of 1972*, HMSO, London.

Department of Health and Social Security (1975a) *Better Services for the Mentally Handicapped,* Cmnd 4683, HMSO, London.

Department of Health and Social Security (1975b) *Better Services for the Mentally Ill*, Cmnd 6233, HMSO, London.

Department of Health and Social Security (1976) *Priorities for Health and Personal Social Services in England, a consultative document*, HMSO, London.

Department of Health and Social Security (1977) *The Way Forward*, HMSO, London.

Department of Health and Social Security (1978) *Report of the Committee of Inquiry into Normansfield Hospital*, Cmnd 735, HMSO, London.

Department of Health and Social Security (1979) *Report of the Committee of Inquiry into Mental Handicap Nursing and Care* (Chairman: Peggy Jay), HMSO, London.

Department of Health and Social Security (1980) *Mental Handicap: Progress, Problems and Priorities: a review of mental handicap services in England since the 1971 White Paper*, DHSS, London.

Department of Health and Social Security (1981a) *Care in Action: a handbook of policies and priorities for the health and personal social services in England*, HMSO, London.

Department of Health and Social Security (1981b) *Care in the Community: a consultative document on moving resources for care in England*, DHSS, London.

Department of Health and Social Security (1981c) *Report of a Study on Community Care*, DHSS, London.

Department of Health and Social Security (1983) *Health Service Development*. Care in the Community and Joint Finance, HC(86) 6, DHSS, London.

Department of Health and Social Security (1988) *Community Care: an agenda for action; a report to the Secretary of State for Social Services by Sir Roy Griffiths*, HMSO, London.

Department of Health and Social Security (1989) *Caring for People, Community Care in the Next Decade and Beyond*. Cmnd 849, HMSO, London.

Economist Intelligence Unit (1973) *Care with Dignity: an Analysis of the Costs of Care for the Disabled*, National Fund for Research into Crippling Diseases.

Employment Gazette (1990) January, pp. 9–19.

Equal Opportunities Commission (1982) *Caring for the Elderly and Handicapped: Community Care Policies and Women's Lives*, Equal Opportunities Commission, London.

Equal Opportunities Commission (1990) *Who Cares for the Carers?*, Equal Opportunities Commission, ch. 4.

Evandrou, M. (1987) 'Challenging the invisibility of carers: mapping informal care nationally', Welfare State Programme, WSP/49, Suntory-

Toyota International Centre for Economics and Related Disciplines, London.

Goffman, E. (1968) *Asylums*, Penguin, London.

Haywood, S. and Alaszewski, A. (1980) *Crisis in the Health Service*, Croom Helm, London.

Hills, J. (1993) *The Future of the Welfare State*, Joseph Rowntree Foundation, York.

Hunt, A. (1978) *The Elderly at Home*, OPCS, HMSO, London.

Hunter, D. (1979) 'Coping with Uncertainty: decisions and resources within Health Authorities', *Sociology of Health and Illness*, 1 (1), pp. 40–88.

Hunter, D. (1992) 'The Move to Community Care with Special Reference to Mental Illness', in Beck, E., Londsdale, S., Newman, S. and Patterson, E. (eds), *In the Best of Health? The status and future of health care in the UK*, Chapman & Hall, London.

Hunter, D. and Judge, K. (1988) *Griffiths and Community Care: meeting the challenge*, King's Fund Institute, London.

Illsley, R. (1981) 'Problems of Dependency Groups: the care of the elderly, the handicapped and the chronically ill', *Social Science and Medicine*, 15A, 3 (Pt. II), pp. 327–32.

Jenkin, Patrick (1980) Speech to the Association of Directors of Social Services.

Klein, R. (1981) 'The strategy behind the Jenkin non-strategy', *British Medical Journal*, vol. 282.

Knapp, M. (1989) 'Private and voluntary welfare', in McCarthy, M. (ed.) The New Politics of Welfare: an agenda for the 1990s? Macmillan, London.

Lonsdale, S. (1992) 'Support and Care for People with Physical Disabilities' in Beck, E., Lonsdale, S., Newman, S. and Patterson, D. (eds) *In the Best of Health: The Status and Future of Health Care in the UK*, Chapman & Hall, London.

McIntyre, S. (1977) 'Old Age as a Social Problem', in R. Dingwall *et al.* (eds), *Health Care and Health Knowledge*, Croom Helm, London.

Ministry of Health (1954) *Report of the Committee on the Economic and Financial Problems of the Provision for Old Age* (Chairman: Sir J. Philipps), HMSO, London.

Ministry of Health (1956) *Report of the Committee of Inquiry into the Cost of the National Health Service* (Chairman: C.W. Guillebaud), Cmnd 9663, HMSO, London.

Moroney, R. M. (1976) *The Family and the State: Considerations for social policy*, Longman, London.

Morris, R. (1993) 'Community Care and the Fundholder', *British Medical Journal*, 306, pp. 635–37.

Nissel, M. and Bonerjea, L. (1982) *Family Care of the Handicapped Elderly: who pays?*, Policy Studies Institute, London.

Oliver, M. (1984) 'The politics of disability', *Critical Social Policy*, 11, pp. 21–32.

Report of the Royal Commission on the National Health Service (1979) (Chairman: Sir Alec Merrison), Cmnd 7615, HMSO, London.

Select Committee on Health (1993) *Community Care: Funding from April 1993*, Third report, session 1992–3, HMSO, London.

Select Committee on Social Services (1980) Third Report, session 1979–80, *The Government's White Papers on Public Expenditure: the Social Services*, HC 702.1, HMSO London.

Select Committee on Social Services (1985) Second report, session 1984/5, *Community Care with Special Reference to Adult Mentally Ill and Mentally Handicapped People*, Cmnd 9674, HMSO, London.

Select Committee on Social Services (1990) Fifth report, session 1989/90, *Community Care: Carers*, HMSO, London.

Taylor, J. and Taylor, D. (1989) *Mental Health in the 1990s from Custody to Care*, Office of Health Economics, London.

Walker, A. (1989) 'Community Care' in McCarthy, M. (ed.), *The New Politics of Welfare: an agenda for the 1990s*, Macmillan, London.

Webb, A. and Wistow, G. (1982) 'The Personal Social Services: incrementalism, expediency or systematic social planning', in Walker, A. (ed.), *Public Expenditure and Social Policy*, Heinemann, London.

Wistow, G. (1982) 'Collaboration between Health and Local Authorities: why is it necessary?', *Social Policy and Administration*, 16 (1), pp. 44–62.

Wolfenden Committee (1977) *The Future of Voluntary Organisations*, Croom Helm, London.

Wolfsenburger, W. (1992) 'The principle of normalisation in the human services', quoted in Hunter, D., 'The Move to Community Care with Special Reference to Mental Illness', in Beck, E., Londsdale, S., Newman, S. and Patterson, D. (eds), *In the Best of Health? The status and future of health care in the UK*, Chapman & Hall, London.

PART THREE

Health and Society

CHAPTER 6

The social bases of ill-health

This chapter aims to explore the trends in the major causes of illness and death in the UK over the last century. The differences in the health status of groups within the population are also examined along the lines of class, gender and ethnicity. The explanations for these differences are analysed as well as the patterns of health service utilisation. Before dealing with trends, explanations and utilisation, an examination of concepts of disease, illness and health are examined and problems of the measurement of these phenomena discussed.

Concepts of disease, illness and health

The concept of disease is rooted in the growth of scientific medicine in the nineteenth century. It was in this period that the disease entities which form the basis of modern medicine began to be classified and recorded. In 1832, the passage of the Anatomy Act had allowed post-mortems to be carried out and the causes of death could be more clearly established. The hospitals, which treated the poor who could not afford the cost of doctors' fees, became the focus for medical practice and the development of clinical knowledge. This knowledge was based on a mechanistic view of the body and normal bodily functioning. Within the medical model, disease categories are based on descriptions of deviations from a norm or the presence of recognisable abnormality. Alternatively, they rest on descriptions of characteristic clusters of symptoms which have been observed by doctors in their clinical practice as leading to particular outcomes and named as a guide to others. The gathering of information either by observation, by examination or by the taking a history from the patient is the first step in the process of diagnosis. The identification of the disease then leads to decisions about treatment. These are based on the body of knowledge and experience developed by clinicians and shared by the medico-scientific community. Document 15 (page 314) describes the medical model.

To some extent the definitions and classifications of disease are social constructs which shift over time. The signs and symptoms of disease tend to be based on concepts of 'normality'. However, normality may be defined in a number of ways in both statistical and social terms. 'Normal' blood pressure, for example, may be defined in terms of a mean or average for the population. Or, it may be defined in relation to a particular person. Normality may also be defined in terms of the ability to carry out particular tasks or to fulfil certain social roles. Again, this may be in relation to what is 'normal' for a population group or in relation to an individual. In other words, what is considered normal may be relative to social groups and involve judgements. In clinical practice, a doctor may take the inability of a patient who is unable to fulfil physical tasks usually carried out by that person, as a possible indication of an underlying pathology. The inability to undertake social roles may also be taken as an indicator of an underlying disease.

Illness is commonly distinguished from disease. Field (1976) uses a now generally accepted definition. He states that:

> Illness refers primarily to an individual's experience of ill health and is indicated by a person's feelings of pain, discomfort and the like.
>
> (Field 1976: 334)

It is thus possible to have an illness without disease and disease without illness. While bio-medical definitions of disease are relatively independent of social behaviour, illness is culturally specific. Individuals draw their ideas about illness from the groups and communities in which they live. Thus, illness has moral, psychological and social dimensions as well as biological. There is of course an overlap between biomedical categories and people's perceptions of illness. Lay people make the decision to consult their doctor on the basis of the symptoms they perceive which will be related to their knowledge, experience, social position and the norms and values of the society in which they live.

Health is an altogether more difficult concept. It can be seen in relation to disease. Thus, a bio-medical definition of health may be the absence of disease or abnormal pathology. It can also be defined as freedom from the symptoms of illness. Thus, for Dubos (1960), health becomes freedom from pain, discomfort, stress and boredom. The World Health Organisation (WHO) definition takes the concept of health a step further to describe it in positive terms, as a 'state of complete physical, mental and social well-being not merely the absence of disease and infirmity'.

However, good health may also be seen in terms of the ability to carry out certain physical tasks or to perform certain social roles. These may be related to age, sex and gender, occupation, ethnicity or other social division, so either doctors or lay people may describe an individual as being 'healthy for their age', or, 'healthy, given a particular disability'. Health can also be seen as the ability to adapt to change and adjust to social circumstances – in terms of the society as well as the individual. For example, for Parsons (1958), a healthy society is one in which there is adaptation to change and this can be conceived in both social and biological terms.

Disease, illness and health are relative and sometimes contested concepts. Theoretical frameworks may be drawn from bio-medicine or social science. Within the latter frame, anthropologists and psychologists as well as sociologists have all made contributions to the literature. Stanton Rogers, in *Explaining Health and Illness* (1991), provides an overview. There has been a variety of empirical studies of the practice of medicine and of lay views of illness and health. The latter are of particular interest as it is lay people who generally make the first decision to consult medical practitioners and thus use health services. How they decide when they are sufficiently ill to consult is therefore of importance.

The concepts discussed so far have been drawn from theories which are then used to examine aspects of behaviour. There have also been studies which collect accounts of people's everyday subjective definitions of health and illness. These have been shown to vary widely. In the 1960s, Herzlich (1976) studied middle-class French women and showed that her subjects had a number of often overlapping views. They talked of 'health-in-a-vacuum', a 'reserve of health' and 'health as a feeling of equilibrium'. Their expectations were high. Blaxter and Paterson (1982) in a survey of attitudes to health among working-class women in Aberdeen, found that they talked about being healthy despite the presence of disease; they had much lower expectations. One respondent commented:

> After I was sterilised, I had a lot of cystitis, and backache because of the fibroids. Then when I had my hysterectomy I had bother with my waterworks because my bladder had a life of its own and I had to have a repair. . . . Healthwise I would say I'm OK. I did hurt my shoulder – I mean, this is nothing to do with health but I actually now have a disability, I have a gratuity payment every six months. . . . I wear a collar and take Valium then, just the headaches – but I'm not really off work a lot with it.
>
> (Blaxter and Paterson 1982: 29)

A more systematic and broader study of attitudes was carried out in 1984–5 (Cox *et al.* 1987) in the Health and Lifestyle Survey where 9000 people were interviewed. In 1991, a second follow-up study was undertaken (Cox *et al.* 1993). A comparison could be made between attitudes in the two periods because a large number of the same people were traced and re-interviewed. It was found that people's own assessment of their physical well-being or health was a fairly accurate reflection of their biological health. The first study recorded people's own assessment of their health in terms of excellent/good/fair or whether they thought their health was poor. The second study found that mortality rates were twice as high for those who described their health as poor or fair. The findings suggest that there is a correlation between subjective views of health and objective measures. People's own self-assessment of their health had tended to predict their own death. We now turn to the measurement of ill-health.

The measurement of death, illness and health

The extent of ill-health in any society can be gauged by both objective and subjective measures. The main measures are mortality – that is, death – and morbidity – that is, illness. The latter can be assessed by 'objective' measures, through clinical assessments or by more subjective self-assessments. In the UK, the Registrar General has kept statistics on death and the causes of death since 1839. These have been used to calculate Standardised Mortality Ratios (SMRs) for groups within the population. The data on deaths for all causes are standardised by age and sex. (Ratios are calculated using 100 as a base, in order to make comparisons over time and changes between populations.)

SMRs can be linked to census data providing a breakdown to the level of an enumeration district (which contains about 200 households). This can be further broken down into postcode districts, consisting of a few streets. Data on death rates can therefore be linked to data on social class characteristics for quite small districts. Researchers have thus been able to look at differential death rates between social classes. Mortality figures for different occupations can also be compared using the Registrar General's decennial supplements.

There are a number of problems with mortality statistics. For example, a social class ranking may be attributed to an enumeration district but this involves an ecological fallacy: that is, all the people living in an enumeration district are assumed to have the same social class. Data on women's mortality rates and their occupations is more flawed than that of men because women's occupations are under-reported (Macfarlane 1990). Data combining mortality and ethnicity are also poor. Official statistics have tended to record country of birth rather than ethnic group. The latter is more useful as it is more likely to reflect lifestyles.

Mortality rates are only a very crude indicator of health status – that is, of the health of people who remain alive. A falling death rate may not mean an improvement in general health and many kinds of chronic ill-health, particularly among adults, which affect the quality of life, may not be reflected in mortality rates. However, the Infant Mortality Rate (IMR) – that is, the number of deaths per thousand births during the first year of life – is generally acknowledged as being a sensitive indicator of a society's general health status. This is because the number of infant deaths tends to be dependent on the social and living conditions and the availability of health services which affect health status at all ages. Butler and Bonham (1963) suggest that IMR is indicative of the number of 'near deaths', which present with defects and deaths at a later stage. They comment:

> Like an iceberg we see only a proportion of the ill results, the deaths. But we must not forget the submerged and larger fraction, the near deaths and the harm they cause.
>
> (quoted in Blaxter 1981: 35)

Data relating to morbidity – the amount of disease and sickness – are a more useful guide to health but the present range of these data are limited. Hospital activity statistics are routinely collected. These record the reason for attendance or admission; discharges and deaths. The data provide only limited information on the socio-demographic characteristics of those attending hospitals. In addition to this routine information, there has been a limited market of one-off national studies which have collected data on health and social characteristics – for example, there have been large periodic sample surveys of general practice.

Most studies have been based on those people actually using health services and this depends upon a willingness to consult. Those studies which have used other methods have found a 'submerged iceberg of sickness' in the community which is never brought to the medical profession. This may be because conditions are defined as 'normal' due to age or occupation, because other remedies are being used or because there is little faith in the efficacy of medical intervention. Community surveys, using house-to-house interview methods, have also been used to establish morbidity in specific areas at particular points in time. Most of the types of study referred to above involve some form of clinical assessment of disease in the population interviewed, although many also collect data on people's views about their health and ill-health.

The main source of regular information on self-reported illness is the General Household Survey (GHS). This survey collects data on 10 per cent of the population annually. It provides information on respondents' own recollections of episodes of ill-health, it makes distinctions between acute illness and chronic illness (where there is long-standing sickness which affects activity) and records consultations with GPs and hospital admissions. Data are also collected on aspects of health behaviour, such as smoking, and the use of services, such as family planning, and aids such as spectacles and contact lenses. Questions have been changed periodically so that there are some difficulties in making comparisons over time, but the GHS nevertheless provides a wealth of data which can be linked to social characteristics. Information on morbidity can also be derived from data gathered for other purposes. Statistics on sickness absence, for example, are collected for the Department of Health for the payment of sickness benefit. However, these data have become less useful since the increase of self-reporting. Also, these data relate only to those who are employed.

Methods for measuring *health* have also been developed. For example, there are methods for assessing functional ability, psychological well-being, the impact of sickness on everyday life and quality of life indicators based on clinical and lay assessments. Bowling critically reviews these in *Measuring Health* (1991). Such methods have been used to assess levels of health in individuals. They may also be used to assess the effects of treatment or to assign costs and benefits to particular treatments. And they are useful in comparing groups in the population to assess relative health status and, for example, how this may vary between age groups.

One of the most interesting sources of data about morbidity and illness, life-styles and health has been provided by longitudinal studies. These indicate how factors related to social position and illness interact over time. An example of this type of study is the Health and Lifestyle Survey referred to above. The survey covered a variety of aspects of life-style such as diet, exercise, smoking and alcohol consumption as well as self assessments and attitudes to health. Eighty per cent of those visited were subsequently examined to establish their physical and mental health (Blaxter 1990). In 1991, more than half of the sample were then traced and re-interviewed. Some of the results are referred to below (Cox *et al*. 1993). Studies as comprehensive as these are important as they can relate particular life-styles and health behaviour to subsequent morbidity and mortality.

In recent years, data on mortality, morbidity and the ensuing impact on disability and the quality of life have been used to assess the burden of disease. This may be used to make comparisons across countries or regions and also to identify how the greatest 'health gains' may be achieved. Interventions by governments or others in specific health policies or health services may be assessed in terms of the greatest benefits which could ensue. Data on mortality can be used to estimate the extent of years of life lost through premature death.

Changing patterns of mortality

The most dramatic improvement in mortality rates has occurred among the very young and this has been progressive since the beginning of the nineteenth century. In the UK, at the beginning of the twentieth century, 10 per cent of children born died within the first year of life. By the end of the 1970s this had fallen to 1.3 per cent and by 1989 was less than 1 per cent. In other words, more than 99 per cent of babies now survive their first year of life.

Table 6.1 **Perinatal Mortality rates in OECD countries 1980–89**

	Perinatal mortality (percentage of live and still births)		Percentage change in perinatal mortality
	1980	*1989*	*1980–89*
Belgium	1.42	1.02*	–28*
France	1.29	0.89	32
Germany	1.16	0.64	45
Ireland	1.48	0.99	33
Netherlands	1.11	0.96	14
Spain	1.44	1.00*	–31*
United Kingdom	1.34	0.90	33

* 1987 or 1980–1987.
Source: OECD Health Systems: Facts and Trends, 1993, Paris.

This is a similar pattern to that of other industrialised countries, although the UK tends to lag behind some other comparable countries. Table 6.1 shows that Germany, the Netherlands and France have slightly better perinatal mortality rates although the rate of improvement for all OECD countries has tended to flatten and close in recent years. Comparisons in infant mortality rates between and within different countries, particularly if expressed as percentages, must be treated with caution as the numbers involved are relatively small.

Overall mortality rates show a gradual improvement, particularly in the age groups under 40. At the turn of the century, expectation of life at birth in the United Kingdom was 48 years for males, and 52 for females. By 1951, this had risen to 66 and 71

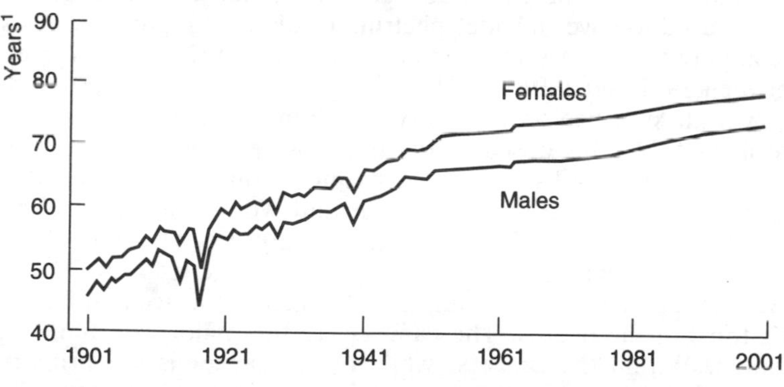

Note:
1 The average number of years which a new-born baby could be expected to live if its rates of mortality at each age were those experienced in that calendar year.

Figure 6.1 ***Expectation of life at birth: by sex, 1901–2001***
Source: Social Trends (1994) HMSO, London.

respectively and by 1993, there was a further increase to 74 years for men and 79 for women (Social Trends 1994). There has been a general slowing down in the improvement in life expectancy; Figure 6.1 shows the life expectancy for males and females in the UK. It should be noted that life expectancy is shorter in Northern Ireland and Scotland.

Changes in the leading causes of mortality and morbidity

The pattern of death and disease in the UK, in line with patterns in other industrialised societies, has changed during this century. In any examination of major causes of death and disease two factors stand out. The first is the relative *decline* in the incidence of infectious diseases and the second is the *relative increase* in diseases of the circulation (including heart attacks and strokes), of the cancers and the respiratory diseases as the major causes of death. The decline in infectious disease has led to increasing numbers of each cohort of births surviving into middle and old age. The largest single factor leading to these improvements has been the greater survival rate of infants in the first year of life. Changes in the pattern of disease have had an impact on the age structure of the population referred to in earlier chapters. As a consequence of this, there has been an overall increase in chronic illness, disability and dependency.

In 1991, coronary heart disease (CHD) accounted for 26 per cent of deaths in England. It also accounted for 2.5 per cent of NHS expenditure (Department of Health 1992). In the same year, almost 12 per cent of deaths resulted from strokes. After CHD, the main cause of death, at 25 per cent, is due to the cancers – a term used to cover a wide spectrum of disease. Figure 6.2 gives a comparison of the selected causes of death in men and women between 1951 and 1991.

Overall, statistics on mortality are dominated by deaths over the age of 70. This obscures the importance of what have been referred to as 'deaths before their time' – that is, early deaths. There are differences between men and women in the leading causes of death as well as between age groups. The two major causes of premature deaths among adults aged 40 to 70 are coronary heart disease among middle-aged men, accounting for one-third of the deaths. The cancers are the major cause among women. Within the cancers, while breast cancer is the primary cause of death among women, it is lung cancer among men. Under the age of 30, accidents, particularly among males, are a major cause of death (Table 6.2), and of these car accidents are the main factor. Accidents involving traffic and poisoning are the most common cause of fatalities among children under 15; they are responsible for approximately 30 per cent of the deaths.

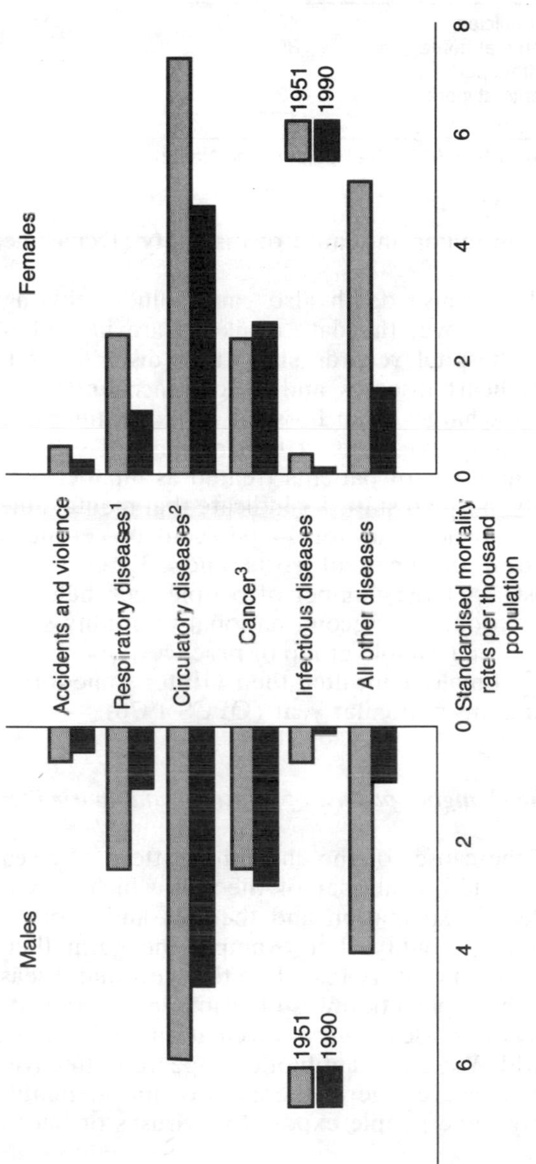

Notes:
1 In 1984 the coding procedure was changed, reducing the number of deaths assigned to respiratory causes.
2 Includes heart attacks and strokes.
3 The figure for neoplasms include both malignant and benign cancers.

Figure 6.2 ***Selected causes of death: by sex, 1951 and 1990***
Source: Social Trends (1992) HMSO, London.

Table 6.2 **Deaths from accidents: all ages England and Wales 1990**

Type of accident	*Percentage in each group*
Motor vehicles	42
Accidents at home	35
Other transport	4
Accidents at work	3
Other	17

Source: DOH (1992) The Health of the Nation, HMSO, London.

Accidents are also an important cause of disability (Department of Health 1992).

The diseases which cause death also cause illness although, for the reason given above, the data available are limited. As one would expect, hospital records show that diseases of the respiratory system, heart diseases and cancers account for the highest number of discharges from hospital after inpatient treatment. Disease may also take a heavy toll in terms of suffering. Looking simply at numbers of patients treated as inpatients and outpatients annually, hospital statistics indicate that mental illness is a major problem. It accounts for 14 per cent of certificated absence, 14 per cent of inpatient costs and 23 per cent of pharmaceutical costs. A large number of people seek help from their GPs for this reason. The second national morbidity survey in 1970–1 found that, in a sample group of practices, one in seven females and one in 14 males consulted their GP for some form of mental illness during this particular year (OPCS 1976).

Explanations for the changing pattern of mortality and morbidity

The debate about the causes of the changing pattern of disease and illness has generated a number of theories which draw on various frameworks of explanation and theories and about the causes of death and morbidity. For example the germ theory popular in the nineteenth century rested on the view that diseases had single causes. The explanation was plausible in the context of a prevalence of infectious disease. Also vaccination, immunisation and, after the World War Two, antibiotics appeared effective in combating disease. However, germ theory was not adequate in explaining why only some people exposed to viruses or bacteria contracted diseases.

In a major contribution, McKeown in *The Role of Medicine* (1979), argues that health improved in the nineteenth century and in turn brought greater resistance to infections. He demonstrated that, from the early nineteenth century onwards, better nutrition and higher standards of living led to a falling mortality rate. This predated advances in medical treatment. Improvements in health status led to changes in reproductive behaviour (fewer children, more widely spaced) which further strengthened resistance to infection. Policies for public health, through modernisation of the water supply and sanitation, lessened the likelihood of the spread of pathogens. As a consequence, McKeown considers that medical intervention through immunisation and vaccination – with the possible exception of diphtheria and poliomyelitis, has had a minimal effect on reduction in the incidence of infectious diseases.

Turning to contemporary disease patterns, McKeown suggests that the causes of the chronic or degenerative diseases, which now predominate, are more complex. People who live longer are more exposed to a range of diseases which have multiple causes. These derive from a combination of genetic, behavioural and environmental factors which may have cumulative effects. Further, as well as being attributable to a range of causes, it may be that these factors create a susceptibility to disease in particular individuals or social groups. We now turn to examine some of the evidence on the difference in disease patterns among particular social groups in order to assess whether this is the case.

Social divisions and ill health

Sex, gender and ethnicity

It has already been indicated that there are differences in men's and women's health. Women have greater life expectancy than men and although the causes of deaths for both groups are similar, they are lower for women in each major category (Moser *et al.* 1988). Women in particular age ranges are also more susceptible to the cancers – in the case of breast cancer, the major cause of premature death in the cancers in women for this age group of diseases, they are uniquely susceptible. And there is little sign of improvement. Women are also twice as likely to be diagnosed as having a depressive mental illness than men. However, men have a higher suicide rate and, once referred to a specialist, are more likely to be diagnosed as having a serious mental illness (Taylor and Taylor 1989).

Patterns in the utilisation of health services are also different for men and women. Women consult health practitioners more. However, this may be due to women's role in reproduction. Pregnancy and childbirth tend to be treated as illnesses. Women also consult for contraception, abortion, fertility treatments and problems associated with the menopause. Macfarlane (1990), in a detailed analysis of women's health, argues that, once the consultations for pregnancy, childbirth and diseases of both male and female genito-urinary systems are excluded, the difference between consultation rates between the sexes virtually disappears.

This bricf summary of men's and women's health cannot do justice to the topic. However, differences are partly due to biology, to exposure to hazards and diagnostic practices. A World Bank report (1993) has estimated that for women between the ages of 15 and 44, one third of the total burden of disease afflicts women exclusively. The report also argues that, because women need to be healthy themselves to fulfil their roles as mothers and household managers, their well-being is particularly important for longer-term improvements to societal health. Other social divisions such as income and occupation also have a crucial effect on health. These are discussed in more detail below.

In relation to the health of ethnic minorities, data are scarce. Routine statistics do not record ethnicity and until 1991, neither did the census. Balarajan and Raleigh (1993), however, provide a useful summary of current data. The 1991 census showed that 94 per cent of the population was white and the next largest group, 1.7 per cent, was from the Indian subcontinent. Ethnic minority populations are not evenly distributed through the country. In Brent, the local authority with the largest ethnic minority population, the proportion is 45 per cent.

Balarajan and Raleigh found that men born in the Indian subcontinent tend to have higher death rates from heart disease than the white population. Both Asian and Afro-Caribbean men are at greater risk of stroke and, for Asians, this is particularly marked for the younger age groups. Figure 6.3 shows the results. Also, babies of ethnic minority mothers are twice as likely to die in the first year of life as the average. Figure 6.4 shows the IMR rates in the 1980s according to the mother's country of birth. Conversely, the death rates from heart disease and cancer for ethnic minority women are lower than the average. In relation to mental illness, small-scale studies suggest that Afro-Caribbean males have higher admission rates to hospital and are much more likely to be diagnosed as having a serious mental illness than the population as a whole (Lipsedge and Littlewood 1982). The causes of these differences can only be speculated upon. For example, it has been suggested that the lower death rates for women in ethnic minorities may be due to lower smoking rates. Higher levels of mental illness have been attributed to a range of factors, such as the stress of migration, the effect of cultural and social mores on behaviour, the response of gatekeepers to particular groups, racism and poor material conditions.

Social class and health status

Most studies which explore the relationship between social class and ill-health use the Registrar General's classification of occu-

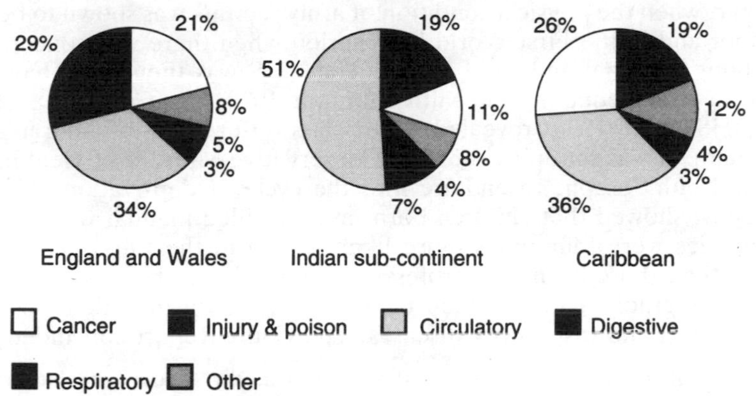

Figure 6.3 **Distribution of cause of death for men aged 20–49 from 1979–1983 by place of birth (England and Wales)**
Source: Dunnel, K. (1993) The Health of the Nation Conference Proceedings, NE and NW Thames RHA.

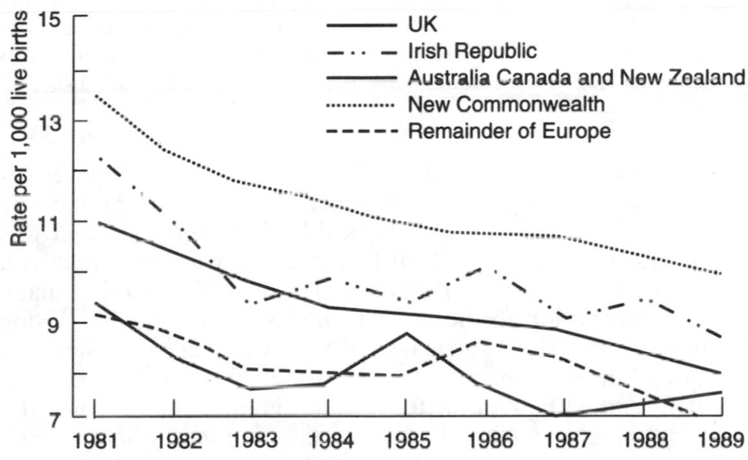

Note:
* Using a 3 year average centred on the year shown

Figure 6.4 **Infant mortality rates by mother's birth (1981–89)**
Source: Dunnel (1993).

pations as a measure of class. Typically, occupations are divided into five broad social classes. The groupings encapsulate a number of variables such as income, poverty, occupation and education which are highly correlated with each other. The issue of class differences in mortality and morbidity had been acknowledged from the nineteenth century [Document 16 page 315]. However, it has only surfaced on to the policy agenda periodically: in the Boer

War, when the physical condition of army recruits was shown to be poor and in the First World War period when there was concern about maternal and child health. The NHS was thought to have dealt with inequalties in health but in the 1970s, the Court Report (DHSS/DES 1976) revealed major class differences in children's health. It was set up by the then Conservative Minister of Health, Sir Keith Joseph, to enquire into the cycle of deprivation. The report showed that children born into unskilled manual workers' families were four times more likely to die in their first year of life than those born into professional families and there was also a class gradient in the main causes of mortality in childhood – accidents and respiratory diseases. The Court Report concluded:

> We have already had occasion to refer repeatedly to the correlations between social class and the prevalence of ill-health and disability in, children. . . . There is now extensive evidence that an adverse family and social environment can retard physical, emotional and intellectual growth, lead to more frequent and more serious illness and adversely affect educational achievement and personal behaviour. . . . In many crucial respects our findings have given us profound anxiety about the state of child health in this country, about the shortcomings of services and those working in them, and about the prospects for new generations if they are to grow up in the same deprived physical and emotional circumstances as many children today have to contend with.
>
> (DHSS/DES 1976: 50 (See Document 10 on page 304))

The next Labour Health Minister, David Ennals, also set up a committee, chaired by Sir Douglas Black, to examine the relationship between class and ill-health. This time, the aim was to look into inequalities in health. Its report was published in a limited edition by the Department of Health in 1980 and has made a major contribution to the debate on class and ill-health. Using 1971 figures, the report showed that there was a class gradient for 68 out of 82 disease categories. Men in social class V between the ages of 15 and 64 had an SMR 1.8 times greater than men of the same age in social class I. Tables 6.3 and 6.4 illustrate the relationships between social class, death rates and morbidity.

Table 6.3 ***Mortality by social class 1931–81 (men 15–64 years, England and Wales)***

Class	*1931*	*1961*	*1981*
I professional	90	75	66
II managerial	94	81	76
III skilled manual/non manual	97	100	103
IV semi-skilled	102	103	116
V unskilled	111	127	166

Source: Adapted from DHSS (1980).

Table 6.4 **Percentage of the population reporting acute and chronic illness who consulted their doctor in the previous two weeks: by socio-economic group 1974 and 1985**

Socio-economic group	*All ages* 1974	*All ages* 1985	*Over 65* 1974	*Over 65* 1985
I	25	27	32	32
II	27	28	31	26
III	31	32	25	30
IV	33	29	26	28
V	33	30	26	28
VI	31	34	28	39
Total	32	31	27	29

Source: Adapted from Le Grand, J. *et al.* (1989)

Subsequent studies have confirmed the class gradient in health status (Townsend *et al.* 1992). Data on morbidity from a variety of studies has also found greater occurrence according to lower social class. For example, the General Household Survey shows double the rates of long-standing sickness among social class V men than those in social class I. The same trends are evident from the longitudinal studies of death rates and morbidity in the civil service (Marmot 1986). Document 20 (page 323) shows the results of this important study and provides a commentary.

Although women's health is more difficult to measure because if they have not worked, they take the occupation of their husband, a class gradient is also evident (Roberts 1990). For example, the study by Moser *et al.* (1988) found that high mortality among women was associated with working in a manual occupation, living in a rented house and having no access to a car. Where these indicators were combined, mortality rates were two to three times higher than for women with none of these disadvantages.

More recently, studies have indicated that in the 1980s, social class differentials are increasing. Davey Smith *et al.* (1990) concluded on the basis of later figures that the gap between mortality rates in social class I and V is widening. The 1993 Health and Lifestyle Survey also found increases in mortality in lower social classes between the first and second survey.

The interpretation of data on class, mortality and morbidity

The major problem with much of the information on the relationship between class and illness is that, of itself, it explains very little. Social class is the most commonly used index of social circumstances. It implies differences in income, education, power of resources and behaviour but measures none of them directly. Partly as a consequence of this, and partly due to prior ideological viewpoints, explanations differ as to why the inequalities occur. There are four major explanations:

1 The results are due to an artefact;
2 That they are a consequence of social selection;
3 That they are related to the health behaviour of individuals;
4 That they are due to inequalities in material conditions.

The issue of explanations is important as these could provide a basis for policy.

The artefact explanation rests on criticisms of the data. For example, Illsley (1986) argues that social class is based on arbitrary groupings of occupations. If comparisons are made between social class and health inequalities over time, as they often are, the occupations which form the basis of the classification have changed so much that they make comparisons meaningless. He suggests that the balance of classes has altered substantially and that the occupations classed as unskilled manual are becoming a smaller proportion of the population.

A social selection explanation suggests that poor health itself leads to downward social mobility and, conversely, those with good health are upwardly socially mobile. This has been demonstrated through studies of the height and birth weight of those in the latter category. It is also thought that this process could occur through selective marriage – less healthy women marrying down the social scale. It has also been shown, in relation to studies of schizophrenia, for example, that the fathers of those suffering from schizophrenia are more equally distributed though the social spectrum than schizophrenics themselves – indicating downward social mobility as a consequence of the illness itself.

The behavioural explanation concludes that inequalities in health are due to differences in behaviour – that is, whether 'risky' practices are followed. For example, it is known that smoking, high blood pressure and high blood cholesterol are associated with CHD. The two latter factors may be associated with poor diet and lack of exercise. Those who take more care of themselves will have better health. The high mortality rates among younger people from accidents, particularly motor vehicle accidents, is also blamed on risky behaviour. In the same way, those with HIV/AIDS may be held responsible for their disease, the cause of which is attributed to sexual behaviour and/or drug abuse. In the 1960s the higher perinatal mortality among social class V mothers was attributed to low take-up of antenatal care.

The materialist explanation attributes differences to poor material conditions and the hazards inherent in society, to which some people have no choice but to be exposed given the present distribution of income and opportunity. There has been a long tradition of research into the association between work and health. Work can bring hazards. The two extracts in the document section [Document 16 page 315] give an example taken from Engels, who describes factory work in the nineteeth century. A recent study of women production line workers is taken from a book by Ruth Cavendish, *Women on the Line* (1982). Both relate illness to production processes and methods of working.

Ill-health has also been attributed to unemployment. At a macro level, Brenner (1977) established a link between levels of production and unemployment and ill-health. He suggests that recessions and wide-scale economic distress exert an impact on health status indicators – IMR, maternal mortality and national mortality rates, especially on deaths ascribed to cardiovascular disease, cirrhosis of the liver, suicide and homicide rates and rates of first admission to mental hospital. Fagin (1981), on the basis of interviews with families suffering unemployment, has argued that the loss of a job is like a bereavement but is not accepted as such. Unemployment, he argues, produces the risk of prolonged stress with implications for physical and mental health [Document 18 page 319]. An Office of Health Economics pamphlet (1993) reviews the literature on health and unemployment.

Low-quality housing has also been shown to be associated with poor health and with higher rates of illness amongst children (Whitehead 1992). Quick and Wilkinson (1991) have focused on income as the major determinant of life expectancy and health. On the basis of international data, they argue that populations in more affluent countries have longer life expectancy. Moreover, those countries with a better record in this (taken as a measure of health) are those where the distribution of income is relatively even, like Sweden and Japan. Quick and Wilkinson also suggest that the experience of Britain between the wars, and during World War Two, confirms their interpretation. The income redistribution, full employment, improvements in diet and attempts to ensure minmum standards for all during the war years had the effect of improving general health. Conversely, the increase in income differentials in the 1980s in Britain (Hills 1993) may lie behind the increasing differentials in health status.

There are problems in disentangling the arguments as the precise linkages may not be apparent. For example, does unemployment *cause* a deterioration in health or are the sick more likely to be unemployed? If the latter is the case, then the association is simply an artefact of the data. If the former is so, then there is support for the materialist explanation. Another example can be taken from the debate about the relationship between ill-health and unemployment. Does unemployment lead to poverty and therefore poor health or, alternatively, are those who live in poor conditions and have poor health more likely to become unemployed? A third example involves women and smoking behaviour. Women in social class V smoke more. They also have poorer health. Are they to blame for this or, as Graham (1987) argues, is smoking a way of coping with living in poor material conditions with small children on a low income?

The arguments tend to become cyclical. This is partly because the phenomena under consideration – ill-health and material circumstances – are so complex and because each explanation has some plausibility. In general terms, the evidence in favour of materialist explanations is strong. Poor living conditions, when linked with environmental hazards, particularly when these are cumulative over time, do lead to poor health. Diseases tend to have a complex aetiology depending on a variety of factors; life-style, behaviour, work, as well as inherited susceptibility. This can be compounded by behavioural habits which have an adverse effect. Document 19 (page 321) shows the effect of ill-health over time.

Both social causality and social selection occur. Occupations affect people's living conditions and their standard of living. Occupations influence people's resources and working conditions involve health hazards. Non-employed people have low incomes and this affects their living standards. Over time there can be a drift down the social ladder due to poor health. Blaxter sums up the findings of the Health and Lifestyle survey thus:

> At the extremes it is of course true that the worst health was found where poverty, an industrial or inner city environment, disturbed social relationships, and a completely unhealthy pattern of behaviour, were all combined. For the great majority, it seems that health is primarily affected by environment and by the characteristics – occupation, income, housing . . . it is among those who are not environmentally vulnerable that harmful behavioural habits such as smoking appear to produce most effect. . . . On the other hand it must be noted that good diet and a high level of exercise were associated with lower illness and better fitness among manual men, especially if they were also non-smokers and non-drinkers . . . lack of stress and an adequate level of social support were particularly protective of those on low incomes.
>
> (1990: 230–1)

Document 17 (page 317) describes people who are most vulnerable to ill-health. As Rainwater (1968) comments, disadvantage may be reinforced by culture:

> Just as lower class people become resigned to a conception of themselves as persons who do not function very well socially or psychologically, they become resigned to bodies which function less well physically.
>
> (quoted in Blaxter 1981: 216)

The distribution of health services

Until now, inequalities in health status have been discussed. These have persisted despite the existence of a national health service. This suggests that health services alone cannot eradicate such inequalities. However, the NHS provided equality of access to health services according to need. So, as Tudor-Hart (1971) suggested, has there been an inverse care law? Do those who are poorest and in worst health either fail to access services at all or obtain ones of poorer quality? The issue is examined in terms of the distribution of services; the differential use of particular services; the quality of services received; and the distribution of resources by social class.

The distribution of services

Health services come in a variety of forms: hospital services, inpatient and outpatient; dental services; preventive services; GP services and so on. Studies carried out touch on some but not all of these. It is known from surveys carried out before or in the early years of World War Two that there was an unequal distribution of services in the UK (Webster 1988). Indeed one of the objectives of the NHS was to achieve a more even spread. A study by Political and Economic Planning in 1944 pointed out that the more affluent areas had a higher ratio of GPs.

> In Hastings before the war there was one GP for every 1,178 persons, whereas in South Shields there was one for every 4,105. . . . Thus the number of residents per GP was twice as great in Kensington as in Hampstead, thrice as great in Harrow; four times as great in Bradford, five times in Wakefield, six times in West Bromwich and seven times in South Shields. The disparity in distribution is even more serious than it appears from these figures because 'under-doctored' districts are usually also poor districts with high rates of sickness and mortality and in special need of a good medical service.
>
> (Political and Economic Planning 1944: 34)

The 1946 Act introduced a system for equalising the distribution, but Butler (1973) concluded that by the early 1970s, there had been no dramatic shift in their location. Certain areas of the country were medically deprived in the sense that existing services were unable to cope with the demands placed upon them, while others had a relative abundance of medical resources in relation to their needs. However, by the mid-1980s, a more even distribution had been achieved and, in comparison with other countries, the UK now has an equitable distribution of GPs (Maynard 1977).

In relation to hospital services, there has been a similar slow progress towards a more even distribution. From 1975, policies have been followed which redistributed the resources going to the different health regions more equitably according to a weighted population. By the early 1980s at the regional level, equity had been achieved, but within regions there were still discrepancies of resources between districts. And even in the early 1990s, hospitals in London are being closed so that those in the Home Counties can be further developed to cater for their local populations.

A more significant question is whether those who needed care most – that is, those in the poorer socio-economic groups – did have access to services according to need. This question has been the subject of much debate. In 1969, Martin Rein, a visiting US academic, argued that:

> the lowest social classes make greater use of hospital inpatient services . . . and . . . they receive what appears to be of as good quality as that secured by other social classes.
>
> (Rein 1969: 807)

However, the Black Report (DHSS 1980) concluded that class differences in need were not fully reflected in health service use.

There appears to be stronger evidence that the higher social classes take greater advantage of preventive health services. Cartwright and O'Brien (1976) comment that:

> There appears to us to be fairly conclusive evidence that the middle class made more use of preventive services, and to suggest that the middle class may in relation to a number of services, receive better care.
>
> (1976: 93–4)

The Black Report cites studies which suggest that women from social class V not only experienced the lowest degree of intensive care during their pregnancies, but were very much more likely to have their babies induced in hospital. Consultation times tended to be longer with higher social classes and there was evidence to show that home visits by consultants to patients in terminal care favoured these groups also.

The use of services by social class

Le Grand, Winter and Wooley (1989) analysed the use of GPs from General Household Survey data. In the two weeks prior to the 1985 survey, 17 per cent of unskilled manual workers and their families (social class VI) and 16 per cent of semi-skilled manual workers and their families (social class V) had visited their GP compared to 14 per cent of the population as a whole and 9 per cent of professionals. This closely reflects assessments of acute and chronic illness in these groups. Self-assessments may not of course equate with illness, people may simply be less stoical. However, the authors conclude that in the use of GPs there is something close to equality of access for equal need. Table 6.4 shows the figures. It also indicates that the gradient in favour of lower income groups steepened between 1974 and 1987. The findings suggest that as far as GPs are concerned, the NHS has been successful in eliminating barriers to access.

Health Service expenditure by social class

Class inequalities may also relate to health service expenditure and logically, if there are inequalities in the two areas already discussed, less is likely to be spent on those in social classes IV and V. Two examples may be given of studies which relate expenditure to social class. Noyce, Snaith and Trickey (1974) analysed the expenditure by local authorities in the three branches of the health service in 1971–2. They found a significant positive correlation between the percentage of the population in professional and managerial socio-economic groups in both community health and hospital revenue expenditure. They concluded:

> evidently as late as 1971/72 no effort was achieving success in directing new capital to deprived regions.

In *Strategy of Equality*, Le Grand (1982) examined NHS expenditure per head by constructing estimates on the basis of patterns of utilisation. He found that the distribution favoured the better off: the higher social groups with professionals, employers and managers receiving nearly 40 per cent more NHS expenditure per person ill than families of semi- and unskilled manual workers. The findings are shown in Table 6.5. However, O'Donnell and Propper (1991) in a similar but later study concluded that there was *no* bias in favour of the better-off.

Overall, the balance of the evidence is that there is an uneven distribution of health and disease along class lines in the UK.

Table 6.5 **Public expenditure on health care by socio-economic group – All persons – England and Wales 1972**

Socio-economic group	*Expenditure per person: percentage of mean*	*Expenditure per person reporting illness: percentage of mean*
Professionals, employers and managers	94	120
Intermediate and junior non-manual	104	114
Skilled manual	92	97
Semi- and unskilled manual	114	
Mean (£) = 100	18.1	103.2

Source: Le Grand, J. (1982).

There is also evidence of an uneven distribution of health hazards in the physical and social environment which again particularly affects the poorer social groups. Risk factors attributable to behaviour and opportunities to adopt a healthier personal life-style are also unequal. The distribution of health services is relatively equitable in the UK in that those who are sicker make greater use of health services. However, in terms of expenditure per head the evidence is more equivocal. In relation to preventive health services, there is some evidence that these are more extensively used by the better-off.

Strategies for health

The discussion of inequalities in health status has indicated that the distribution of income, adequate housing, access to employment, a hazard free environment and a healthy life-style are critical factors in determining health status but also that inappropriate life-styles can damage health. However, it should not be forgotten that, although the benefits are difficult to measure, health services themselves can contribute to improved well-being and a reduction of suffering. Some studies have shown direct links. For example, Blaxter (1981) argues that reductions in infant mortality rates in Aberdeen in the 1950s and South Wales in the 1970s showed that:

> despite a situation in which the environmental and social characteristics of the population are by no means ideal (for example the social class distribution and the physique of mothers was considerably less advantaged to good results than those in the south of England), improvements have been achieved in terms of indices such as the perinatal mortality rate which compare with the best in the UK.
>
> (Blaxter 1981: 193)

During the 1980s, Conservative governments have reduced emphasis on social policies which provide access to a range of material benefits. Indeed, there is evidence that the distribution of income and access to housing has become more unequal. In 1979, 1.7 million people had incomes 40 per cent below that year's average. By 1990–1, this had increased to 7.7 million (Hills 1993). The proportion of the population living on less than average incomes has risen while the psycho-social stress caused by high unemployment has added to differential experiences for particular groups. These factors may have contributed to the widening differentials in mortality and morbidity in the late 1980s in the UK (Wilkinson 1992). Conservative governments have tended to concentrate on policies for health education to change life-styles. In the 1990s, the government developed a health strategy designed to develop healthy alliances to combat the diseases causing the greatest burden of ill-health. These policies will be discussed in the next chapter.

Conclusion

In the UK, various groups have put forward a more radical agenda for social and health policy. Examples are Hills' (1993) discussion of policy options in *The Future of Welfare*; *Health, Wealth and Poverty* (1993) by Webster *et al.* and Pond and Popay's (1993) discussion of policy options in *Dilemmas in Health Care*. The World Bank in *Investing in Health* (1993) has a number of key messages for all governments. First, it argues that governments should pursue sound macro-economic policies which aim to reduce poverty. They also need to expand basic schooling, especially for girls, because the way in which households – particularly mothers – use information and financial resources to shape their diet, fertility, health care and other life-style choices has a powerful influence on the health of household members. Second, they should give priority to a number of basic public health programmes such as immunisations and AIDS education and a package of essential clinical services which focus on sick children, maternity and obstetrics and the major causes of mortality and morbidity. Third, it argues for some form of funding for universal coverage for basic health services, competition between those supplying health care and strong government regulation. The World Bank proposals refer to countries with widely different levels of income and wealth but there are important pointers for UK health policy. These are discussed further in the final chapter.

References

Balarajan, R. and Raleigh, S. (1993) *Ethnicity and Health: a guide for the NHS*, Department of Health, London.

Blaxter, M. (1981) *The Health of Children. A Review of Research: the place of health in cycles of disadvantage*, Heinemann Educational Books, London.

Blaxter, M. (1990) *Health and Lifestyles*, Tavistock/Routledge, London.

Blaxter, M. and Paterson, E. (1982) *Mothers and Daughters: a three-generational study of health attitudes and behaviour*, Heinemann Educational Books, London.

Bowling, A. (1991) *Measuring Health: a review of quality of life measurement scales*, Open University Press, Milton Keynes.

Brenner, H. M. (1977) 'Health Costs and Benefits of Economic Policy', *International Journal of Health Services*, 7, pp. 581–623.

Butler, J. (1973) *Family Doctors and Public Policy*, Routledge & Kegan Paul, London.

Butler, M. R. and Bonham, D. E. (1963) Perinatal Mortality: the first report of the 1958 British Perinatal Mortality Survey, in Blaxter, M. (1981) *The Health of Children. A Review of Research: the place of health in cycles of disadvantage*, Heinemann Educational Books, London.

Cartwright, A. and O'Brien, M. (1976) 'Social Class Variations in Health Care and the Nature of GP Consultations' in Stacey, M. (ed.), *The Sociology of the NHS*, Sociological Review Monograph No. 22, Keele University.

Cox, B. *et al.* (1987) *The Health and Lifestyle Survey*, The Health Promotion Trust, Cambridge.

Cox, B. *et al.* (1993) *The Health and Lifestyle Survey: Seven Years On*, Dartmouth, Aldershot.

Davey Smith, G., Bartley, M. and Blane, D. (1990) 'The Black Report on Socioeconomic Inequalities in Health 10 Years On', *British Medical Journal,* 301, pp. 373–77.

Department of Health (1992) *The Health of the Nation*, HMSO, London.

Department of Health and Social Security and Department of Education and Science (1976) *Fit for the Future. Report of the Committee on Child Health Services*, Chairman: Sir Donald Court, Cmnd 6684, HMSO, London.

Department of Health and Social Security (1980), *Inequalities in Health: a report of a research working group* (Chairman: Sir Douglas Black), DHSS, London.

Dubos, R. (1960) *The Mirage of Health,* Allen & Unwin, London.

Fagin, L. (1981) *Unemployment and Health in Families*, DHSS, London.

Field, D. (1976) 'The Social Definition of Illness', in Tuckett, D. (ed.), *An Introduction to Medical Sociology,* Tavistock, London.

Graham, H. (1987) 'Women's Smoking and Family Health', *Social Science and Medicine,* 25, pp. 46–56.

Herzlich, C. (1976) *Health and Illness: a social psychological analysis*, Academic Press, London.

Hills, J. (1993) *The Future of Welfare: a guide to the debate*, Joseph Rowntree Foundation, York.

Illsley, R. (1986) 'Occupational Class, Selection and the Production of Inequalities in Health', *Social Affairs*, 2:2, pp. 151–65.

Le Grand, J. (1982) *Strategy of Equality: redistribution and the social services*, George Allen & Unwin, London.

Le Grand, J., Winter, D. and Wooley, F. (1989) 'The National Health Service: safe in whose hands?' in J. Hills (ed.), *The State of Welfare: the welfare state in Britain since 1974*, Clarendon Press, London.

Lipsedge, M. and Littlewood, R. (1982) *Aliens and Alienists*, Penguin, London.

Macfarlane, A. (1990) 'Official Statistics and Women's Health', in Roberts, H. (ed.), *Women's Health Counts,* Routledge, London.

McKeown, T. (1979) *The Role of Medicine: dream, mirage or nemesis?* Blackwell, Oxford.

Marmot, M. (1986) 'Social Inequalities in Mortality: the social environment' in Wilkinson, R. (ed.), *Class and Health: research and longtitudinal data*, Tavistock, London.

Maynard, A. (1977) 'Avarice, inefficiency and inequality: an international health care tale', *International Journal of Health Services*, 7, 2.

Moser, K., Pugh, H. and Goldblatt, P. (1988) 'Inequalities in women's Health: looking at mortality differences using an alternative approach', *British Medical Journal*, 296, pp. 1221–4.

Noyce, J., Snaith, A. and Trickey, J. (1974) 'Regional Variations in Allocation of Financial Resources to Community Health Services', *The Lancet,* 1, 554.

O'Donnell, O. and Propper, C. (1991) 'Equity and the Distribution of NHS Resources', *Journal of Health Economics*, 16, 1–10.

O'Donnell, O., Propper, C. and Upward, R. (1989) 'An Empirical Study of Equity in the Financing and Delivery of Health Care in Britain', Centre for Health Economics, University of York, Discussion Paper, 85.

Office of Health Economics (1981) *Accidents in Childhood*, Briefing No. 17, September, Office of Health Economics, London.

Office of Health Economics (1993) *Impact of Unemployment on Health*, Office of Health Economics, London.

OPCS (1976) *Morbidity Statistics from General Practice: Second National Study 1970–1971*, HMSO, London.

Parsons, T. (1958) 'Definitions of Health and Illness in the Light of American Values and Social Structure', in Jaco, E. (ed.), *Patient, Physicians and Illness*, Free Press, New York.

Political and Economic Planning (1944) 'Medical Care for Citizens', *Planning*, no. 222.

Pond, C. and Popay, J. (1993) 'Poverty, economic inequality and health', in Davey, B. and Popay, J. (eds), *Dilemmas in Health Care*, Open University, Milton Keynes.

Rainwater, L. (1968) 'The Lower-class: health, illness and medical institutions' in Deutscher and Thompson, E. J. (eds), *Among the People: encounters with the poor*, Basic Books, New York.

Rein, M. (1969) 'Social Class and the Health Service', *New Society*, 14, 807.

Roberts, H. (ed.) (1990) *Women's Health Counts*, Routledge, London.

Social Trends (1993) Central Statistical Office, 23, HMSO, London.

Stanton Rogers, W. (1991) *Explaining Health and Illness: an exploration of diversity*, Harvester Wheatsheaf, London.

Taylor, J. and Taylor, D. (1989) *Mental Health Services in the 1990s: From Custody to Care?* Office of Health Economics, London.

Townsend, P., Whitehead, M. and Davidson, N. (1992) *Inequalties in Health* (new edition), Penguin, London.

Tudor-Hart, J. (1971) 'The Inverse Care Law', *The Lancet*, 1.

Webster, C. (1988) *The Health Services Since the War: problems of health care: the NHS before 1957*, vol. 1, HMSO, London.

Webster, C., Whitehead, M., Wilkinson, R., McAuslan, J., Parker, H. and Benn, T. (1993) *Health, Wealth and Poverty*, Medical World/ Socialist Medical Association, London.

Whitehead, M. (1992) 'The Health Divide' (2nd edition) in *Inequalities in Health*, Penguin, London.

Wilkinson, R. (1992) 'Income and Health', in Webster, C. *et al.*, *Health, Wealth and Poverty*, Medical World/Specialist Medical Association, London.

World Bank (1993) *Investing in Health: World Development Report* 1993, Oxford University Press, New York.

CHAPTER 7

Doing better and feeling worse: critiques of health care

By the mid-twentieth century most advanced industrial societies had developed state-financed health care systems and health expenditures were rising along with growth rates. There was an expansion of investment and spending on health care facilities and in increase of professionals and others involved in health work. The belief was that medicine had made, and was making, a significant contribution to the health and happiness of individuals. Dollery, writing in the late 1970s, sums up the mood:

> Some of the early achievements in the treatment of infectious disease were so miraculous as almost to surpass belief. They literally changed the world. The watch and wait while the pneumonia of the young adult progressed through crisis to lysis or death. The agony of a child with otitis media or worse still osteomyelitis, the long-drawn-out vigil of the patient with pulmonary TB coughing away his life. Anti-bacterial chemotherapy made the cure of such scourges almost a matter of routine. It was a time of optimism. Science appeared to have the salvation of the world in its hand and mankind could look forward to an era of healthy ease and modest luxury. The budgets of the Medical Research Council and the National Institutes of Health increased exponentially and journalistic comment about medical research was almost always eulogistic.
>
> (Dollery 1978: 1)

A greater scepticism developed during the 1970s and 1980s which was not simply related to less lusty growth rates but also awareness that in most Western industrial societies increased spending did not necessarily bring improvements in health. Despite the existence of state-financed health services, problems persisted. Research had shown that there were continuing inequalities in the distribution of resources and therefore access was not universal. The burden of ill-health, furthermore, was greatest among the population of certain regions and among members of particular groups such as ethnic minorities, the lower social classes and those working in hazardous occupations. Life-style has been shown to have a profound effect on health status.

It was also apparent that health systems were resistant to change and had frequently failed to adapt to meet new demands created by the increased burden of dependency characteristic of advanced industrial societies. The World Health Organisation in its 1978 Alma Declaration had pointed out the importance of primary care, community health programmes and the prevention of ill-health – all representing a different model of health care from that embraced by the NHS (Document 22, page 327). Furthermore, health care was criticised for being bureaucratically organised and alienating for the individual. Despite improvements in services, the contribution of medicine to the relief of suffering, the lengthening of life expectancy and increases in the numbers of patients treated, there was a sense of, in Wildavsky's (1980) phrase, 'doing better and feeling worse'.

In the 1970s, against the background of immediate policy concerns described in previous chapters, a number of criticisms developed which are the focus of this chapter. These had different starting points and drew on different frameworks of analysis. Here, they have been grouped into a number of critiques. Although this tends to oversimplfy the work of particular writers, the aim is to clarify the assumptions on which the critiques rest.

The professional dominance critique

During the 1970s, a number of social scientists (Freidson 1970a, 1970b; Johnson 1972; McKinlay 1977; Mackenzie 1979) had argued that the medical profession and the medical model of care had dominated health care legally, politically, administratively and morally. This was the analytical key to understanding the distribution of resources and power in health care. Freidson – whose books *Professional Dominance* (1970a) and *The Profession of Medicine* (1970b) laid down the foundations of the argument, was particularly influential in generating further work. His criticisms were not new. G. B. Shaw, for example, launched a scathing attack on the medical profession in the preface to *The Doctor's Dilemma* in 1911 [Document 24, page 331]. Freidson, however, took a more critical stance than that which had prevailed during the age of optimism in the 1950s and 1960s.

As a sociologist, he stressed the autonomy of the medical profession in making decisions about patient care and their dominance in the division of labour and their influence on policy-making. In his view, this derived from political activity which was legitimised by political and social elites through a system of state licensing. Medical practitioners, organised around their discipline, he suggested, give Western systems of medical care their basic and characteristic structure. Although this role was mediated by the state in Britain (Johnson 1972), the control of the basic core of skills, an increasing division of labour and a structure of institutionalised contacts enabled doctors to consult and be consulted about a wide range of health policies. Furthermore, they had a key position in the delivery of health services. Through the exercise of clinical autonomy – the right to decide what was best for the patient – they acted as gatekeepers in the distribution of material goods and resources. In Freidson's words the profession could:

> drive a wedge into other zones of practice to maintain control over facilities, the organisation of service delivery and training. All the work done by other occupations and related to the service of the patient is subject to the order of the physician. The profession alone is held competent to diagnose illness, treat or direct the treatment of illness and evaluate the service. Without medical authorisation little can be done for the patient by para-professional workers. The client's medication, diet, excretion and recreation are all subject to medical orders. So is the information given to the patient about what his illness is, how it will be treated, and what are the chances of improvement.
>
> (Freidson 1970a: 252)

As Freidson suggests here, medical dominance did not stop at the boundaries of the health system but extended to other personal service workers outside the health system, to teachers, social workers and the like. Its influence and power is strongest at the level of the doctor-patient relationship where, Freidson declared:

> . . . the medical profession had the first claim to jurisdiction over the label illness, and anything to which it might be attached, irrespective of ability to deal with it effectively.
>
> (Freidson 1970a: 251)

To argue that doctors exercised this control over an area of knowledge and set of ideas came to be referred to as the 'medicalisation thesis'. Zola concluded that:

> . . . medicine is becoming a major institution of social control, nudging aside the more traditional institutions of religion and law. It is becoming the repository of truth, the place where absolute and final judgements are made by supposedly morally neutral and objective experts. And these judgements are made, not in the virtue of legitimacy, but in the name of health.
>
> (Zola 1972: 170).

All kinds of problems were brought to the doctor; from obesity to unwanted pregnancy; from childnessness to contraception; from laziness to crime. It was argued that medicine has the tendency to 'make' diseases – such as child-battering, alcoholism, schizophrenia – as well as to dominate the institutional mechanisms which have been developed to cope with them. Conrad and Schneider (1980: 33) concluded that:

> By naming the spirit that underlines the deviance, authority places the deviant under control of language and customs and turns him from a threat to a support of the social system.

Kennedy, in *The Unmasking of Medicine* (1981), argued that the practice of medicine is a moral exercise as well as a technical one and that doctors act in a paternalistic way, taking away the autonomy of the patient. The medical profession's jurisdiction in the giving and withholding of treatment – in relation to abortion, mental handicap, as well as in the designation of diagnostic categories such as alcoholism or depression, conceals judgements about the person and the person's status. Thus, choices are made which should rightly be left to the individual.

Oakley's study of childbirth, *Women Confined* (1980), is an account of the medicalisation of childbirth, where technical expertise and therefore medical choices overtake personal ones. The study was based on interviews with women at different stages of pregnancy and postpartum and gives a graphic picture of doctors' and mothers' view of pregnancy, and the fundamental difference in their perspectives on the meaning of childbirth. Doctors, she suggests, have the following viewpoint. They:

- define reproduction as a specialist subject in which only doctors are experts in the entire symptomatology of child-bearing;
- define reproduction as a medical subject, as exactly analogous to other pathological processes as topics of medical knowledge and intervention;
- select limited criteria of reproductive success, i.e. perinatal and maternal mortality rates;
- divorce reproduction from its social context, pregnant patient-hood being seen as a woman's only relevant status;
- restrict their definition of women to their pregnant status therefore typifying them as 'by nature' maternal, domesticated, family-orientated people.

This failure of the medical profession and the medical model of illness to recognise patients as persons in scientifically based medical systems has been underlined by the work of some anthropologists and other social scientists who examined the handling of illness in cultures different from our own (for example, Maclean 1971). These studies showed that other health systems might be more successful in dealing with social dimensions of illness which involve pain and suffering and readjustment. Thus in less industrialised societies, physical and behavioural changes in people's illness may be coped with through particular rituals which are meaningful in terms of the culture and help to reintegrate the individual within it.

Young, an anthropologist who worked with the Amhara people, describes the process through which the group deals with an illness episode. He says:

> A sickness episode begins when the principal [actor] or his relative decides the range of symptoms into which his signs could be translated.

> Next they must obtain the services of someone, whose medical powers are appropriate to this range of symptoms; under certain circumstances, they may have power enough themselves to translate the signs. Their choice of diagnostician decides what set of rules will be played, what individuals (including therapists and pathogenic agents) and audiences can be mobilised, and what sort of social states will be involved. The therapist's task is to communicate and legitimize the episode's outcome, and this too, takes place according to rules shared by sick persons, healers, and audiences.
>
> (Young 1976: 149)

Rules and rituals can help to provide an answer to the fundamental questions raised by all illness. Why is this happening to me and how do I cope with this? It also involves the group in an episode which is potentially threatening to its stability. The medical or disease model represented by the medical profession with its concentration on the individual acted on by biological forces, underestimates the importance of the circumstances leading to illness, the social relations involved and the importance of other health workers in the equation.

Perhaps the best-known polemic on the medicalisation thesis is Illich's *The Limits to Medicine* (1976) where the author argues that institutionalised medicine has become a threat to health through social, clinical and structural 'iatrogenesis', or damage done by the provider. These terms are described and illustrated in Document 26 (page 339). As a Christian socialist, Illich mounted a moral crusade against many aspects of modern industrial and professional society which he saw as attacking the autonomy and sense of responsibility of the individual. His critique was directed mainly at curative medicine and its limitations. Although few would fully endorse his emphasis on the destructive power of modern medicine, he has helped to encourage a greater scepticism about its benefits.

The professional dominance critique can account for the political influence and power of the medical profession in terms of its control over an area of knowledge. It is less able to explain why that knowledge has been and is so highly valued. After all, Cochrane in *Effectiveness and Efficiency* (1971), McKeown in *The Role of Medicine* (1979) and a number of other medical and sociological studies have shown how the 'scientific' bases of medical practice have been exaggerated and they have pointed to the fashionable nature of many therapies. Why is it then that medical knowledge continues to hold such sway? The link with science and high technology may be important in mystifying the public. It may also be that the public has a vested interest in attributing the power to care and heal to the profession. After all, those who mediate in the process of illness and death in any society have always had an influential position. Moreover, it may be that the critics of medicine have underestimated its achievements in alleviating suffering and disability (Strong 1979: 199). The ambivalence of the role of the medical profession is illustrated by the extracts in Document 24 (page 331). A further criticism of the professional dominance approach is that it fails to relate medical influence to the wider distribution of power in society and to the reasons as to why political and social elites should support medicine's claims.

The political economy critique

The focus of the political economy critique is on the political and economic circumstances which create particular patterns of illness and disease and secondarily on the lack of appropriateness of societal responses to these. In 1974, McKeown and Lowe argued that the significant improvements in health which had occurred during the nineteenth and early twentieth centuries were due to improvements in the standard of living and not primarily to medical intervention:

> It [the modern improvement in health] began in the eighteenth century and was reflected in a decline in mortality which has continued, with interruptions, until the present time. The improvement was initiated by an increase in food supplies which resulted from the Agricultural Revolution that spread throughout Europe after 1700. From about 1870 this influence was powerfully supported by improved hygiene, particularly in respect of water supplies and sewage disposal. In the twentieth century, further advance followed the introduction of effective preventative and therapeutic measures (immunisation and drugs). The contribution of the last influence to the total decline in mortality was relatively small and the improvement in human health was therefore due predominantly to a change in reproductive behaviour and to modification of the environment by provision of food and protection from physical hazards.
>
> (McKeown and Lowe 1974: 20)

Thus, the improvement of health was primarily due to economic factors and social changes, secondarily to political factors, through social intervention, and thirdly to medical intervention.

Research on the effect of social factors on ill-health underlined the importance of societal structure and organisation. For example, those working at the Centre for Studies in Health Policy argued that we live in an 'ill-health promoting economy' and commented on the values which supported the pursuit of ill-health:

> The pinnacle of achievement in health has come to be equated with the spectacle of men and women becoming overstressed and under-exercised, indulging in excessive consumption of food, cigarettes and alcohol for a number of years before being rushed to an intensive care

unit and submerged in expensive technology only when acute symptoms have prevented them from indulging in further consumption.

(Draper, Best and Dennis 1976: 28)

It was argued that a collective response was necessary to counter such factors. McKeown (1979) declared that social action and inaction in the societal arrangements for the provision of food, shelter, transport and work bore the responsibility for certain classes of causes of ill-health. He said:

The physical environment which we have constructed, high rise housing, the extensive use of petrol-driven vehicles, the change in eating habits, methods of processing, manufacturing and distributing food, the manufacture and production of new products, all have brought new and unanticipated hazards.

(McKeown 1979)

The social organisation of providing for the necessities of life, whether in the public or private sector, played a part in the aetiology of physical illnesses as well as being a factor contributing to stress-related illnesses, depression and neuroses.

The Black Report on *Inequalities in Health* demonstrated effectively that the impact of hazardous social and environmental factors fell heavily on particular groups (DHSS 1980). Social deprivation, measured by occupational class, was associated with ill-health, and the use of and availability of health services tended to reinforce inequalities through lack of adequate services. There was also evidence to suggest that particular occupations and life-styles increased exposure to health hazards. The social causes of ill-health were shown to be complex and varied. It was argued that they remain embedded in the socio-economic structure, but affected smaller groups more than was the case with the nineteenth-century infectious diseases, along the lines of gender, ethnic group, occupation and geographical area, as well as class. The effects of deprivation and hazard were cumulative. Poor growth and physical development in adolescence and childhood were likely to influence susceptibility to disease throughout life and these in turn were affected by the social position, circumstances, health and habits of parents.

A political economy critique has often, both now and in the nineteenth century, been effective in explaining inequalities in health care and social conditions associated with ill-health. It generated many policy proposals and strategies for the amelioration of conditions – the Beveridge proposals and the post-war welfare legislation among them. However, proponents of these views paid less attention to the underlying power relationships which inhibited change. Marxist scholars tackled this question, arguing that both the patterns of illness and disease and the arrangements for health care, with its division of labour, professional and bureaucratic dominance, was characteristic of the mode of, and relationships within, production in advanced capitalist society.

The Marxist critique

According to the Marxist critique, the organisation and practice of medicine and the provision of health services supported capitalist organisation and the interests of the modern state. This accounts for inequalities, medical dominance and the ill-health – promoting economy. Engels declared that the ruling ideas of each age have ever been the ideas of its ruling class. A contemporary Marxist, Navarro (1978) in *Class Struggle, the State and Medicine,* explicitly rejected the view that the structure of medical services and its inequalities in the use of health services could be explained in terms of forces within the medical profession or that they result from lack of societal responsiveness to change. He aimed to demonstrate that class relations, and the class structure of British society, determined all the significant aspects of health policy and health care. Thus, Navarro argued that more was spent on the health care of the middle class and that wealthier regions attracted a greater share of health resources. The provision of a national health service with its concentration on curative medicine rather than on the care of dependent groups and prevention of ill-health was seen to reflect bourgeois ideology. Curative medicine and the medical establishment served the interests of capital by concentrating attention on individual ill-health. This depoliticised health issues. It diverted attention from the illness-generating conditions in the social structure - from polluted and polluting environments, dangerous working conditions and the like.

The Marxist critique also emphasised the social control functions of medicine. It saw the emphasis on the individual's responsibility for health as diverting attention away from structural factors and the importance of political action in changing the structural balance of power. Marxist writers often embraced the medicalisation thesis, arguing that medical knowledge was ideological. McKinlay declared that:

> Starting with a relatively simple set of possibly effective procedures fulfilling some uncontrived human needs, medical care under capitalism has become transformed into an increasingly sophisticated, yet ineffective body of unnecessary values with increasing bio-technology, ancillary testing, ritualistic surgery, over-utilisation of hospital and superfluous appointments.
>
> (McKinlay 1977: 479–80)

The argument is reminiscent of Marcuse's commentary on the state's role in the creation of false needs in industrial societies (Marcuse 1972).

McKinlay (1979) links these arguments to the analysis of the health care system as a large and profitable enterprise which is part of, and linked to, the business sector. The example he and others base their arguments on the 'health care empire' in the US. The argument has been less developed in relation to the UK which has a national service, except in relation to the drug industry. This industry is part of an international network of capitalist enterprise and about one-tenth of health spending in the UK is on pharmaceuticals, even though in the UK, the NHS is a monopoly buyer and has in some cases negotiated price reductions from international companies (Abel-Smith 1976). However, Collier (1990) argues that there has been poor central control of prices and profits.

The seemingly inexorable rise of health spending in welfare states has led to a further variant of the Marxist thesis. O'Connor (1973), Gough (1979) and Offe (1984) have argued that the crisis in health care spending in welfare states in the 1970s was the result of an inevitable conflict between the need for the state to legitimise its position by spending on health to satisfy the desires of the electorate and the requirement of capitalism for profit.

The Marxist critique has been used in a further dimension to analyse and explain the division of labour within the NHS itself. Both Doyal in *The Political Economy of Health* (1979) and Navarro (1978) regard the rigid division of roles between strata of health workers along class and ethnic lines, with little interchange between them, as well as the reduction of the patient to the object of the labour process, as reflections of wider social divisions.

A socialist-feminist critique of health care is also partially developed by Doyal in highlighting the role of women in the division of labour in health care. She pointed out that the position of women in the health system reflected their place in the social structure. The caring and less powerful role of nurses, who were mainly women, is compared to the curing and leadership role of doctors, who were mainly men. Within medicine itself, the hierarchy in status also followed gender lines, from male-dominated surgery to the more female-dominated specialisms such as community and child health. Oakley (1980) and Ehrenreich and English (1979), in different contexts, argue that contemporary health care demotes women's expertise as healers as well as medicalising many areas of female experience in the interests of male careers. Women play a large role in the health care of their families. They assume, and are expected to assume, prime responsibility for well and sick children and for dependent relatives. They are involved in pregnancy and childbirth. They take the main responsibility for contraception and are uniquely susceptible to particular health problems, for example, depressive illness. It was argued that the contribution of women as health workers, and their particular needs within health care, were neglected or distorted. These authors conclude that a capitalist and patriarchal social structure and the social status and relationships stemming from it are the explanation for the inadequacies of contemporary health care.

One of the areas where it was argued that the medical mandate had operated in favour of the concerns of doctors and hospitals was in relation to childbirth. For example, by the 1980s, almost 99 per cent of births took place in hospital. As Chapter 12 will show, by the beginning of the 1990s, many of these assumptions outlined in the critiques outlined above, which share a scepticism about modern medicine, had been challenged, sometimes successfully.

The radical right critique

The final 1970s critique to be examined is that which came from the radical right. While agreeing with many of the criticisms of modern health services, the radical right differed in embracing what modern medical care had to offer. Its focus was on enhancing the ability of the consumer to buy medical care in the marketplace. It also put forward a practical agenda for policy change.

In Britain, the views of the radical right were promoted by the Institute of Economic Affairs, the Centre for Policy Studies and, when they had gained power in 1979, the right wing of the Conservative government. *The Litmuss Papers* (Sheldon 1980) represented a contemporary view of the NHS. According to the radical right, the NHS was underfunded, bureaucratic and unresponsive to patients because it was a large, centrally-provided organisation. Covert rationing, queuing, inertia, resistance to change and appalling industrial relations were, according to the radical right, the result of public sector management. Professionals were prevented from providing the service they wished to offer. Facilities were inadequate – both in terms of the availability of up-to-date technology, equipment, trained manpower, and on the 'hotel' side of health care. Hospital buildings were old and ill-equipped. Waiting lists for relatively simple but not critical operations such as hernias, varicose veins or hip-replacements were long and, although these are not life-threatening conditions, they caused considerable discomfort and impaired the quality of life. Health institutions and procedures were bureaucratic, alienating, time-consuming and the patient became an object rather than being treated as a human patient. Managers were powerless to run their hospitals due to lack of the power to deal with groups of staff. Wage inflation, which drove up costs, was caused by the Byzantine arrangements with unions and the professions. Moreover, freely available health care under the NHS did not encourage an individual sense of responsibility for health, nor regular surveillance and preventive measures.

Sheldon declared:

> The NHS must fail, because it does not supply the British people with the best medical care they want because it prevents them as individual consumers from paying for the services that suit their personal family circumstances, requirements and preferences.
>
> (Sheldon 1980)

The arguments of the radical right rested on the idea of the rational sovereign consumer and a belief in a remedy for the problems of the NHS on the demand side. On the supply side, competition would drive down prices. The aim was to reduce the role of government in health care which, they believed, should be treated as a good like any other and supplied by the private rather than the public sector.

A number of ideas were put forward to fund health care. While *The Litmuss Papers* favoured a system involving a combination of private and state insurance with measures to encourage private sector supply, a Centre for Policy Studies paper (1988) favoured vouchers or health credits which could be used to purchase private insurance or treatment in private or NHS hospitals. Compulsory insurance on the French or German model was also considered in the early 1980s. The Adam Smith Institute (1988) proposed Health Maintenance Units. These Units would be run by a partnership of doctors and for an annual subscription, payable by the NHS, patients would receive total care. There was, however, a secondary reason for promoting private health care. The private market is an export earner. It could attract foreign capital, and therefore take its place as part of the business revival promised to follow from the 1979 Conservative government's electoral victory.

The views of the radical right were based on the assumption of the existence of a group of well-endowed, intelligent, healthy and rational consumers with an ability to protect their health and avoid illness through their individual actions. Social and economic factors in the causation of disease were ignored and so were the collective benefits accruing from a healthier population. It was assumed that individuals would be able to evaluate the health care they received and that individual decisions would affect the standard and efficiency of this care. Neither assumption was necessarily valid. The problem of evaluation of technical and professional activities remained, despite 'consumer choice'.

Final comment

There is no doubt that all the critiques mentioned above have presented a challenge to the NHS and to government policy in health care. Each contains a partially valid analysis. Their main contribution was that they showed that existing health policy rested on a particular set of assumptions. The critiques foreshadowed the paradigm shifts which were to occur in health policy during the 1980s. One shift was the challenge to the medical model of illness.

The second shift was a political one. The politics of the New Right gained ascendancy with the Thatcher governments of the 1980s. The political shift was not simply ideological but was a policy response to a period of low growth and high unemployment when the increasing demands on public spending were seen to pose a threat to economic policy.

References

Abel-Smith, B. (1976) *Value for Money in Health Services,* Heinemann, London, ch. 6.

Adam Smith Institute (1988) *The Health of Nations*, London.

Centre for Policy Studies (1988) *Britain's Biggest Enterprise – ideas for radical reform of the NHS*, London.

Cochrane, A. L. (1971) *Effectiveness and Efficiency: random reflections on health services*, Nuffield Provincial Hospitals Trust, Oxford.

Collier, J. (1990) 'A Policy for Medicines and the Pharmaceutical Industry', in Carrier, J. and Kendall, I. (eds), *Socialism in the NHS*, Avebury, Aldershot.

Conrad, P. and Schneider, M. (1980) *Deviance and Medicalisation: from badness to sickness*, Mosby, St Louis.

Department of Health and Social Security (1980) *Report of a Research Working Group on Inequalities in Health* (Chairman: Sir Douglas Black), DHSS, London.

Dollery, C. (1978) *The End of an Age of Optimism*, Nuffield Provincial Hospitals Trust, Oxford.

Doyal, L. (1979) *The Political Economy of Health*, Pluto Press, London.

Draper, P., Best, G. and Dennis, J. (1976) *Health, Money and the National Health Service*, Unit for the Study of Health Policy, London, p. 28.

Ehrenreich, B. and English, D. (1979) *For Her Own Good: 150 years of the experts' advice to women*, Pluto Press, London.

Freidson, E. (1970a) *Professional Dominance: the social structure of medical care*, Atherton Press, New York.

Freidson, E. (1970b) *The Profession of Medicine*, Dodd Mead, New York.

Gough, I. (1979) *The Political Economy of the Welfare State*, Macmillan, London.

Illich, I. (1976) *Limits to Medicine. Medical Nemesis: the expropriation of health*, Marion Boyars, London.

Johnson, T. (1972) *Professions and Power*, Macmillan, London.

Kennedy, I. (1981) *The Unmasking of Medicine*, Allen & Unwin, London.

Loudon, J. B. (ed.) (1976) *Anthropology in Medicine*, Academic Press, London.

Mackenzie, W. (1979) *Power and Responsibilty in Health Care*, Oxford University Press, Oxford.

McKinlay, J. (1977) 'The Business of Good-Doctoring or Doctoring as Good Business: reflections of Freidson's view of the medical system', *International Journal of Health Services*, 7 (3), pp. 459–83.

McKinlay, J. (1979) 'A Case for Refocussing Upstream: the political economy of illness', in Jaco, E. G. (ed.), *Patients, Physicians and Illness,* Free Press, New York (3rd edn).

Maclean, U. (1971) *Magical Medicine,* Penguin, London.

Marcuse, H. (1972) *One Dimensional Man*, Abacus, London.

McKeown, T. (1979) *The Role of Medicine: dream, mirage or nemesis?*, Blackwell, Oxford.

McKeown, T. and Lowe, (1974) *An Introduction to Social Medicine,* Blackwell, Oxford.

Navarro, V. (1978) *Class Struggle, the State and Medicine: an historical and contemporary analysis of the medical sector in Great Britain*, Robertson, Oxford.

Oakley, A. (1980) *Women Confined: towards a sociology of childbirth*, Robertson, Oxford.

Oakley, A. (1982) *Subject Woman,* Penguin, London.

O'Connor, J. (1973) *The Fiscal Crisis of the State*, St Martins Press, New York.

Offe, C. (1984) *The Contradictions of the Welfare State*, Hutchinson, London.

Shaw, G. B. (1956) *The Doctor's Dilemma* (originally published 1911), Penguin, London.

Sheldon, A. (ed.) (1980) *The Litmuss Papers*, Centre for Policy Studies, London.

Strong, P. (1979) 'Sociological Imperialism and the Profession of Medicine', *Social Science and Medicine*, 13a, 2, pp. 199–215.

Wildavsky, A. (1980) *The Art and Craft of Policy Analysis*, Macmillan, London.

Young, A. (1976) 'Some Implications of Medical Beliefs and Practices for Social Anthropology', *American Anthropology*, 78 (5), pp. 147–156.

Zola, I. K. (1972) 'Medicine as an Institution of Social Control', *Sociological Review*, 20 (3), pp. 487–504.

PART FOUR

New Directions for Health Policy

CHAPTER 8

New directions: Conservative government policies in the 1980s

In the 1980s, Conservative governments drew selectively on the critiques of health care discussed in the previous chapter to restructure welfare institutions. Although ideas from the New Right which emphasised monetarist economics, reductions in public spending and personal responsibility were predominant, the monopoly power of large public bureaucracies and the power exercised by welfare professionals within them were also a target of Thatcherism. The latter were seen as forces which inhibited change. This chapter examines the principles expounded by Conservative politicians and the policies adopted in the lead up to the 1990 reforms. The NHS was the last welfare institution to be restructured. This was because of its popularity, the power of interest groups within it and also uncertainty about how to proceed.

The economic and political ideas of the Thatcher governments

The Conservative Party manifesto for the 1979 election presented Britain as a failure – its values eroded, its economy disabled and its public services a burden on the taxpayer. The first priority of government was to create an enterprise economy. It was believed that this could be achieved by maintaining tight control of the money supply to reduce inflation. This involved cutting public expenditure and, in what remained of the public sector, pursuing value for money. There were a number of other themes which ran through the rhetoric and policies of the Thatcher administrations. As political confidence grew and ways of achieving political aims were identified, changes became more radical.

While the first and predominant theme was to reduce public expenditure, a second theme was a belief in the benefits which would accrue if principles of private sector management were applied to government. An aspect of this was the empowerment of managers at the expense of other groups supplying labour in the public sector (whether unionised or professional). Like Bernard Shaw (see Document 24, page 331), Conservative governments believed that the professions with their monopoly power constituted a conspiracy against the laity.

A third theme was the encouragement of self-help and the transfer of the burden of provision from the state towards the community and the family. In the health arena, this was manifest in the encouragement of private insurance and the increase in charges for NHS services, which came out of household income.

A fourth theme was the encouragement of competition on the supply side of health care. This took a number of forms, from deregulation to the encouragement of competition within the public sector. The public sector was also opened up to competition from private firms in similar areas of work.

The search for economy

The question was one of restricting resources to the NHS and seeking gains in both efficiency and effectiveness. This theme has already been addressed in Chapter 5 and will only be briefly referred to here. In the early years of the first Thatcher governments, Patrick Jenkin wrote in the Foreword to *Care in Action* (DHSS 1981: 1):

> I'm sure you do not need reminding that the Government's top priority must be to get the economy right; for that reason, it cannot be assumed that more money will always be available to be spent on health care.

This promise was borne out. During the 1980s, the funding available was often significantly less that the 2 per cent considered necessary for growth. The effect was cumulative. Despite the annual efficiency savings, by the second half of the 1980s there was growing public dissatisfaction. A tax-funded NHS was known to be popular. For example, various British Social Attitudes surveys (for example, 1988) showed that although the public wished to reduce taxation, nevertheless there was strong support for a tax-funded service. Table 8.1 shows the findings.

By the mid-1980s, there was a sense of crisis in the NHS. In 1986, the Social Services Select Committee (1986) concluded that the 'underfunding' of the health service had risen to almost £1.3 billion. Public dissatisfation with health care was also rising, as indicated in Table 8.1. Despite a media campaign highlighting the plight of the NHS, the Conservatives won a mandate for a third term of office in June 1987. However, by the end of the year, as Butler reports (1992) a survey conducted by the *Independent* newspaper showed that 3000 beds had been closed that year through lack of money and personnel. The Royal Colleges of Physicians, Surgeons and Obstetricians appealed to the Secretary of State:

> . . . patient care is deteriorating. Acute hospital services have almost reached breaking point. Morale is depressingly low. . . . An immediate review of acute hospital services is mandatory. Additional and alternative

Table 8.1 **Attitudes towards the NHS in Britain 1983–1987**

	Percentage of respondents	
	1983	1987
First priority in public spending to the NHS	37	52
First of second priority	63	79
Support for a tax-funded NHS:		
Top 25%	72	68
Middle 50%	64	72
Bottom 25%	57	66
Very satisfied with the NHS	11	7
Very dissatisfied with the NHS	7	15

Source: Adapted from Bosanquet, N. (1988).

resources must be found. We call upon the government to do something now to save our Health Service, once the envy of the world.

(quoted in Butler 1992: 4)

In January, the Prime Minister annouced that a review was under way. The result was published in January 1989 as the White Paper, *Working for Patients* (Secretary of State for Health 1989). This laid out the radical agenda for the NHS described in the next chapter.

Improving NHS management

Pollitt, at the start of his book on *Managerialism in the Public Services* (1990), suggests that it has been a commonly held assumption from the 1970s that better management would solve a range of social and economic problems. Conservatives took no exception to this belief. They looked to management theorists, particularly those from the US, for ideas about how to run the public sector in Britain. Among those whose ideas were influential were Drucker (1990), who argued that in order to survive the 1990s, large organisations needed, in stock-market language, 'to unbundle'. This meant dividing core from peripheral functions: the latter should be hived off or contracted out to separate agencies. Organisations should have fewer layers, be knowledge-based and smaller and leaner. Good information systems were essential for assessing markets and performance. The command and control model of a large, centralised agency was perceived as both inefficient and ineffective. A centralised 'strategy' was important but 'production' could be decentralised to smaller peripheral agencies.

Osborne and Gaebler (1992) were also influential. They declared that, on the basis of US studies, public sector managers freed from bureaucratic constraints became innovative and entrepreneurial. They were able to exercise greater autonomy in changing and adapting their organisations to respond to what local communities wanted. Instead of accepting the status quo, they could find solutions to problems if they were given sufficient freedom to do so.

Conservative politicians brought in successful private sector businessmen to advise them on how to run public services. Derek Rayner – a director of Marks and Spencer, now Lord Rayner – was appointed to scrutinise aspects of public services to find efficiency savings while Roy Griffiths – then a director of Sainsbury's, the food retailer, now Sir Roy – headed an inquiry into the management of the NHS (DHSS 1983). He concluded that the NHS suffered from 'institutionalised stagnation'. Changes were difficult to achieve in the hospitals and districts because no one was responsible for leading the organisation and setting objectives related to meeting the needs of patients. He declared:

> . . . business men, have a keen sense of how well they are looking after their customers. Whether the NHS is meeting the needs of the patient and the community, and can prove it is doing so is open to question.
> (DHSS 1983: 10)

Griffiths' solution was to change the organisational culture of the NHS by introducing features of business management. At the top, the NHS was to be freed from political constraints by the appointment of a supervisory board with an independent chairperson. Within the regions, districts and units, a single general manager would replace the management team. The general manager's task was to provide a driving force for developing management plans, taking personal responsibility for providing appropriate levels of service; ensuring the quality of care; meeting budgets; achieving cost improvements; increasing productivity; monitoring performance and rewarding staff; ensuring research and development; and initiating measures to assess health outputs. The report recommended the appointment of directors of quality assurance in each district to improve performance. Other private sector practices such as the introduction of performance-related pay were also recommended.

During 1984, although strongly opposed by the British Medical Association on behalf of doctors, general and other management, the changes recommended by Griffiths were introduced into the service. At a national level, a Supervisory Board and the NHS Management Executive (NHSME) were established. As its title suggests, the role of the Board was to supervise the NHSME. The intention was to distance the Department of Health from the running of the service. Their role was simply to provide a policy steer. However, there were difficulties in achieving the change of culture desired by Griffiths; and it proved impossible to separate the NHS from political influence. Following the resignation of the first post-holder as Chair of the Supervisory Board, the Minister of Health took over the chairmanship of what became the Policy Board – thus the politicians were back in the driving seat.

It also proved difficult for the new general managers to lead their organisations positively. There were a number of reasons for this. The dominant group in health care was doctors. Clinical autonomy was rooted in the political and financial structure of the NHS. It required time to develop new techniques necessary for the tight management of resources envisaged by Griffiths: for one thing, it required time to introduce the necessary information systems to collect and analyse data in order to manage activity against budgets. Training was also required in new skills to produce a cadre of general managers. Griffiths had hoped that doctors would be drawn into management but most were reluctant to leave clinical practice. Moreover, the early 1980s (as Chapter 4 has outlined) was a period of severe cuts in the expenditure of many units, and required efficiency savings thus dominated management agendas. A number of research studies of general management undertaken in the mid-1980s concluded that the influence over doctors had been slight.

In the early 1980s further attempts were made to devise methods of achieving greater value for money. A system of annual review was introduced. Performance indicators covering clinical activity, staff, finance and estate management was tested in the Northern Region. These revealed enormous variations in costs. The total cost per inpatient case, for example, varied by as much as 50 per cent and the cost of medical support services by 100 per cent (*The Times Health Supplement*, 26 March 1982).

Up-to-date information systems were also being introduced. In 1980 the Social Services Committee had argued that the DHSS should:

> give a high priority to developing a comprehensive information system that would permit this committee and the public to assess the effect of changes in expenditure levels of patterns on the quality and the scope of services provided.
>
> (Social Services Select Committee 1981)

This theme was reiterated in subsequent years by the Public Accounts Committee (PAC 1981).

Banyard (1991) concluded that although managers had more control over setting clinical targets, there had been little impact at the front line. Strong and Robinson (1990), in their ethnographic study of health managers, found considerable puzzlement among managers about their role and concluded that many felt trapped between central directives and doctors who still gave the day-to-day orders. Harrison, Hunter, Marnoch and Pollitt (1992), who undertook their research in 1987–8, found growing cohesiveness among managers. However, they concluded that although many managers were remarkably successful in containing conflicts, few were positively leading their organisations.

Flynn (1991), who conducted interviews with 43 managers in six districts in 1988, found that the cumulative consequences of a number of years of underfunding had led managers to take a lead in order to manage the severe cuts in expenditure. With the widening shortfall between resources and demand, he concluded that managerial influence over clinicians had increased. One District General Manager summed up the change in attitudes when he said:

> Now we are setting the priorities. . . . The more that finance is a problem, the more important is management's role in the manipulation of resources. Until recently doctors protected their areas, but now they have seen that resources are capable of being redistributed.
>
> (Flynn 1991: 221)

It is ironic that it appeared to require resource starvation for a shift in power from doctors to managers to occur. However, it is also the case that resource management was bringing clinicians into the field. In some hospitals a partnership between clinicians and managers had developed; Hunter (1992) discusses the implications of this as doctors form alliances with managers or become managers themselves.

Curbing professional monopolies

In 1983, an advisory policy paper on the professions, although not published, was widely leaked to the press (*The Guardian*, 19 February 1983). It argued that professionals had monopoly power in a number of public services and that this went against the interests of consumers. A number of examples can be found of the way in which policy developed.

In 1984, the optical services were deregulated. Lenses and spectacles could be sold by anyone. By implication, this meant that the professional skill of the optician was unnecessary. This action followed an Office of Fair Trading report (Department of Trade 1982) which suggested that the restrictions on outlets for the sale of lenses and spectacles had allowed excess profits to be made by international optical companies. It was argued that it was not necessary for the public to be protected from unqualified practitioners:

> . . . inaccurate spectacles could not cause permanent damage to the eyes, but there exists the possibility of minor discomfort.
>
> (Allsop and May 1986: 95)

In effect, this undermined a professional monopoly on dispensing. Other measures were also introduced to encourage 'fair trading' generally (Miller 1992). For example, in 1989, the Monopolies and Mergers Commission recommended a liberalisation of the rules over advertising. The General Medical Council, the profession's regulatory body, agreed to the production of leaflets which practices were now expected to provide for their patients. GPs could also provide information for the public and the media. The production of practice leaflets was made mandatory with the introduction of the new GP contract in 1990.

In 1994, the Monopolies and Mergers Commission (MMC) inquired into the BMA's fee guidelines for private patients. It saw these as an attempt to manage the market in their own interest and concluded that guidelines should be abolished. The report stated:

> . . . we believe that price competition is not inimical to quality.
> (Monopolies and Mergers Commission 1994)

Nonetheless, the MMC also concluded that BUPA's scale of prices could continue because, as insurers, BUPA (a private, non-profit making medical insurance company) were distanced from the doctors who supplied the service.

Encouraging self-reliance – increasing choice

One of the themes of Thatcherite Conservatism was to encourage individuals and families to take more responsibility for their own welfare. The other side of the coin was that, as individuals took on this new role, they would have to be given the opportunity to exercise choice. Both these aims were pursued in relation to the prevention of ill-health and are discussed in a later chapter. Here, policies to increase the take-up of private insurance and increased payments for health commodities are discussed.

Private medical insurance

From the second half of the 1970s, for a variety of reasons discussed below, private medical insurance increased dramatically. Figure 8.1 shows the trends. The Royal Commission on the NHS (1979) estimated that in 1976, 3 per cent of the total expenditure on health could be attributed to private insurance. Between 1979 and 1981, the private insurance market increased from 5 per cent of the population to 7.3 per cent (Laing and Buisson 1992). By 1989, according to the Association of British Insurers, 13 per cent of the population were covered (quoted in Higgins 1992). By 1991, this had fallen back to 12 per cent (OHE 1992, Laing and Buisson 1993).

Since the 1970s, the private health insurance market has grown

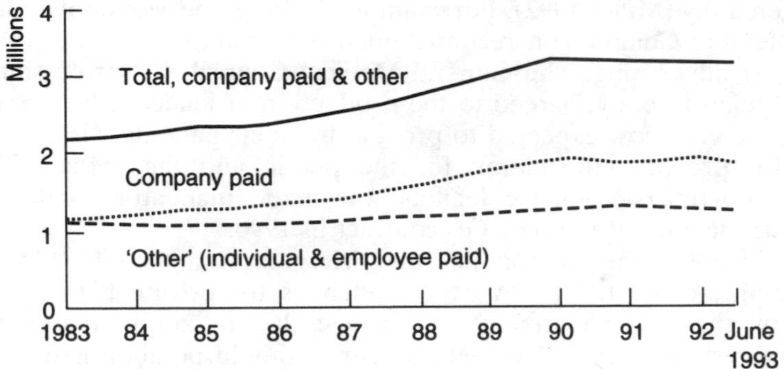

Figure 8.1 **Private health insurance subscribers at 31 December by purchase category, UK 1983–93**
Source: Laing, W. and Buisson, R. (1993).

overall, although there have been occasional fluctuations. Growth is attributable to both demand and supply factors. On the demand side, the majority of subscriptions were taken out by employers for their employees as fringe benefits. In 1980, tax concessions were introduced for employers who make contributions on behalf of their staff with incomes below £8,500. By the early 1980s, to remain competitive in the labour market, most large employers were offering health insurance to their senior managers (Higgins 1992). And since the early 1980s, white collar unions have taken out subscriptions on behalf of their members. This created some difficulties for insurers as the number of claims rose because insurance cover had been extended to those in poorer health. The costs to private insurance companies went up while at the same time there was greater competition.

Also on the demand side, private insurance has grown as a consequence of increased take-up from individuals. Although the rate of growth of individual subscriptions was slower in the early 1980s, it increased by the late 1980s. In 1990, new forms of tax relief for elderly people for health insurance were introduced. This reduced resources for the Exchequer and therefore the NHS. Propper (1989) has estimated that the loss of tax revenue was between £5.2 and £148 million per year. Those who take out private insurance generally do so for convenience – to fix a date for hospital admission in advance or in order to get treatment quickly (Higgins 1988).

Calnan, Cant and Gabe (1993) investigated some of these issues in a study of subscribers and non-subscribers to health insurance. Their findings tended to confirm earlier studies. People had private insurance most often because it was a perk from employment. Once insured, people decided to take advantage of private care. People preferred individualised care, they felt it minimised the risk of loss of work-time through not being treated immediately. However, those insured continued to support a publicly funded NHS:

> Our respondents were pro-NHS in principle but took out private health insurance for practical reasons, while resenting that they had to pay twice and wishing that they could get the service they wanted from the NHS.
>
> (Calnan, Cant and Gabe 1993: 91)

However, although the majority of respondents said that private insurance had given them more choice in terms of the timing of hospital admissions and the comfort of surroundings, they did not feel more empowered or knowledgeable. For example, they gave little indication of having shopped around. Table 8.2 shows that household contributions to private medical insurance have more than doubled during the 1980s.

On the supply side, therefore, people appear to take out private insurance because NHS care is insufficiently flexible to meet their needs. For example, waiting times present a problem. Although the number of people on waiting lists has decreased during the 1980s, waiting times, especially for non-urgent surgery, have increased. Minor but irritating conditions such as hernia operations and varicose veins are often dealt with by the private

Table 8.2 ***Household expenditure on health in real terms 1981–92***

	£ per week at 1992 prices[1] and percentages			
	1981	*1986*	*1991*	*1992*
National Health Service				
Prescription charges and medical appliances	0.17	0.18	0.19	0.18
Payments for dentist, amenity hospital bed	0.19	0.16	0.35	0.39
Non-National Health Service				
Medicines, lotions, dressings, appliances	0.80	1.09	1.40	1.43
Medical, dental, nursing and optical fees (except spectacles)	0.56	0.64	0.86	0.55
Spectacles	0.28	0.55	0.63	0.80
Medical insurance premiums	0.19	0.37	0.58	0.56
Total weekly expenditure on above	2.17	2.99	4.01	3.91
Expenditure on above items as a percentage of total household expenditure	*0.9*	*1.2*	*1.5*	*1.4*

Note:
[1] Adjusted to real terms using the retail prices index.

Source: Social Trends (1994) HMSO, London.

sector. But so are conditions where speedy treatment is either required or reduces discomfort. For example, in 1985, over a quarter of the hip replacements, hysterectomies and coronary artery by-pass grafts were carried out in the private sector. Furthermore, 50 per cent of all abortions are carried out privately. Another reason for the increase in the take-up of health insurance may be related to the better facilities in private wards and hospitals.

As Calnan, Cant and Gabe's findings suggest, those who have private health insurance tend to have professional and managerial jobs. In 1987, 29 per cent of those with degrees and 41 per cent of those with incomes above £26,000 a year had taken out insurance. This compared to 7 per cent of the least well-qualified and 4 per cent of those in the lowest income group. Middle-aged professionals at 34 per cent were the group most likely to have insurance (OPCS 1986–7, Bosanquet 1993).

The private sector is essentially parasitic on the NHS. It draws on staff who were trained in NHS hospitals at public cost. Higgins (1992) estimated that 2 per cent of medically trained staff work full time in private hospitals, as do 7 per cent of nursing staff. The private sector depends upon part-time consultants who have contracts within the NHS. There may be difficulties in maintaining quality in these circumstances. The private sector has not adopted the stricter audit procedures used within the NHS.

Increased charges

Charges for particular items have been part of NHS financing since the 1950s. However, the increases were greater in the 1980s than in previous periods. In 1991–2, payments from patients were £954 million. More than half of this amount was due to increases in dental charges and a quarter came from prescription charges (OHE 1992). Although prescription charges have risen sharply, between 1979 and 1994 there has been an increase from under £1 per item prescribed to almost £5. However, exemptions cover about 80 per cent of prescriptions issued, so this reduces the revenue forthcoming. In the early 1980s, charges for sight-testing (with some exemptions) and a withdrawal of subsidies on spectacles increased household expenditure, although the full effect on different levels of family budget is not known.

The expenditure of households on health commodities as shown in Table 8.2 is not large, but the doubling of expenditure between 1981 to 1992 is nevertheless significant. Epsing Anderson (1990) refers to this as the 'commodification of welfare'. Such shifts may bring more revenue for government but they also increase the share of household expenditure on goods which previously cost less. The burden of sickness falls most heavily on those with low incomes; it is increased with charging policies which may not be off-set by exemptions. Charges may thus reduce take-up and this, in turn may cause delay in seeking treatment. In the longer term they may add to costs.

Competitive tendering

In 1983, following Health Circular HC(83)18, health authorities were required to put their catering, domestic and laundry contracts out to tender so that these public services could be tested against market prices. Market theory suggests that competition increases innovation in the search for cost-effectiveness. The aim was to ensure provision at the lowest possible cost with the savings being passed back to fund patient services. In 1980, competitive tendering had been introduced in local government. Its extension to the health service was resisted by trade unions. They argued that many health service staff were already low-paid and that the competitive process would drive down labour costs still further. The policy was also criticised by the Labour Opposition who argued that the NHS required an especially dedicated workforce. Catering and cleaning staff often had contact with patients and could be seen as part of the health care team. They also believed that private sector provision would bring factory methods of work which were inimical to patient care. A further argument was that the complexity of tasks in hospital was greater than in similar services in the private sector. Hospital laundry, for example, needed highly specialist equipment for processing and there were unlikely to be sufficient firms to create competition.

The circular required health authorities to complete the tendering process by 1986. By that date, 55 per cent of catering contracts and about three-quarters of the domestic and laundry services had been put out to tender and agreed (National Audit Office (NAO) 1987). Milne (1992) found that there were differences between the three areas in the extent to which the in-house tenders were accepted. In catering, the number going to the private sector was small. In the case of domestic services, most contracts initially went to the private sector, but by 1990 this had fallen back to about a third. In the case of laundry services, in 1984, 45 per cent of contracts went to the private sector, but by 1990 this was only 20 per cent. In general, the larger contracts tended to go to the private sector (Milne 1992).

By 1987, the NAO estimated that competitive tendering brought cost savings of around 20 per cent. It had also brought greater flexibity in responding to local labour market conditions than was possible under the Whitley Council agreements. In their 1987 report, the NAO recommended that senior managers should be brought in to specify and monitor contracts as the process of tendering could thus encourage a general service review. In 1988, a further move to encourage hospitals to be more entrepreneurial was made possible following the Health and Medicines Act. Guidelines for tendering were relaxed so that NHS providers could bid for service contracts by selling their own services either to other hospitals in the NHS or to the private sector. This allowed income to be generated which could be spent on patient services.

In *Competing for Quality* (Treasury 1991), the then Chancellor of the Exchequer, Norman Lamont, spelt out some general operational principles for the public services. These echoed the views of the US management theorists referred to earlier. The White Paper states that in the 1990s, large parts of the public sector must be 'market-tested' to ensure that they are being provided in the most effective way [Document 25, p. 337]. It says:

> . . . private sector businesses have increasingly chosen to concentrate on their core business. They stick to what they know best. And they buy in specialist contractors to provide new ideas, more flexibility, and a higher level of expertise than could exist in a purely in-house operation. The benefits of competition are great. [Public sector] managers have to account for their performance against financial and quality targets. Their responsibility requires them to look for the best deal for users of their services, whether the task is done in-house or bought in from outside.
>
> (Treasury 1991: 1)

As a consequence of the White Paper, each health authority will have to set out plans for market testing and there will be a national database maintained on the contracts awarded and to whom. In early 1994, one Welsh Health Authority put out a tender for its cardiology services as an alternative to developing their own (*Health Services Journal*, 24 February 1994: 7).

Encouraging the private sector

As well as trying to make the NHS more 'business-like', the Conservatives took steps to increase the role of the private health care sector. In 1948, the existence of the NHS did not preclude private health care. There have been a number of ways in which private practice has been interconnected with the NHS.

First, anyone could receive private treatment by a private doctor in a private hospital financed by private health insurance or by direct payment. As recently as 1975, 40 per cent of bills were paid directly by patients rather than by insurance companies. Following the establishment of the NHS, the number of private beds was small. Higgins (1992) estimates that in 1979 there were 6700 private beds outside NHS hospitals and most of these were owned by non-profit-making religious organisations or charities. However, between 1982 and 1988, encouraged by the rise in the numbers of people covered by private health insurance, government subsidies and demand from overseas visitors, the total number of beds in the private acute sector increased by almost a quarter. In particular, a number of US-owned companies moved into the British market and by the end of the period had a bigger share than the non-profit-making hospitals (Busfield 1994). However, by the end of the 1980s, there was excess capacity in private acute hospitals, particularly in London. This was due to shortening lengths of stay in NHS hospitals and the decline in overseas patients seeking treatment in Britain. In the early 1990s, Higgins (1992) notes that the US hospitals have tended to sell out to European non-profit-making organisations.

Second, under an agreement reached between Bevan and the hospital consultants, patients could be treated privately for payment in NHS hospitals. In 1971, there were 4500 pay beds in NHS hospitals in England. By 1986, this had fallen to 3000 (*Social Trends* 1994). Despite the relatively small numbers, the issue of pay beds provoked political controversy. In the mid-1970s, Barbara Castle, when Secretary of State for Social Services, attempted to phase out pay beds and introduce controls over the development of private hospitals. These policies were reversed by the incoming Conservative government in 1979. Pay beds were again authorised. In the 1980s, pay beds have tended to decline, possibly because of the increase in the number of private hospitals. This is despite the efforts of NHS hospitals to expand their private beds in order to raise revenue.

A third aspect of private care is that from 1948, consultants could hold part-time contracts with the NHS so they could maintain a private practice. As Labour Secretary of State for Health between 1974–6, Barbara Castle altered consultants' contracts to encourage a full-time commitment to the NHS. In 1979, this policy, too, was reversed. Consultants were allowed to earn up to 10 per cent of their NHS salary from private practice while still remaining on full-time NHS contract (there is no limit for those on part-time contracts.) Griffiths *et al.* (1987) estimated that in 1984, 85 per cent of NHS consultants undertook some private work. Some also had a share in the private hospitals which developed during the 1980s (Mohan and Woods 1985). In 1994, the Monopolies and Mergers Commission reported that in 1991–2, 86 per cent of consultants undertook private work. Forty per cent earned less than £10,000 per annum, while 4 per cent earned more than £100,000 per annum from this work.

Fourth, and this was particularly encouraged in the 1980s, NHS patients could be treated in private hospitals, nursing homes and residential institutions. As indicated in Chapter 5, in the early 1980s the growth in bed numbers in private residential homes was rapid. In the 10 years between 1979 and 1989, there was a fourfold increase in private residential homes and nursing home beds multiplied two-and-a-half times. In the late 1980s, NHS managers were also encouraged to take out contracts for the treatment of NHS patients in private hospitals to clear the waiting list. Since 1980, controls over private hospital development had been relaxed and cooperation between the NHS and the private sector encouraged. The sale of NHS land to the private market is also now allowed.

As indicated earlier in this chapter, aspects of public service delivery will be increasingly tested against alternative private sector provision. This may also apply to large capital projects. For some years, health authorities have been encouraged to enter partnerships with the private sector in capital schemes. In 1993, the Treasury rules were relaxed still further to encourage private sector investment for viable projects held back by a lack of public money. Willetts (1993) describes a variety of options for private financing.

The lead up to the NHS reforms

While these changes were occurring, the government appeared reluctant to alter the funding or core activities of the NHS itself. A number of right-wing think-tanks and Conservative politicians had produced their prescriptions for the NHS. These ranged from voucher systems to a shift towards insurance funding. In 1985, a visiting US economist, Alain Enthoven (1985) had declared that the NHS was in a state of 'gridlock' or 'pluralistic stagnation'. His analysis found immediate support among the government advisers. Eager to storm the last bastion of the welfare state, they advocated the salutary discipline of the free market. Enthoven's prescription was based on the model of an enlarged Health Maintenance Organisation. He suggested that health agencies should have budgets to purchase services for populations from competitive providers. The proposal was attractive to politicians and civil servants. David Willetts, then director of the Centre for Policy Studies, claims to have shown an *Economist* article about Enthoven to Margaret Thatcher (Allsop and May 1993). This, he declared, led to the setting up of a Prime Ministerial policy review. The then Chancellor of the Exchequer wrote in his memoirs that he found the NHS 'highly inefficient and fundamentally flawed' (Lawson 1992: 614). He too claims credit for initiating the subsequent Thatcher review.

At about the same time as Ministers were reviewing the health service, the Prime Minister's Efficiency Unit had embarked on a critical review of the civil service which resulted in the report known as *The Next Steps* (Efficiency Unit 1988). This declared that senior management in the civil service was dominated by people whose skills lay in policy formulation but who had relatively little experience of how services were delivered. *The Next Steps* advocated a change in the attitudes and behaviour of Whitehall civil servants. This was to be effected by setting up quasi-autonomous self-regulating agencies responsible for fulfilling contracts and meeting performance targets set by Ministers.

The Next Steps criticised the civil service on two counts. First, it argued that:

> There is too little emphasis on the results to be achieved from resources . . . the Government is judged by what money goes in [to public services] and not what comes out.
>
> (Efficiency Unit 1988: 26)

Second, it went on to argue that the National Audit Office and the Public Accounts Committee, whose remit it was to scrutinise public expenditure, spent too much time finding fault with what happened in the past rather than applying pressure for improvement in the future. In a revealing comment, *The Next Steps* remarks that this was occurring:

> at a time when taxpayers were becoming increasingly conscious of what they should expect from public expenditure on health, education and other services and hold Ministers to blame for their deficiencies.
>
> (pp. 3–4)

It was clear that the Thatcher government wished, ultimately, to distance itself from responsibility for public services.

Finally, the political context provides a further explanation for the timing of the Prime Minister's Review and the subsequent reforms. The Conservatives, embarking on their third term of office, decided to gamble. One week afterwards The *Independent* newspaper reported that David Willetts, asking a senior civil servant what he would do about the NHS, had received the reply:

> I'd either leave it entirely alone, because it is too politically dangerous. Or I'd destabilise it, and see what happened.
>
> (Timmins 1989)

The next chapter describes the NHS reforms and assesses the changes.

References

Allsop, J. and May, A. (1986) *The Emperor's New Clothes: Family Practitioner Committees in the 1980s*, King Edward's Hopital Fund for London, London.

Allsop, J. and May, A. (1993) 'Between the Devil and the Deep Blue Sea: Managing the NHS Act in the wake of the 1990 Act', *Critical Social Policy*, 38, 5–22.

Banyard, R. (1991) 'How do UGMs Perform?' *Health Services Journal*, 21 July, pp. 824–5; 'Management Mirrored', *Health Services Journal*,

28 July, pp. 858–9; 'More Power to Units' *Health Services Journal*, 4 August, pp. 882–3; 'Watching the revolution', 4 August, pp. 916–17.

Bosanquet, N. (1988) 'The Ailing State of the National Health' in Jowell, R., Witherspoon, S. and Brook, L. (eds), *British Social Attitudes, the 5th Report*, Gower Publishing, Aldershot.

Bosanquet, N. (1993) *Interim Report: the national health* in Jowell, R., Brook, L., Prior, G. and Taylor, B. (eds), *British Social Attitudes, 9th Report*, Dartmouth Publishing Company, Aldershot.

Busfield, J. (1994) 'Medicine and Markets: power, choice and the consumption of private medical care', in Burrows, R. and Marsh, C. (eds), *Consumption and Class: divisions and change*, Macmillan, Basingstoke.

Butler, J. (1992) *Patients, Policies and Politics*, Open University Press, Milton Keynes.

Calnan, M., Cant, S. and Gabe, J. (1993) *Going Private: why people pay for their health care*, Open University Press, Milton Keynes.

Department of Health and Social Security (1981) *Care in Action: a handbook of policies and priorities for health and personal social services*, HMSO, London.

Department of Health and Social Security (1983) *NHS Management Inquiry*, DHSS, London.

Department of Trade (1982) *Opticians and Competition – a report by the Office of Fair Trading*, HMSO, London.

Drucker, P. (1989) 'Peter Drucker's 1990s: the futures that have already happened', *The Economist*, 21 October, pp. 27–30.

Drucker, P. (1990) *The New Realities*, Mandarin, London.

Efficiency Unit (1988) *Improving Management in Government: the next steps*, HMSO, London.

Enthoven, A. (1985) *Reflections on the Management of the NHS*, Nuffield Provincial Hospitals Trust, London.

Epsing Anderson, G. (1990) *The Three Worlds of Welfare Capitalism*, Polity Press, Cambridge.

Flynn, R. (1991) 'Coping with Cutbacks and Managing Retrenchment in Health', *Journal of Social Policy*, 20 (2), pp. 215–36.

Griffiths, R. (1983) *The NHS Management Inquiry Report*, DHSS, London.

Griffiths, R. (1991) *Seven Years of Progress – General Management in the NHS*. The third annual Audit Commission lecture, *Health Economics*, 1 (1), pp. 61–70.

Griffiths, H., Iliffe, S. and Rayner, R. (1987) *Banking on Sickness, commercial medicine in Britain and the USA*, Lawrence & Wishart, London.

Harrison, S., Hunter, D., Marnock, G. and Pollitt, C. (1992) *Just Managing, power and culture in the NHS*, Macmillan, London.

Higgins, J. (1988) *The Business of Medicine: private health care in Britain*, Macmillan Education, London.

Higgins, J. (1992) 'Private Sector Health Care', in Beck, E., Lonsdale, S., Newman, S. and Patterson, D. (eds), *In the Best of Health?* Chapman & Hall, London.

Hunter, D. (1992) 'Doctors as Managers: Poachers turned gamekeepers?' *Social Science and Medicine*, 35, 4, 567–66.

Laing, W. and Buisson, R. (1992) *Laing's Review of Private Health Care 1991/2*, Laing & Buisson Publications, London.

Laing, W. and Buisson, R. (1993) *Private Medical Insurance: market update*, Laing & Buisson Publications, London.
Lawson, N. (1992) *The View from Number 11: memoirs of a Tory Radical*, Bantam Press, London.
Miller, F. (1992) 'Health Policy, Competition and Professional Behaviour', in Harrison, A. (ed.), *Health Care UK*, King's Fund, London.
Milne, R. (1992) 'Competitive Tendering for Support Services', in Beck, E., Lonsdale, S., Newman, S. and Patterson, D., *In the Best of Health?*, Chapman & Hall, London.
Mohan, J. and Woods, K. (1985) 'Restructuring Health Care: the social geography of public and private health care under the British Conservative government', *International Journal of Health Services*, 15, pp. 197–215.
Monopolies and Mergers Commission (1989) *Services of Medical Practitioners: A Report on the Supply of Services of Registered Medical Practitioners in relation to Restrictions on Advertising*, Cmnd 582, HMSO, London.
Monopolies and Mergers Commission (1994) *Private Medical Services*, Cmnd 2452, HMSO, London.
National Audit Office (1987) *Competitive Tendering for Support Services in the NHS*, session 1986/7 HC318, HMSO, London.
Office of Health Economics (1992) *Compendium of Statistics*, Office of Health Economics, London.
OPCS (1986–7) *Social Survey Division General Household Survey*, No. 19, HMSO, London.
Osborne, D. and Gaebler, T. (1992) *Reinventing Government*, Addison Wesley, Mass.
Peters, T. and Waterman, R. (1982) *In Search of Excellence*, Harper & Row, New York.
Pollitt, C. (1990) *Managerialism in the Public Services: the Anglo-American experience*, Blackwell, Oxford.
Propper, C. (1989) *Working for Patients, the Implications of the White Paper for Private Patients*, Centre for Health Economics, York.
Public Accounts Committee (1981) *Financial Control and Accountability in the NHS*, 17th Report, Session 1981 HC 255, HMSO, London.
Secretary of State for Health (1989) *Working for Patients*, Cmnd 555, HMSO, London.
Social Services Select Committee (1981) *Public Expenditure on the Social Services*, Third Report, Session 1980/81 324, HMSO, London.
Social Services Select Committee (1986) *Public Expenditure on the Social Services*, 4th Session 1985/6, vol. 1, HMSO, London.
Social Trends 24 (1994) Central Statistical Office, HMSO, London.
Strong, P. and Robinson, J. (1990) *The NHS under New Management*, Open University Press, Milton Keynes.
Timmins, N. (1989) 'Is the Health Service Safe in Their Hands?', *Independent*, 9 Feb.
Treasury (1991) *Competing for Quality, Buying Better Public Services*, Cmnd 1730, HMSO, London.
Willetts, D. (1993) *The Opportunities for Private Funding in the NHS*, Social Market Foundation, London.

CHAPTER 9

The 1990 NHS reforms

In 1989, the Prime Minister's Review of the NHS, *Working for Patients* (WFP) was published (Secretary of State for Health 1989). The government proposed to maintain the public financing of the NHS but on the supply side of health care, an internal market was to create greater efficiency through increased competition. After legislation, in the 1990 NHS and Community Care Act, the reforms were implemented in April 1991 in the NHS. The community reforms, discussed in Chapter 5, were implemented in April 1993.

The reforms have been seen by most commentators (Butler 1992, Day and Klein 1991, Le Grand and Bartlett 1994) as the most crucial since the start of the NHS. They signified a shift from the command and control economy to a managed market within the service. In so doing the incentives for those working in the service, the relationships between different levels of authority as well as the politics within the NHS were changed fundamentally. Whereas previously, the hospital and community services and the separately administered family practitioner services operated within vertical lines of authority leading to the NHS Management Executive (NHSME) (from mid-1994 this became known as the NHSE, the NHS Executive) and the Department of Health (DOH), in the new structure, the stronger relationships were horizontal – between purchasers and providers at the district level. Furthermore, purchasers and providers had different roles and functions and this was the most crucial element of the health reforms. Purchasers had a budget to buy services. They drew up a contract for the services needed by their population and bought these from hospitals and community service units. Providers' units were to compete annually for funded contracts which had to be sufficient to maintain their financial viability. Although vertical relationships with the DOH and the NHSME remained, these were less dominant than the market relationships at the local level.

In other respects, the reforms are not a radical departure. The principles of comprehensiveness, universality and equity were reaffirmed. Greater choice for patients was added as a principle. The service remained funded from taxation. Furthermore, the reforms incorporated many of the beliefs about public service management already introduced into the NHS, such as the need to contain public expenditure, the value of competition and the lessons learnt from private sector management. Also, the main theme running through WFP, that of greater efficiency and value for money, was not new. The main aim of the health reforms, like others before, was to achieve 'better health care' – that is, health care interventions which combined low price with quality and health gain. Document 13 (page 310) provides an extract from WPF including the key changes.

The assumption behind the government's approach was that the introduction of market incentives would change the micro-economics and politics of health provision using new sets of incentives. This chapter will describe the NHS reforms and discuss the advantages and disadvantages which are claimed to have resulted. These are discussed in terms of general principles. The reforms have added efficiency and choice to the original NHS aims of equity, comprehensiveness and accountability. The question of whether a new NHS politics has developed alongside managed competition will be discussed in the final chapter.

There are three major difficulties in reaching conclusions about the health reforms. First, the 1990 Act set in motion a series of further changes. Some of these were anticipated – for example, the increasing numbers of hospital and health care Trusts. Others were not – such as the repercussions of GP fundholding which gave faster access to hospital care for fundholding patients at the expense of non-fundholders. In 1994, further changes are planned in NHS structure along with a fourth and fifth wave of GP fundholders. The reforms are akin to a continuing revolution. This makes assessment difficult as there are no beginning and end points for comparison.

A second problem is that the government decided not to evaluate the reforms. The changes were based on beliefs about the value and impact of competition and the need for total systemic change. Subsequently, although a few studies have been carried out by academic researchers, these have been limited in scope (Drummond and Maynard 1993, Le Grand and Bartlett 1994, Robinson and Le Grand 1994). A third problem is that too little time has elapsed for the reforms to take effect, so any conclusions reached by these studies are tentative.

The internal market

The reforms introduced in 1991 were based on three main principles. First, the large public hospitals, if they opted to become Trusts, while they remained still publicly owned, were freed from the main rules governing their activity. Their main purpose was to remain financially viable and they were able to raise both income and capital for this purpose without seeking permission from the Department of Health. They could also determine the pay scales of employees as well as the remuneration of individual staff. Second, each district became a buyer of services rather than a provider and could look for services from the private as well as the public sector. Only a small core of staff and services were retained at district level. Third, larger general practices could hold budgets to purchase services. The funding for this was top-sliced from district budgets. These GP fundholders (GPFHs) could buy certain services from providers for their practice population and were thus encouraged to consider carefully the services they wanted and to choose the most cost-effective options.

As the reforms were implemented, a variety of patterns of service developed, based on local circumstance. This meant that there was no standard pattern – indeed the intention had been to encourage local enterprise and innovation. Another potentially confusing aspect of the reforms as they have evolved was the changing terminology. At the time this book was written, the DHAs have become Health Authorities (HAs), the term 'purchasing' is being replaced by 'commissioning', although some texts refer to 'contracting'. They all mean the buying of services. Providers have now become Trusts, although there is a small residue of directly managed units. The changes are now examined in more detail.

The role of Health Authorities in commissioning contracts

In 1991, there were 190 HAs in England. Subsequently, mergers between authorities reduced this number so that by 1993 there were 145. Figure 9.1 shows the structure. There were also 90 Family Health Service Authorities (FHSAs) responsible for family practitioner services. By April 1994, there were 108 HAs. Some had merged to cover larger populations and others had merged with an FHSA covering the same area. By 1996, it is envisaged that all HAs and FHSAs will be merged to make all-purpose agencies which commission for the full range of hospital, community and general practitioner services for their population. In many areas, authorities already work closely together. These changes will bring England and Wales into line with Scotland and Northern Ireland. Ironically, the merging of functions fulfils one of Bevan's dreams – to unify the management of hospitals, community services and GPs. At the same time, it confounds another. Bevan wanted a seamless web of care. In fact, the purchaser/provider split has created a patchwork quilt of agencies.

Since 1990, HAs, which continue to have a Chair and an appointed Board made up of executive and non-executive members, have been allocated budgets. These are based on a weighted capitation formula. The level of funding is determined by the population of the area with a weighting for age, sex and social

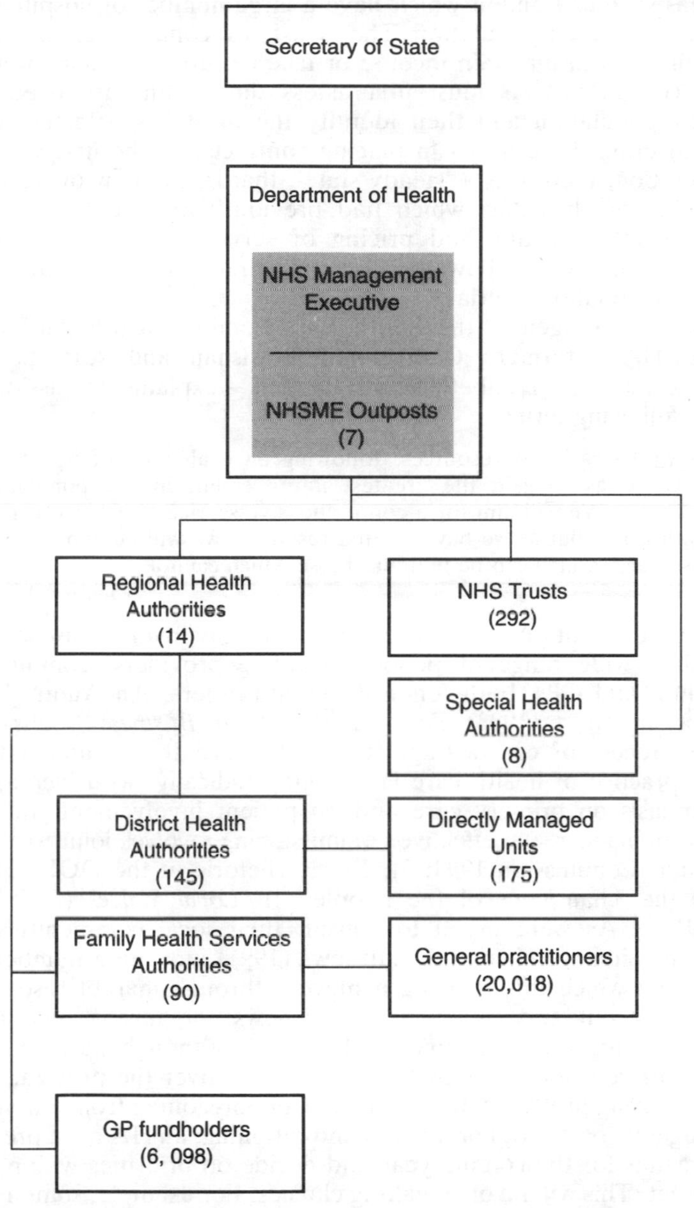

Figure 9.1 ***Structure of the NHS 1993***
Source: Department of Health (1993) HMSO, London.

deprivation. The formula has created problems for metropolitan areas such as London which have a large number of hospitals in relation to their population. They must now compete for contracts to fill beds to maintain income or face closure. In order to draw up contracts, HAs must first assess the health care needs of their population and then identify the most cost-effective way of meeting those needs in placing contracts. In the first year of operation, there was a 'steady state', that is, the flow of patients was to the hospitals which had previously treated them. This allowed the costing and pricing of services to be established before HAs were allowed to place contracts freely according to price or quality criteria.

One new agency, the South East London Health Authority (SELHA) – formerly Camberwell, Lewisham and North Southwark and West Lambeth health districts – explains its mission in the following terms:

> [we will] target our resources, following an evaluation of health care needs, so as to gain the greatest improvement in our population's health . . . We will aim for a comprehensive service to achieve genuine health gains, but as we have limited resources we will be explicit about those needs which can be met and those which cannot.
>
> (Sabin 1992: 54)

The process of drawing up contracts typically involves discussions with a wide range of people including providers, community groups and GPs, both fundholders and others. An Audit Commission report (1993) *Their Health, Your Business*, spells out the process of contracting. It puts forward the argument that the practice of health care is changing radically, with increasing emphasis on primary care and on patient involvement. In this environment, really effective commissioning involves joint working (Audit Commission 1993: 3). In the rhetoric of the DOH, HAs are the 'champions of the people'. In *Local Voices* (NHSME 1991), HAs were urged to consult their local communities in commissioning. Ham and Matthews (1991) indicate a number of ways in which this is being achieved: through market research; carrying out surveys of patients' views; organising meetings; undertaking life-style surveys. However, although participation was offered, local groups had little power over the process; this could bring problems in the future. Commissioning from a limited budget involves both prediction and rationing: an HA must predict demands for the coming year and decide on priorities within the budget. This will involve making choices. For example, some HAs have decided not to purchase treatment for tattoo removal and to fund only a limited number of fertility treatments. Ham (1993) describes priority setting in six districts, and Stockford (1993) reviews the development of purchasing during 1993.

Contracts can be placed on a block, cost per case or cost and volume basis. The first form of contracting is most common. A Health Authority will place a block contract with a hospital for a set number of patient episodes over a period of a year for a global sum. Two elements remain outside the contracting process: Extra Contractual Referrals (ECRs), individual patient referrals outside the contract, and the treatment of patients who come in through Accident and Emergency and who require further hospital care treatment. In both cases bills for care must be met by the HA where the patients live. A principle of *Working for Patients* was that money should follow the patient. This, it was believed, would create an incentive to hospitals to provide high-quality, specialist services. Also, if a patient needed emergency or specialist care, which is essentially unpredictable, they could be treated appropriately.

In 1993, the role of directors of public health was clarified in relation to assessing the health needs in order to improve health status. The directors had to hold specialist qualifications in public health and were expected to develop and promote a health strategy as well as coordinate activity relating to clinical care (NHSME 1993).

GP fundholders as commissioners

Fundholding GPs (GPFHs) are also purchasers of services and funding for them is top-sliced off HA budgets. They may place a contract for their patients or refer to hospital as necessary. In both situations, providers are paid on a cost per case basis. From 1991, GPs with practices over a certain size, 11,000, then 9000 and now 7000, may hold budgets for their practice populations and can commission a range of services, including diagnostic services, outpatient services and certain elective surgical procedures. Initially, very generous budgets and financial inducements were offered to GPs to become fundholders. They received per capita allowances and additional assistance to help improve information technology and practice management. GPs may retain any savings which result to put back into their practice. In some areas, GPFHs have grouped together with other practices to form consortia to share management costs. In some respects, fundholding has been unexpectedly popular with GPs. Glennerster, Matsaganis and Owens (1992) report a range of innovations. In 1994, there were further fundholders and in 1995 a fifth wave.

Views of the long-term value of fundholding remain divided. There is a conflict between the principles of HA commissioning and GP fundholding. HAs commission on a population basis and have an incentive to build stable relationships with providers over the long term. Contract switching has the potential for creating a chaotic health care market which cannot benefit patient care. The

GP, on the other hand, buys services for a practice and individual patients and has greater flexibility to change the patient flow. Furthermore, the more GPFHs there are in an area, the less the HA can plan services through commissioning as it loses control and its budget to the fundholder. Ham (1993) reports on a variety of methods of joint commissioning between fundholders and the HA. These aim to obtain the benefits of both methods.

Other criticisms of fundholding have been that it creates incentives for GPs to save money by treating patients themselves rather than referring them to hospital (Abel-Smith 1992). Iliffe (1993) believes that GPs are not equipped with the necessary skills for fundholding in terms of management and financial accounting. He argues that it encourages cost-cutting without assessments of the effect of this on the quality of care. He concludes that fundholding needs proper evaluation because the only demonstrable advantage at present relates to a reduction of prescribing costs. General practice is discussed further in the next chapter.

The purpose of commissioning

In the rhetoric of the current reforms, commissioning is seen as 'the engine of change' and managers in HAs have been portrayed as change masters. There are examples of waiting times being cut, day surgery increased and outpatient services transferred to GP surgeries, and these are attributed to the purchaser-provider split. As was argued in Chapter 4, there are wide variations in the costs of treatment in the NHS. A recent report from the Chartered Institute of Public Finance and Accountancy (1993) showed that differences remain wide. The costs per day for orthopaedic patients were shown to vary from £70 to £430. If all hospitals provided these services at average costs, the NHS could achieve savings of more than £87 million per year. Arguably, the main purpose of the internal market is to bring about these savings.

The financial circumstances in which HAs found themselves following the health reforms has varied considerably and so have their relationships with local providers. Some HAs have to rely on one provider who is therefore in a monopoly position. Others have used competition between a number of local hospitals to drive down costs, yet others have built up collaborative relationships.

It is acknowledged that commissioning poses many problems for which managers, let alone GPs, were ill-prepared. Osborne and Gaebler, whose text on entrepreneurial public sector management, *Reinventing Government* (1992), is acknowledged by the head of the Home Civil Service, Sir Robin Butler, as a major influence on current UK government thinking, spells out the pitfalls. While contracting is a common method of injecting competition into public services, it is one of the most difficult methods a public organisation can choose. Writing and monitoring contracts requires a great deal of skill (Osborne and Gaebler 1992: 87).

Data on health needs and current service utilisation are often poor and are intrinsically difficult to collect while methods for assessing needs are in their infancy. Questions also arise about how prices set by providers can be tested; how quality and health outcomes and health gains should be assessed as well as about how authorities should make decisions and who should be involved. Currently, routinely available information on activity, quality, outcomes as well as costs is inadequate (Rafferty and Gibson 1994, Bartlett and Le Grand 1994). However, they are also a necessary part of priority setting. In the commissioning system, rationing can become much more transparent, at least within the system. In general, commissioning brings the power to determine what services are bought which have little accountability. This is discussed further below.

In 1993, a survey of purchasing in 100 health authorities concluded that the HAs did not yet set priorities or make rationing decisions explicitly. The authors, Redmayne, Klein and Day (1993), comment that at present there are too many government directives which have added to the list of 'priorities'. This has led to available resources being spread too thinly. For example, *The Health of the Nation* (DOH 1992a) has set a number of targets in relation to improving health status and the NHSME has urged HAs to improve charter standards, cut waiting times, expand day surgery and develop healthy alliances.

NHS Trusts

Before 1990, nearly all hospitals and community services were managed by DHAs. The reforms allowed hospitals and community units to draw up business plans to opt for status to become self-governing Trusts. Their income would come from winning contracts for patient services. In order to become a Trust, assets had to be costed to include an estimation of capital value with a 6 per cent return on that capital. This was to put the NHS on a par with the private sector. To be awarded Trust status, financial viability had to be demonstrated as a non-profit agency. WFP declared explicitly that an application for Trust status would not be accepted if it meant keeping an otherwise financially unviable hospital open (Secretary of State for Health 1989: para 3.17).

Trusts were to be run by Boards of Directors which included a Chair, the chief officers of the provider unit and appointed non-executive members. They were to have freedom to determine rates of pay for staff, make capital investments and could rationalise or alter their services to reflect judgements about market movements. Thus Trusts gained a larger degree of autonomy and financial freedom.

In WFP, the government argued that:

> . . . self government . . . will encourage a greater sense of local ownership and pride. . . . It will stimulate the commitment and harness the skills of those who are directly responsible for providing services . . . it will encourage local initiative and greater competition. All this will ensure a better deal for the public, improving the choice and quality of the services offered and the efficiency with which those services are delivered.
>
> (Secretary of State for Health 1989: 22)

By August 1992, there were 156 'first wave' Trusts, or 35 per cent of all hospital and community units, fully operational. A further 129 followed during 1993. By April 1994, there were approximately 440 Trusts providing 90 per cent of all hospital and community health services (Figure 9.1 above; DOH 1993).

The creation of Trusts, leaving behind them a small residue of directly managed units (DMUs), has spawned a varied pattern of agencies with more specific and narrower functions. These agencies are not only more numerous but the way in which they are structured varies. In some districts, FHSAs have combined with community units; in others there has been a split between acute, community and the family health services and their geographical boundaries may have changed. Indeed, FHSAs are both purchasers and providers. They may be said to commission services from their GPs but may also act on their behalf to commission services from Trusts.

The main role of Trusts is to provide the services which purchasers want. They may compete for either block, cost and volume or cost per case contracts. In addition, they may earn income from ECRs and for treating the patients of GP fundholders. The latter two categories are attractive because they bring additional income outside the block contract. This is why Trusts may give priority to these cases and thus extend waiting times for their local population who will be covered by the block contract. Financial transactions form the basis of relationships between health authorities and from the outset, it was intended that competition between providers would be a mechanism for driving down unit costs.

In provider agencies, whether Trusts or DMUs, managers and doctors are now compelled to join in the common pursuit of winning contracts for their services. In some instances, doctors have been drawn into management as heads of clinical directorates, making decisions about what they can provide within the financial targets of annual business plans. A 1990 survey by the NHSME showed that 40 per cent of units had clinical directorates, whilst 80 per cent had at least some clinicians holding budgets (Salter 1992). Increasingly, clinical directorates must make rationing decisions to keep within the targets, as well as choices about levels of activity and new developments. Doctors are learning to be more aware of the costs of what they provide and are making choices accordingly. Computerised financial and patient activity systems are starting to make it possible to track costs and activity more closely. Senior managers, working alongside the more market-orientated non-executive members, are determining pace and strategy while clinicians are developing new skills of business management (Ashburner, Ferlie and Fitzgerald 1993).

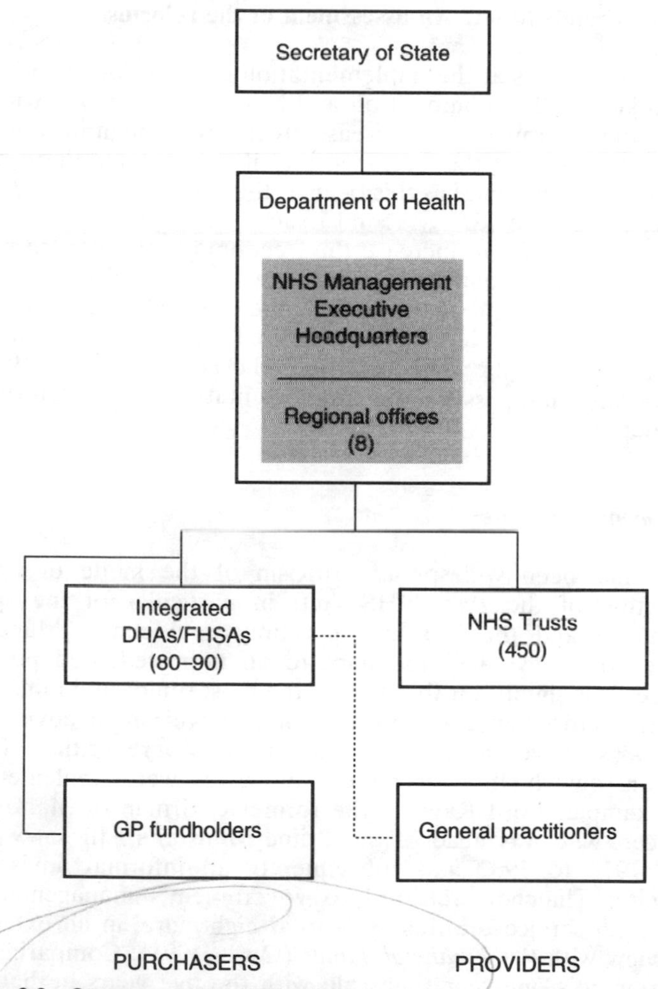

Figure 9.2 ***Structure of the NHS 1994***
Source: Department of Health (1993) HMSO, London.

Changes at the centre

In late 1993, a further change was proposed with the merger of regions, to leave eight in all. By 1996, these will be abolished in favour of eight regional offices within the NHSME. The stated aim of *Managing the New NHS* (DOH 1993 and 1994) is to continue the decentralisation of the service. In effect, the NHSME will become absorbed into the DOH but the two will have different roles. The former will be the operational arm of the service with the responsibility for managing purchasing, while the DOH will determine general strategy. Figure 9.2 shows the structure.

Managed competition? An assessment of the reforms

This section looks at the implementation of the reforms and then at two key issues – competition and NHS management. A major aim of the reforms was to increase efficiency through introducing market forces. Has this occurred and if it has, have there been gains in efficiency and has this been at the expense of equity? And who exercises choice? A second issue is the management of the NHS. The aim was to increase the freedom of managers to make decisions without central controls. How has the division between central planning and management and allowed entrepreneurial forces at the local level been resolved? What have been the consequences of the reforms for public accountability? Before considering these, issues, the implementation of the reforms is considered.

Implementation issues

There has been widespread criticism of the mode of implementation of the 1990 NHS Act, in particular of the speed of change and the lack of operational guidelines. Managers in the NHS have had to adapt to an unprecedented pace of change. It is significant that two of the most senior and influential private sector managers, brought in as government advisers in the 1980s, have been among the most severe critics of the way the new NHS management processes were implemented. For example, Lord Rayner, the former chairman of Marks and Spencer, who was head of the Prime Minister's Efficiency Unit from 1979 to 1982 and subsequently an informal adviser to Margaret Thatcher, referred to government's management of the health service reforms as 'a total nightmare' in an extended interview with the *Financial Times* (Owen 1991). Comparing the government's one-year timescale with the five years he had felt necessary to introduce major changes in Marks and Spencer, he deplored the lack of allowance made for starting-up costs and the consequent strain on management and financial resources. He declared:

> There is no way we would do it without making the necessary resources available to manage the change. There is no way we would do it without proper experiment and evaluation.

However, from the Government's perspective, piecemeal change was out of the question. The aim was to alter the culture and habits throughout the system.

Competition between HAs and Trusts: does it exist?

A major problem in answering this question is the lack of evaluation. Some commentators on the health reforms argue that there is, as yet, little competition between providers in the new NHS. This may be because purchasers and providers enter into a comfortable alliance with each other or because the local geography results in a monopoly position for one or the other. For example, Le Grand and Bartlett (1994) suggest that it may be particularly difficult to maintain the distance necessary for market transactions when individuals dealing with each other may only recently have been colleagues in the previous system. Harrison and Bartlett (1993) conclude from their study of the Bristol and Weston area where one HA was faced with a single supplier:

> The absence of a range of suppliers and the likelihood of services being purchased from a single provider, suggest that competition does not exist in any real sense of the word.
>
> (Harrison and Bartlett 1993: 88)

It has also been argued that Trust markets could not be truly competitive because of patients' reluctance to travel long distances. A large patient catchment area is needed to cover the high fixed costs. Local hospitals are therefore likely to be protected and will in effect be local monopolies. The high set-up costs would in any case put off competitors.

In other areas, where there are a number of alternative providers, commissioning authorities are in a monopoly position. They are then in a position to threaten the viability of a hospital by removing contracts to a lower-cost source of supply. In 1993, University College Hospital was threatened in this way and the Secretary of State for Health intervened to maintain the status quo. The HAs were required by the Secretary of State to retain their contracts as the hospital was a valued centre of teaching and research.

Ferlie, Cairncross and Pettigrew (1992) have argued that there is a variety of different forms of market in the business world;

in many cases, alliances are built up to stabilise relationships. There was a range of behaviour from cooperation through to cut-throat competition. In the US where *public* services have adopted a purchaser-provider split, in many cases contracts were not typically subject to competition. And where they were, it was often difficult to compare bids directly. In other words, in both the private and public sector, perfect competition rarely applies. Agencies work for stability and there is a degree of trust.

The discussion above suggests that market forces within the NHS are likely to be 'managed' by local-level actors, particularly given the history and values within the service. Many of those working in the NHS, particularly if they have professional allegiances, believe that competition between Trusts is antithetical to the values of the NHS. They argue that hospitals can have a number of roles – training staff and carrying out research as well as treating patients. These functions need to be protected. So too does the quality of patient care and equity of access. Allowing Trusts to fail as a consequence of market forces would put these into jeopardy. In practice, since 1991, market forces have been regulated. As in the old NHS, increments for teaching and research have been funded from the centre; measures have been introduced to protect particular hospitals. Trusts have also had limits set on their ability to borrow capital as well as being shielded from financial collapse. To date, no Trust has faced bankruptcy – although, particularly in London, there have been managed closures.

Similar arguments against competition can be applied to the unleashing of competitive forces *within* Trusts through the relaxation of pay and salary scales. For example, Le Grand (1992) argues that one consequence of the creation of independent Trusts will be to convert the NHS from a monopoly purchaser of labour. In the past it was able to bargain nationally with the relevant professional associations. Now, there will be local-level bargaining. Each Trust may be faced with a staff group with expert skills who may be in a monopoly position to raise their labour costs. Drawing on the US experience, he predicts that this shift will serve to push up wage and salary costs. In particular, it may increase still further the differential between those who have scarce skills and those who do not.

Osborne and Gaebler (1992: 88) make a similar point when they argue that 'privatising to a monopoly is not only senseless but extremely expensive'. They give the example of commissioners in the US who dispense with their own in-house equipment and services to reduce to a 'core' function but find themselves 'over a barrel' when contractors raise their prices.

The impact of GP fundholding

There is evidence that fundholding in general practice has led to considerable innovation and to benefits to the patients and GPs of these practices. This is partly due to the additional funds provided but also that GPs have been able to achieve changes in the way in which services are supplied to them. Trusts, eager for GP contracts, have provided the kind of services which GPs want. Some examples are a speedier analysis and transmission of test results, shorter waiting times for outpatient services and the transfer of consultant services to the GP surgery (Glennerster *et al*. 1994).

The disadvantages of GP fundholding have been mainly in terms of lack of geographical spread. Fundholding has been most extensively taken up by the better organised practices in more affluent areas of the country. Poor inner city GPs are least likely to be fundholders. There is also evidence that in some Trusts, waiting times for elective surgery for fundholders' patients is significantly less than for patients generally (Whitehead 1994). This raises further issues of equity.

To date, fundholding is limited to about 25 per cent of the population. Glennerster *et al*. also point out that, in 1993, the share of the total hospital and community budget taken by fundholders was only 2 per cent. Most hospital procedures and major episodes of hospital care, those which cost over £5000, remain outside fundholding. These limits could, however, change over time.

The effect of managed competition on costs and efficiency

In relation to the question of efficiency within Trusts, there has been little research. Newchurch and Company Ltd (1993), in a study of 57 first-wave Trusts, found that all had demonstrated an ability to stay within financial limits, and concluded that this demonstrated a remarkable ability on the part of managers to adjust to significant change. In their study of the early years of the health reforms, Le Grand and Bartlett (1994) examined the unit costs of similar hospitals applying for Trust status in the first and second waves. They found that their unit costs were lower than the average but concluded that this was not due to market forces but to the fact that they were a self-selected group and already had low unit costs. The NHSME has also claimed increasing patient activity since the introduction of the reforms. However, it is not possible to separate the effect of the reforms themselves from the additional funding which has been allocated to the service.

However, against these possible gains must be set the upheaval within the NHS and the problems of learning to work a new system. For example, some Trusts have used their budgets and fulfilled their contracts by January of the financial year so patients must wait for treatment until the following year. Overall, waiting lists have not reduced. Although there is some evidence that the numbers waiting more than two years has fallen, the numbers waiting a shorter length of time have increased. Waiting lists may be manipulated in a number of ways and in any case are a poor measure of unmet need.

GP fundholding was intended to create incentives for practices to reduce costs to improve services in other ways. In a matched study in the Oxford region, which compared the prescribing costs of GPs from fundholding and non-funding practices, Bradlow and Coulter (1993) showed that fundholders' prescribing costs have risen less than those of practices as a whole. Overall in 1992–3, the projected drug overspend by non-fundholding practices was 9 per cent and for fundholders 1.4 per cent (Glennerster *et al.* 1994). However, in relation to referrals to hospital, there is no evidence that these have been affected by fundholding (Coulter and Bradlow 1993). Nor, indeed, is there any evidence that fundholders are selecting lower-cost patients, as many had feared. There have, of course, been costs as well as benefits to fundholding. GP fundholding has high administrative costs and, with a large number of small units, the costs are duplicated. Some practices offset this by combining into larger consortia.

In conclusion, given the limited evidence available it can be argued that Hudson is not alone in arguing that benefits of a quasi-market in health and social care have tended to be asserted rather than demonstrated (Hudson 1992). Maynard and Hutton (1992) and Le Grand (1992) point out that while Enthoven's ideas (1985) on managed competition (referred to in the last chapter) have stimulated policy debates and institutional changes in three continents, analysis of their effect on resource allocation and cost control remains incomplete. The little evaluation available, they note, suggests that price competition is difficult to create and sustain and that the effects of managed care remain unproven.

Equity and choice

There has been little assessment of the consequences on equity of the NHS reforms. Whitehead (1994) considers the available evidence. Other things being equal, the greater diversity of health care is likely to have increased further the scope and type of health care available in different areas. Whether this is any greater than in the 'old' NHS is not known. In the case of GP fundholding, and access to day surgery, there are examples of preferential treatment (Mahon, Wilkin and Whitehouse 1994). WFP also emphasised the importance of patient choice. There is no evidence of increased choice in the new NHS. GPs exercise choice *on behalf of* their patients, particularly if they are fundholders. Commissioners buy services *on behalf* of patients. It may be that health care has become more complicated for patients themselves to understand and there is little or no information on the services to which they are entitled.

Managing the NHS in the wake of the reforms

The reforms have undoubtedly had a profound effect on NHS management. They were intended to encourage enterprise and the entrepreneurial spirit. Within the Trusts, there is clear recognition that an enhanced capacity to measure and understand and therefore control costs and activity is essential. New management systems have been introduced and business plans for clinical directorates enable activity to be planned and monitored more effectively. In some cases this has brought clinicians into senior management roles and in other cases a new partnership between managers and clinicians has developed. The security of consultants' jobs now depends more directly on the performance of their Trust. This has led Bartlett and Le Grand (1994) to discuss the future of Trusts in terms of labour-managed cooperatives.

Across the country, some imaginative schemes have developed, often led by individuals with a vision. For example, an innovative community project in the Wirral, where there is a severe drug abuse problem, involves inter-agency collaboration, a multi-professional team and extensive user-participation (May 1992). Layzell (1994) describes ways of involving local people in service purchasing in Derbyshire. Consumer audit has also developed as a method of finding out the views of service users (Bradburn, Kershaw and Allsop 1994).

But there is a price to pay for the reforms. Introducing costing and market mechanisms have brought a variety of operational problems. In 1992, Maynard and Hutton (1992) argued that these require heavy investment in data collection and in utilisation and the associated human capital. They suggest that while administrative costs have been inflated, there is less money available for patient care and managers still lack essential information. Two years later, Rafferty and Gibson (1994) pointed out that essential data on which contracting depends is still lacking. It is difficult to acquire good data on patient activity and the cost of that activity. This then requires to be analysed and interpreted. Developing measures of quality and outcome then present further challenges.

Since the health reforms, there have been large increases in the numbers of administrative, clerical and managerial staff in the NHS. The edition of *Health and Personal Social Service Statistics for England* issued in September 1992 (DOH 1992b) records that spending on general managers' salaries increased ten-fold in the five years between 1987 and 1991: from £25.7m to £251.5m. Between 1989 and 1992, the number of managers has increased from 46,000 to 167,000 – that is by more than 260 per cent. Administrative and clerical staff increased by 15 per cent in the same period (Hansard, Written Answer. 4 November 1993 cols 458 and 460).

By the 1990s, it is possible to identify two divergent trends in the relationship between the Department of Health at the centre and the Health Authorities at the periphery (Paton 1992). Responsibility now lies with a large number of smaller agencies. The rhetoric is about devolution, local autonomy and diversity, but central government nevertheless continues to dictate the agenda. Health care remains finance-led while a stream of directives from the NHSME and circulars from the Department of Health impose tight timetables for implementation and rules for commissioning. This leaves little opportunity for evaluation, learning from mistakes and local enterprise.

Furthermore, the NHS cannot become a learning organisation when news management is the order of the day. The Department of Health is obsessed with secrecy, while the Management Executive actively discourages public debate. An increasing number of Trusts and other authorities are employing public relations consultants to put a gloss on their activities, and imposing 'gagging clauses' on their employees.

A further downside of the more competitive environment in the NHS has been some cases of serious mismanagement as HAs have tried to privatise services and introduce new financial systems to cope with new tasks. One example is the loss of £10 million for patient services in the West Midlands region in an attempt to privatise the supplies service. Another is the failure of Wessex RHA to control costs in its computerisation plans. In both cases, Public Accounts Committee inquiries highlighted issues of control and accountability (Public Accounts Committee 1993 and 1994). The Public Accounts Committee commented on the dangers of a more entrepreneurial approach in the management of public services. It declared:

> . . . there is no reason why a proper conduct of public business and care for the honest handling of public money should not be combined with effective programmes for promoting honesty and efficiency.
>
> (PAC 1994: iv)

The policy vacuum

Despite the number of directives from the centre, there are also signs of a policy vacuum. This may reflect a lack of commitment to a managed NHS and a greater concern to increase competition:

alternatively it may simply reflect a lack of leadership. While the NHS remained a national service committed to particular values of meeting need on demand in an egalitarian manner, the commitment to provide for a range of health needs became less important. In a situation where each commissioning authority is deciding individually what it will fund, and where providing authorities are deciding what they can afford to offer, the absence of a central commitment to plan priorities is more critical (Allsop and May 1993, Ham 1994b).

Perhaps the most remarkable aspect of the health service changes is the way in which the identification of long-term objectives has lagged behind the structural changes. For example, the White Paper, *The Health of the Nation* (Secretary of State for Health 1992) was published nearly two years after the NHS Act. Furthermore, although this document sets targets for the reduction of mortality and morbidity, it does not offer any commitment to the policies and resources needed to achieve these targets. Minogue has commented that the ideology of better management was all too frequently offered as a solution to what was simplistically diagnosed as bureaucratic inadequacy. The real issue, he argued, was policy failure (Minogue 1983). Although for the first time an inter-departmental committee now has the remit to look at health issues, so far silence has been a more conspicuous output than activity (Hunter 1991). The committee does not have a dedicated budget, and so its deliberations are unlikely to be high on anyone's agenda.

Sir Roy Griffiths, a former chairman of the retail grocery chain, Sainsbury's, made clear in his 1991 Audit Commission lecture that he would have preferred different implementation priorities:

> Major policy issues were left uncovered. There was no attempt to establish objectives at the centre and no concentration on outcomes.
>
> (Griffiths 1992: 64)

A number of groups have called for a more effective planning framework for the NHS. For example, Liddle and Parston (1993) argue that a consistent and coherent framework of health and quality objectives is needed to guide purchasing. Unless all purchasers are signed up to the wider framework, it will be impossible to develop strategies to meet those objectives consistently and equitably. They also believe that if value and quality are going to improve, robust, long-term relationships between purchasers and providers need to be developed.

From the comments of both politicians and NHS managers it is possible to discern two approaches to the new NHS. There are those who embrace competition and who see the market as an effective way of reducing the costs to the public of NHS care. Conversely, there are those who see in the reforms an opportunity to build more collaborative relationships to plan for a more effective service without losing the traditional values of the old NHS.

Accountability

Major concerns have arisen in relation to accountability as a consequence of the reforms. One of the problems is a lack of clarity about which part of the Department of Health (DOH) and the NHSME is responsible for what. In a discussion of the Next Steps programme, Bogdanor (1990) explained that when agencies are involved, ministers will be responsible to Parliament for policy as opposed to operational matters. But who defines 'policy', and who distinguishes it from matters of operational management? It is likely, he claims, that ministers will take the credit for successes, while the chief executives of agencies will be blamed for failure. This is even more likely when a strong policy commitment is lacking at the centre.

At local level, the policy vacuum raises issues of accountability to local populations. The culture of the NHS has always been inward-looking, and now Trusts, in particular, run the risk of promoting their own corporate values and identity at the expense of collective goals. Managers and professionals may collude to shut out public scrutiny. Members of Trust Boards and commissioning agencies, both of which are modelled on private sector boards of directors, are political appointments. Recent research has shown that the majority are run by white, male businessmen from private sector backgrounds (Cairncross and Ashburne 1992).

At the level of the HAs which commission for services, there is also a lack of accountability. Many managers, uncertain of their role and remit, are anxiously searching for a magic formula that will cloak the decisions they make on behalf of their populations in some semblance of what they hope will be value-neutral rationality (May 1992). Sabin, an American doctor on sabbatical in the UK, found purchasers to be worried about their lack of legitimacy in the eyes of their local populations (Sabin 1992). And even though they were trying to 'cultivate legitimacy' by doing surveys, attempting to create some form of dialogue with their local communities and establishing links with general practitioners, he warns that their position is highly vulnerable. When shrouds begin to wave and real needs cannot be met, he says, purchasers will be in the front line. But there are no structures for local accountability and the public debate on issues of 'rationing' and priorities has scarcely begun.

Even if managers running commissioning authorities are driven by a concern for consumer interests, it is far from clear how they will know what these interests are. The increasing diversity of provider agencies makes it difficult to assess whether there is an accessible and adequate range of basic services. While commissioning authorities have confidently declared their intention to meet health care needs within available resources, making choices involves major ethical issues. So far, political debate has been minimal, and mechanisms for consulting and informing individuals and communities have yet to be developed.

Many of the new agencies now cover far larger geographical areas than the district health authorities they have replaced. And unlike US members of Health Maintenance Organisations, who can make the choice to buy into a particular scheme, individuals in the UK have no choice between purchasers. As the former controller of the Audit Commission, Howard Davies, points out, it will be some time before NHS users appreciate the implications of the purchaser/provider split with its new structure of responsibilities (Davies 1992).

Another issue related to accountability is regulation. Who regulates the Boards of the various agencies within the patchwork quilt? Will the new arrangements for scrutiny by regional offices be sufficient? At their best, the Boards of provider units and Trusts may achieve greater value for money and good quality services for their patients. But who will take action where standards are poor? Patients often cannot judge whether or not they are receiving appropriate health care. Those working within the organisation have an incentive to collude. The accountability of commissioning agencies is altogether more nebulous, and it is here that the policy vacuum is the most serious. Some managers have attempted to fill this by developing principles on which to base policy. For example, East Anglian region uses accessibility and equity among its criteria while focusing on particular disease categories where mortality and morbidity rates are high. But how can the users of services be involved in the decisions being made on their behalf?

The question of accountability throws up yet another issue. Where should citizens turn for redress of their grievances: to the Minister, to their MP, to the manager? It is part of the enduring legacy of Thatcherism that citizens have become consumers, with all the loss of rights which that means (Wilding 1992). While what the *Financial Times* referred to as 'a raft of charters' floats out from Whitehall, and while every local unit appears to be producing its own individual Patient's Charter with a confusing mixture of citizen's rights and customer service standards, the result is ultimately a diffusion of responsibility. In addition, these charters are already placing enormous pressure on junior and frontline staff (Paton 1992). They are expected to cope with nationally imposed criteria and raised consumer expectations without the allocation of additional resources for training or increased investment in facilities. These issues are discussed further in Chapter 12.

The politics of the new NHS

It has been suggested above that governments have aimed to steer a course between competition and regulation – although they have been accused of achieving neither. This attempt to balance both approaches may reflect the high regard with which the public holds the NHS. The Major governments have been unwilling to let the market operate to destabilise the service.

At the local level, the greater diversity of agencies and circumstances has brought a parallel variety in local NHS politics. A crucial factor is the extent of monopoly or competition as well as personal relationships between those on either side of the commissioner/provider divide. Future researchers will have a rich vein to tap in observing and accounting for local practice. So far, there has been limited research indicative of the changing relationships between the main groups of providers rather than specific local circumstances.

A number of commentators have suggested that the financial crisis in health service funding at the end of the 1980s and the uncertainty as well as the opportunities created by the NHS reforms have forged a more cohesive cadre of managers who have taken the lead in their organisations (Barrett and McMahon 1990; Hoggett 1991; Flynn 1992; Harrison, Hunter, Marnoch and Pollitt 1992). It is argued that managers now determine the agenda of change and negotiate strategy. But the role and task of managers in Trusts and those in commissioning agencies are now very different. Within Trusts, clinicians must work within business plans laid down by Boards: within directorates they work alongside managers to determine priorities. Decisions about patient care once patients are in hospital and issues of standards of care remain the terrain of clinicians who work through a process of medical audit. The degree to which there is management domination probably varies with local circumstances. Clinicians who are skilled and also good managers probably have greater rewards and autonomy in the new NHS. However, the contraction of services in many metropolitan areas, particularly London, will create redundancies in the profession on a scale not experienced hitherto.

There are those who are concerned with the greater dominance of the managerial agenda and believe that a concentration on competition will drive out commitment to the ethic of socially responsible management which has been part of the tradition of the NHS. Stewart (1991) argues, in the context of local government, that the main challenge for public sector managers in the 1990s is to provide services which meet the needs of local populations and are also responsive to individual requirements. He sees the solution to this as managers working closely with professionals. The management task will be to design the conditions in which the professionals can operate – helping them to update and adapt their knowledge and skills to meet changing conditions. Stewart goes on to warn that if an organisational balance is not maintained, there is a danger of management itself becoming too rigid. The public sector, he claims, may turn into a series of fragments, each with its own defined purpose and its own performance measures.

Problems of funding

The issue of underfunding has been a continuing theme in the history of the NHS. The official NHS historian, Charles Webster, claims that 'the problem of the early NHS was not profligacy but resource starvation' (Webster 1988).

Successive governments have pinned down health expenditure to unrealistically low levels. This, he argues, has been a false economy. Questions of finance have always dominated the agenda and they continue to do so. Although health care expenditure has risen rapidly, in 1990 the UK's total health spending still remained among the lowest in the developed world, one quarter below the EC average. Document 29 (page 345) provides comparative figures. And while market mechanisms may make efficiency gains at the margins they cannot compensate for underfunding. It is possible that the costs of change have taken funding away from patient care with little real benefit in organisational efficiency.

Conclusion

The main aim of the 1990 NHS reforms was to contain costs and achieve greater value for money, by introducing competition on the supply side of services. Although it was claimed that the principles of the NHS were unchanged, in the rush to implement the changes, the pursuit of other goals took second place. What research has taken place is inconclusive as to the effects of the reforms on measures such as costs and efficiency and equity. What governments have attempted to do is bring about a balance between regulation and competition. There is evidence of some successes and some failures on both counts. An overall evaluation is not possible in the continuing climate of change.

The serious problems which have dogged the NHS throughout its history still remain. Government continues to strike a balance between cost-containment and adequate funding and the pros and cons of medical and managerial decision-making, although the roles and tasks of each have been fundamentally altered in the reforms. Issues of public accountability remain and have yet to be resolved.

The break-up of the NHS into a variety of sometimes competing agencies with both commissioning and providing roles suggests that the politics of the NHS is now more localised and more volatile. The split between the Department of Health headquarters in London where strategy is determined and the Management Executive in Leeds which leads operational management diffuses the locus of power and makes structured corporate politics less likely. What is not clear is how strongly the Department of Health will lead on issues of policy and planning in the future, how much they will impose prescriptions and how far they will prevent market forces from driving out unviable hospitals.

Government has pledged to retain a commitment to the core values of the NHS, spelt out in Chapter 2. However, there are no easy answers to how these obligations can be met. Osborne and Gaebler, who are advocates of a strong steering role for government, argue that government must structure the market-place to meet social needs (1992: 312–13). Mintzberg (1989), an American writer on management, argues that we have to 'trust' managers in this respect because we have little alternative. Nevertheless, as citizens and users of the NHS, we must be prepared ceaselessly to apply pressure; to try to democratise decision-making, regulate where necessary and induce change where possible.

References

Abel-Smith, B. (1992) 'Cost containment and new priorities in the European Community', *The Milbank Quarterly*, 70 (3), pp. 393–416.

Allsop, J. and May, A. (1993) 'Between the Devil and the Deep Blue Sea: managing the NHS in the wake of the 1990 Act', *Critical Social Policy*, 38, pp. 5–22.

Appleby, J. (1993) 'NHS Purchasing Decisions are Still Not Explicit', *British Medical Journal*, 307, p. 1376.

Ashburner, L., Ferlie, E. and Fitzgerald, L. (1993) *Boards and Authorities in Action*, NHS Paper II, National Training Directorate, Bristol.

Audit Commission (1993) 'Their Health, Your Business: the new role of the District Health Authority', Audit Commission, London.

Barrett, S. and McMahon, L. (1990) 'Public Management in Uncertainty: A Micro-Political Perspective of the Health Service in the UK', *Policy and Politics*, 4, 18, 257–68.

Bartlett, W. and Le Grand, J. (1994) 'The Performance of NHS Trusts: what does the early research tell us?' in Robinson, R. and Le Grand, J. (eds) *Evaluating the NHS Reforms*, King's Fund Institute, London.

Bogdanor, V. (1990) 'The Problem of Making Whitehall Accountable', *Financial Times*, 8 March.

Bradburn, J., Kershaw, M. and Allsop, J. (1994) 'Eye-opener,' *Health Service Journal*, 4 August.

Bradlow, J. and Coulter, A. (1993) 'Effect of Fundholding and Indicative Prescribing Schemes on General Practitioners' Prescribing Costs', *British Medical Journal*, 307, pp. 1186–9.

Butler, J. (1992) *Patients, Policies and Politics: Before and after Working for Patients*, Open University Press, Milton Keynes.

Cairncross, I. and Ashburne, R. L. (1992) *NHS Trust Boards: the first wave, – the first year*, Centre for Corporate Strategy and Change, Warwick University.

Chartered Institute of Public Finance and Accountancy (1993) *Health Service Statistics*, 1992, CIPFA, London.

Coulter, A. and Bradlow, J. (1993) 'The Effect of the NHS Reforms on General Practitioners' Referral Patterns', *British Medical Journal*, 306, pp. 433–7.

Davies, H. (1992) *Fighting Leviathan: building social markets that work*, The Social Market Foundation, London.

Day, P. and Klein, R. (1991) 'Political Theory and Policy Practice: the case of general practice 1911–1991', Paper presented at the Political Studies Association Conference, University of Lancaster.

Department of Health (1992a) *The Health of the Nation*, HMSO, London.

Department of Health (1992b) *Health and Personal Social Services Statistics for England, 1992 edition,* HMSO, London.

Department of Health (1993) *Managing the New NHS,* DOH, London.

Department of Health (1994) *Managing the new NHS: functions and responsibilities in the new NHS*, DOH, London.

Drummond, M. and Maynard, A. (eds) (1993) *Purchasing and Providing Cost-effective Health Care*, Churchill Livingstone, London.

Enthoven, A. (1985) *Reflections on the Management of the NHS*, Occasional Paper 5, Nuffield Provincial Hospitals Trust.

Ferlie, E., Cairncross, I. and Pettigrew, A. (1992), 'Understanding Internal Markets in the NHS', in Tilley, I. (ed.), *Managing the International Markets*, Chapman & Hall, London.

Flynn, R. (1992) *Structures of Control in Health Management*, Routledge, London.

Glennerster, H., Matsaganis, M. and Owens, P. (1992) 'A Foothold for Fundraising', Research Report, no. 12, King's Fund Institute, London.

Glennerster, H., Matsaganis, M., Owens, P. and Hancock, S. (1994) 'GP Fundholding: wild card or winning hand?' in Robinson, R. and Le Grand, J. (eds), *Evaluating the NHS Reforms*, King's Fund Institute, London.

Griffiths, R. (1992) *Seven Years of Progress – general management in the NHS*. The third annual Audit Commission lecture, 1991, *Health Economics*, 1 (1), pp. 61–70.

Ham, C. (1993) 'The Odd Couple', *Health Services Journal*, 23 September, pp. 28–9.

Ham, C. (1994a) 'Think Globally and Act Locally', 13 January, pp. 27–8.

Ham, C. (1994b) 'Priority Setting in the NHS', *British Medical Journal*, 307, pp. 435–8.

Ham, C. and Matthews, T. (1991) 'Locality Purchasing', King's Fund Institute, London.

Hansard (1993) *Written Answer*, Dr Mawhiney, 4 November, London.

Harrison, S., Hunter, D., Marnock, G. and Pollitt, C. (1992) *Just Managing: Power; and Culture in the NHS*, Macmillan, London.

Harrison S. and Bartlett, W. (1993) 'The NHS Reforms' in Le Grand, J.

and Bartlett, W. (eds), *Quasi-Markets and Public Policy*, Macmillan, London.

Hill, A., Milne, R. and Hawke, C. (1993) 'Waits and Measures', *Health Service Journal*, 12 August, pp. 24–5.

Hoggett, P. (1991) 'A New Management in the Public Sector', *Policy and Politics*, 4 (19), pp. 243–56.

Hood, C. (1991) 'A Public Management for All Seasons', *Public Administration*, 69 (Spring), pp. 3–19.

Hudson, B. (1992) 'Quasi-markets in Health and Social Care in Britain: can the public sector respond?', *Policy and Politics*, 20 (2), pp. 131–42.

Hunter, D. (1991) 'The Health Strategy and the Hole at the Centre', *British Medical Journal*, 303, p. 1350.

Illife, S. (1993) 'General Practitioners and Incentives', *British Medical Journal*, 307, pp. 1156–7.

Layzell, A. (1994) 'Local and Vocal', *Health Services Journal*, 20 January, pp. 28–30.

Le Grand, J. (1992) 'Paying for or Providing Welfare', Paper for Social Policy Association Annual Conference, University of Nottingham, July.

Le Grand, J. and Bartlett, W.L. (1994) *Quasi-markets and Social Policy*, Macmillan, London.

Liddle, A. and Parston, G. (1993) *Effective Management of the NHS*, IPPR, London.

Mahon, A., Wilkin, D. and Whitehouse, C. (1994) 'Choice of hospital for elective surgery referrals: GPs' and patients' views' in Robinson, R. and Le Grand, J. (eds) *Evaluating the NHS Reforms*, King's Fund Institute, London.

May, A. (1992) 'Smack, crack and prop', *The Health Service Journal*, 22 October, p.15.

Maynard, A. (1991) 'The New NHS: towards a better outcome?', *Health Direct*, NAHAT, Birmingham.

Maynard, A. and Hutton, J. (1992) 'Health Care Reform: the search for the holy grail', *Health Economics*, 1 (1), pp. 1–3.

Minogue, M. (1983) 'Theory and Practice in Public Policy and Administration', *Public Policy*, 11 (1), pp. 63–85.

Mintzberg, H. (1989) *Mintzberg on Management: inside our strange world of organisations*, Collier Macmillan, London.

Newchurch and Company Ltd (1993) *The Third Newchurch Guide to NHS Trusts*, Newchurch & Company, London.

NHSME (1991) *Local Voices*, NHSME, Leeds.

NHSME (1993) *Public Health: responsibilities of the NHS and the roles of others*, HSG (93)56, Leeds.

Osborne, D. and Gaebler, T. (1992) *Reinventing Government*, Addison Wesley, Mass.

Owen, G. (1991) 'Twin-track Talent at the Top – the Monday Interview', *Financial Times*, 4 February.

Paton, C. (1992) 'Firm Control: creeping centralisation in the NHS', *The Health Service Journal*, 6 August, pp. 20–2.

Public Accounts Committee (1993) *West Midlands RHA, Regionally managed services organisation*, 57th Report of the PAC, HMSO, London.

Public Accounts Committee (1994), 8th Report of the PAC, HMSO, London.

Rafferty, J. and Gibson, G. (1994) 'Banking on Knowledge', *Health Service Journal*, 10 February, pp. 28–30.

Redmayne, S., Klein, R. and Day, P. (1993) 'Sharing our Resources: purchasing and priority setting in the NHS', NAHAT, Birmingham.

Robinson, R. and Le Grand, J. (1994) *Evaluating the NHS Reforms*, King's Fund Institute, London.

Sabin, J. (1992) '"Mind the Gap": reflections of an American health maintenance organisation doctor on the new NHS', *British Medical Journal*, 305, 29 August, pp. 514–16.

Salter, B. (1992) 'Policy Paradox and the Rationing Issue; managing the tensions', Medway Research Programme, Centre for Health Services Studies, University of Kent, Canterbury.

Secretary of State for Health (1989) *Working for Patients*, Cmnd 555 HMSO, London.

Stewart, J. (1991) 'Professionalism, Politics and Public Service', in *Managers and Professionals: Report on a one day conference organised by the Office of Public Management*, Office of Public Management, London.

Stockford, D. (1993) 'Perspectives on Purchasing', *Health Service Journal*, 9 December, pp. 20–3.

Timmins, N. (1989) 'Is the Health Service Safe in their Hands?' *Independent*, 9 February.

Webster, C. (1988) 'Confronting historical myth', in May, A. (ed.), *What future for the NHS? Thoughts for the Prime Minister's Review* in *The Health Service Journal*, 19 May.

Whitehead, M. (1994) 'Is it Fair? Evaluating the equity implications of the NHS reforms', in Robinson, R. and Le Grand, J., *Evaluating the NHS Reforms*, King's Fund Institute, London.

Wilding, P. (1992) 'The British Welfare State; Thatcherism's enduring legacy', *Policy and Politics*, 20 (3), pp. 201–12.

CHAPTER 10

General practice in the new NHS

After years of relative neglect, since the mid-1980s general practice has become a focus for government policy. Following the White Paper, *Promoting Better Health* (DHSS 1987), a new contract of employment was negotiated in 1989. With the health reforms of 1990 and the introduction of GP fundholding and its planned extension during the 1990s, general practice has become a central rather than a peripheral platform for health care delivery. This chapter aims to examine the factors which have led to this policy shift, its new direction and its consequences. It is argued that more support needs to be provided for general practice for it to fulfil its potential.

What is general practice?

General practice is a term covering the services provided by medical practitioners in the community. Unlike many other health systems, the UK has retained GPs as generalist doctors for first-line care. Since 1970, qualified doctors wishing to enter general practice must undertake vocational training – that is, postgraduate training in this area of medicine. GPs may take further examinations to become members of the Royal College of General Practitioners. In 1994, almost half of them have done so (personal communication RCGP).

Since 1948, GPs have provided services under contract to the NHS. This has allowed them considerable autonomy to practise. For patients registered with them, GPs have provided access to 24-hour care. A GP may maintain night-time cover personally or make arrangements with another doctor or a deputising service to do so. GPs are available for consultation in the surgery or, if necessary, they will visit the patient at home. They are first-line diagnosticians – referring the patient to hospital for further specialist treatment or to health or social workers in the community for other needs. In this way, they are an avenue to caring services in the community.

Since 1990, general medical services have been managed by FHSAs which are also responsible for the other family practitioner services provided by dentists, pharmacists and opticians. Additional community services such as district nursing, health visiting, health education and so on are currently managed by community trusts. Together, the FHSA and community service supply what is known as primary health care (DHSS 1986a).

In the UK, general practice is a collection of small businesses providing comprehensive and continuing care. About 93 per cent of the population is registered with an NHS GP. Patients may choose their doctor although this choice is dependent on geography (for patients in remote areas, it is theoretical). Doctors also have the freedom to decline to take a patient on to their list or may remove one from it. The arrangement is based on the view that because the relationship between the doctor and patient is special there should be an element of mutual compatibility. A minority of patients have difficulty in registering with a GP. As a last resort, the FHSA may assign them to a practice for a period of six months.

A small percentage of the population is not registered at all. Among these are those who are most vulnerable to ill-health – homeless people or those living in temporary accommodation. GPs do not have an obligation to take on people with no fixed address, but some FHSAs and GPs have made special arrangements to deal with this problem.

Continuity of patient care is maintained through the patients' medical record – this moves with the patient if they change practices. Most people have a long-term relationship with their practice. Although the majority of consultations take place in the doctor's surgery, patients may request a visit in their home and the doctor must decide whether the patient's condition warrants such action. Home visits constitute about 15 per cent of consultations. Most GPs do not continue to care for their patients in hospital unless they have access to a community hospital which offers nursing care and rehabilitation. Continuity between those involved in the patient's treatment is maintained by letter or telephone.

GPs deal with most illness in the community and are responsible for about 90 per cent of the overall number of patient contacts. On average, patients visit their GP between four and five times per annum. Although this has changed little over the years the rate at which GPs refer their patients to hospitals has tended to increase. By 1991, the average GP had 7000 consultations a year of which 240 involved referral to a specialist (Coulter 1992a).

Trends in general practice

Patterns of practice and team-working

The number of GPs in England and Wales has been rising slowly. In 1993, there were about 30,000 GP principals – almost twice the

Table 10.1 **Trends in general practice in England and Wales, 1980–1990**

	1980	*1990*
Number of GPs	25 000	30 000
and av. list size	2 150	1 900
Number of practice nurses	1 000	8 000
Other employed staff	22 000	48 000
Number of prescriptions	345 million	395 million

Source: Adapted from *Audit Commission* (1993).

number of hospital doctors at consultant grade. The doctors' list size has been falling, as Table 10.1 indicates. Practices have tended to increase in size. In 1990, almost 60 per cent of practices contained four or more doctors, about 30 per cent had two to three doctors and less than 10 per cent were single-handed. In 1952, by contrast, almost 50 per cent of GPs were single-handed. During the 1980s, there were also large increases in the numbers of staff employed by GPs, particularly in the figures for practice nurses (Audit Commission 1993).

Team-working: Efforts have also been made to develop team-working in general practice. The Harding Committee defined this in the following way:

> . . . the primary health care team is an interdependent of general medical practitioners and secretaries and/or receptionists, health visitors, district nurses and midwives who share a common purpose and responsibility, each member clearly understanding his or her own function and those of other members, so that they all pool skills and knowledge to provide an effective primary health care service.
>
> (DHSS 1981: 2)

The development of the primary health care team was first recommended by the Gillie Committee on the role of the family doctor (Ministry of Health 1963). It was hoped that the 1974 re-organisation would facilitate the development of primary health care teams and greater integration of GP services by establishing structures and mechanisms for planning and coordination. This, like many aspects of the reorganisation, proved to be over-optimistic. Changes in structure did not alter intrinsic difficulties. As independent contractors, GPs choose their own mode of operation for their patients and the geographical area they cover. The attachment of staff brought GPs into a relationship with the organisational structure of community nurses and raised questions of the management and the leadership of the resulting teams. As

Styles (1994) points out, with the NHS reforms, team-working has become increasingly important but nevertheless remains a challenge.

Attachment could either be achieved through the employment of staff in the practice or through arrangements made with the community health services to second nursing and other staff to the practice. There have been many obstacles to developing team-working in the latter case, not least because community staff work to different goals and within different organisational structures. For GPs a particular problem in urban areas was the lack of overlap between the practice population and the areas covered by community staff. In 1981, the Harding Committee (DHSS 1981), which was set up to investigate the primary care team, found evidence of wasteful overlap as well as poor service coverage. For example, in one urban Area Health Authority it was estimated that 10,000 children out of a target population of 70,000 were not receiving visits when nurses were attached. The discontinuities between community services and general practice remain. The difficulty of reconciling the different modes of primary care organisation presents a stumbling block particularly in meeting the needs of elderly and chronically disabled people.

The role of general practice

The organisation of general practice in the UK has been generally considered to have a number of advantages, such as its efficacy and cost. Because it is organised around illness in individuals, families and communities – rather than along the lines of medical specialisms – it has the potential for embracing the curative, caring and preventive aspects of medicine. It is also claimed that general practice is holistic. Thus, it provides care by someone who knows the patient (Gillie 1963), and the illnesses which individuals present can be seen in the context of their lives and their health behaviour. The disadvantage of generalist practice is that inevitably, the GP knows a little about everything but has special expertise in nothing. However, the essential skill of GPs lies in being able to recognise serious illness and refer. They can be said to protect the patient from unnecessary hospitalisation.

Because general practice is provided in small units, at least in urban and suburban areas, there is usually a practice within 'pram-pushing distance'. In rural areas, GPs may overcome the necessity for patients to travel by holding surgeries in village halls or even people's living rooms. Since 1948, a central Medical Practices Committee has had a remit to review the spread of GPs within areas of about 30,000 population to ensure an even distribution throughout the country. Areas have been designated in categories from 'open' where any GP can set up a practice, to 'restricted', where there are already sufficient doctors. By 1984, there were no severely under-doctored areas; about 10 per cent were relatively under-doctored; another 10 per cent were over-doctored where no new practices could be set up; the remaining districts had an appropriate 'balance'.

General practice is flexible and relatively inexpensive as it requires only a low-level technology – making it a cost-effective form of delivery care. While treating the vast majority of illnesses, it absorbs only about 15 per cent of the NHS funding. Until the end of the 1980s, the family practitioner services were demand-led and not cash-limited. In 1991, their share of the NHS budget devoted was about 24 per cent, of which expenditure on family doctors and the drugs they prescribe was about 70 per cent. In the 1990s, the slice of expenditure taken by general practice has been rising relative to other areas of the NHS (Taylor 1991, Audit Commission 1993). Table 10.2 shows the figures.

General practice provides a screening device for more expensive hospital care. But for patients, the GP may be perceived as a barrier as well as a gateway. Indeed there are inherent tensions in the GP–patient role. While GPs can be in touch with the needs of individuals in a way which few other health workers can, they may restrict entry to other forms of care. Cartwright (1967) and

Table 10.2 **NHS expenditure in England and Wales on family health services 1991–92**

	Percentage	*Cost: millions of £*
Pharmacists' renumeration	9	631
Dental	19	1 298
Opthalmic	2	152
Medical	34	2 382
Pharmacist	36	2 522
Total	100	5 254

Source: Adapted from *Audit Commission* (1993).

Table 10.3 **Aspects of primary care seen in need of improvement 1987–91**

% saying that each is in need of 'a lot' or 'some' improvement	*1987*	*1989*	*1990*	*1991*
GP appointment systems	47	45	41	44
Amount of time with each patient	33	34	31	29
Waiting time at GP's surgery	na	na	28	27
Being able to choose which GP to see	29	30	27	26
Quality of medical treatment by GPs	26	27	24	26

Source: Adapted from Bosanquet, N. (1993).

Cartwright and Anderson (1981) have explored the concerns of patients and GPs through national surveys and identified areas where the priorities of GPs and patient differ. Table 10.3 shows the results of a more recent study of patients' concerns.

The status of GPs

GPs are a key professional group in the functioning of the modern welfare state. Their role goes beyond dealing with the sick in the community and acting as gatekeeper to more costly hospital care – it also includes certification of unfitness for work. In common with the medical profession as a whole, GPs have benefited from the social and cultural authority accorded to medical practitioners and from the institutions which limit competition and provide self-regulation. For example, they were guaranteed a long career as there was, until 1990 when it was set at 70, no statutory retirement age. They were, and are, a powerful structured-interest group well represented at national level through the British Medical Association. An effective network of local committees can quickly bring matters of regional concern on to the national agenda.

Unlike other doctors employed in the NHS, GPs are self-employed – a status they negotiated in 1946. Subsequently, this status has been a symbol of independence from NHS management and is a jealously guarded privilege. From 1948 to the mid-1980s, the bodies administering GP contracts, the Executive Councils and then the Family Practitioner Committees (FPCs), by and large played a limited 'pay and rations' function. This began to change in the mid-1980s and is discussed below.

Although GPs are paid by the state, the level of remuneration is determined nationally through a review body which negotiates on the basis of a target average income. Since 1966, the level of GP income has been equivalent to that of a hospital consultant. The remuneration received is tantamount to a salary based on a mixture of capitation, fees for certain services and reimbursement of costs. Practice premises are regarded as private property; they may belong to the GP and represent a capital investment or be rented. The FPC/FHSA must gain permission to inspect premises. Perhaps more important, from the point of view of managing the service, are the practical implications of the way GPs practise. The large number of small units makes surveillance of activity difficult. Decision-making takes place in the intimacy of the surgery or home in the light of what the doctor perceives to be the needs of the patient. There are considerable variations between practitioners in the way they work.

In many ways, GPs had made a favourable bargain with the state. Until the mid-1980s, there was virtually no knowledge about, or scrutiny of, the day-to-day work of GPs apart from some monitoring of prescribing from peers or others. The type of practice, who was employed, the decisions made about treatment and care were matters for individual decision and judgement and GPs did not have to consider the financial consequences of their clinical decisions to refer. Moreover, GPs' patients have been slow to exercise 'voice' in relation to the service received and the lack of information given to them has made 'exit' from one practice to another difficult. In effect, GPs have acted as small monopolistic suppliers of primary care as they have determined what was available and have dominated the division of labour in the practice.

General practice and health policy in the 1980s

The policy shift to primary care

A number of factors contributed to the shift towards primary care during the 1980s. First, there were general socio-demographic factors. General practice was well placed to provide clinical leadership for the care of elderly and mentally ill people in the community.

Second, there were the findings of studies and research which showed that the standards of GP practice were sometimes low, the more so in already deprived areas. In 1981, the Acheson Report on inner London showed that general practice was poor in areas of higher social deprivation in the capital. For example, a high number of very elderly GPs were still practising; compared to other parts of the country, there was also a large proportion of single-handed GPs; there were many premises with poor telephone-answering services, and low numbers of additional staff were employed. In essence, primary care teams had not developed sufficiently and there was a perceived need to improve standards overall. (London Health Planning Consortium 1981.)

A third factor which encouraged a policy shift was external to the NHS. In 1978, the World Health Organisation in its Alma-Ata declaration stressed the importance of health for all (Document 22 p. 327). By 1985, targets had been set in order to achieve 'health for all by the year 2000' (WHO 1985). There were six major themes; the need to reduce inequalities in health status and the importance of health promotion and the prevention of disease, of motivating people in a concern for health, of multi-sectoral cooperation, of the primary health care sector and of international cooperation. Although the UK was relatively slow to respond to the WHO initiative (see Chapter 11), it saw the logic in strengthening primary care as this was cost-effective.

Over the years, there had been a drift towards hospital medicine. Many activities which could be undertaken in the community had shifted to the hospital (Honigsbaum 1985). Yet a few general practices showed what could be done – some offered clinics for diabetes and asthma patients, some had developed methods of screening elderly populations to identify those at risk (Taylor 1991), others enlarged a range of staff including those with counselling or paramedical skills such as physiotherapy.

A fourth element was the increasing emphasis on the prevention of ill-health. The GP was well placed to extend services in this way because most of the population were registered with them. In addition, the FHSA held the registration data for a larger area and this provided a basis for the practice of 'population medicine'. At-risk groups could be identified and contacted for screening or health surveillance. The local general practice could carry out the tests or checks and provide feedback for the patient, giving health advice.

A final factor explaining the shift to primary care was that it fitted comfortably with neo-liberal Conservative values. General practice, with its large number of units, could compete for patients, if they could be made more business-like. FHSAs, through monitoring and regulation, could raise service standards. In the US, health maintenance organisations (HMOs) had developed along these lines.

Conservative policies for primary care

The above account may suggest that Conservative policies towards primary care progressed according to a preconceived design. It is much more likely that policy evolved as Conservative thinking developed the programme to introduce market forces into public services. It is suggested, for example, that GP fundholding was introduced into *Working for Patients* (Secretary of State for Health 1989) as an afterthought (Butler 1992).

In 1985, the first step was taken by Kenneth Clarke, the then Minister for Health, to give additional powers to Family Practitioners Committees (FPCs) to 'manage' as opposed to 'administer' the contracts of family practitioners. FPCs were required to 'plan' the provision of primary care service for their populations. The change revealed that although FPCs had the responsibility for so doing, they had little power. While a few FPCs were working alongside their GPs to improve the service, many continued to play a traditional 'pay and rations' role (Allsop and May 1986).

In the mid-1980s, two reports provided alternative policy options for primary care reform. The Cumberledge Report on Neighbourhood Nursing (DHSS 1986b) proposed that a senior community nurse should provide the leadership for locally based community nursing services. In the same year a Green Paper, on improving primary health care (DHSS 1986a), recommended that general practice should become the focus for its provision. The prevention of ill-health could develop from general practices using nurses employed by them. The Green Paper also floated the idea of 'health care shops', places where a range of health practitioners and associated goods could be found. The idea was coolly received and dropped from the subsequent White Paper.

Following a period of consultation, the White Paper, *Promoting Better Health* (DHSS 1987), proposed a strong leading role for general practice in dealing with illness and promoting health. In a crucial step, which undercut community nursing, additional resources were made available to encourage GPs to employ practice staff to increase their activity and carry out more health surveillance. *Promoting Better Health* also contained a range of measures to make general practice more susceptible to market forces. GPs were to produce practice leaflets to provide information for patients. FPCs were asked to carry out consumer surveys. It was made easier for patients to change their doctor – patients no longer had to get the doctor to sign their medical card before transferring to another GP.

One of the stumbling blocks to change was the GPs' contract of employment. Drawn up initially in the 1940s, this had changed little since the 1960s. In 1990, despite opposition from the GPs – more than 70 per cent rejected the revised version presented by their negotiating body – a new contract (DOH 1989) was introduced. The stated aims were to give consumers more choice by providing information; to make the terms of service more specific so that all practices were encouraged to provide services already available from the best practices; to make the system of payment more performance-related; and to strengthen the role of the FHSA in monitoring this performance and to ensure greater value for money. The most important aspects of the new contract are summarised in Document 28 (page 343).

GPs were to become more accountable to the FHSA. They had to provide more data on practice activity and produce annual reports; prescribe within indicative budgets; offer an annual home visit to patients over 75 and assess their needs; offer a health check for new patients; meet targets for vaccination, immunisation and cervical cytology; and if providing child health surveillance, they were required to follow locally determined protocols. Additional payments were made conditional on meeting targets for prevention and money was available for health promotion clinics. Changes to the payment system created incentives to attract increased numbers of patients. The amount which could be earned through capitation rose by 60 per cent. At the same time, GPs came under greater surveillance from FHSAs.

The other side of the coin was increased responsibility for FHSAs. They had to monitor activity and assess whether targets had been met to qualify for additional payments. They had a carrot in the form of a budget to allocate funds for practice staff, computers and premises differentially. About 10 per cent of the allocated budget could be used for discretionary payments – for instance, to persuade practices to develop new services. FHSAs could also appoint independent professional advisers to support practices and to encourage medical audit. The composition of FHSAs was changed. Members were still appointed by the Secretary of State but, like the District Health Authorities, they were now chosen for their business and management skills. Professional representation, which had previously constituted half the membership, was drastically reduced; for example, there was only one doctor on the committee.

To summarise, the regulation of GP activity was increased and GPs were required to provide more services. The method of payment was changed to introduce financial incentives to carry out more medical work within the practice – such as minor surgery or specialist clinics. There was an implicit emphasis on planning and providing a range of health care services for a practice population. The FHSA was expected to assess population needs, decide on priorities and develop a plan of action. By implication, primary care was to be more actively managed to ensure that practices were responding to the health needs of the community.

The 1990 reforms and general practice

The 1990 reforms have already been described in the previous chapter. Under these arrangements, GP fundholders play a role in commissioning services from hospitals. They are also providers of primary care and are commissioned by the FHSA on the basis of an assessment of the health needs of the area. The aim in introducing fundholding was to give a 'kick-start' to the NHS reforms.

In 1991, GPs in practices with populations of more than 9000 could opt to become general practice fundholders (GPFHs). This gave them the ability to purchase certain hospital services, such as elective referrals to hospitals, outpatient visits and diagnostic services, up to a cumulative cost of £5000 per patient. There was an additional allowance for prescribing, management and computing costs. The funding made available to GPFHs was deducted from the DHA budget at regional level. In 1993, the minimum size of practice qualifying for fundholding status fell to 7000. Also, additional funds were made available to GPFHs to purchase community care services. This puts GPs in a pivotal position to buy the whole range of services for their practice populations and therefore to manage primary care delivery. Morris (1993) describes how this can be done.

GPs who are not fundholders may also be able to influence the commissioning process. DHAs have developed a variety of methods for involving practitioners. However, their influence is less direct as it does not involve monetary transactions. Some GPs have developed alliances with other practices to apply greater pressure in the contracting process.

There are clearly incentives for GPs to become fundholders in terms of the autonomy which this gives. Fundholders are proxy buyers on behalf of their practice and hold a strong bargaining position on behalf of their patients (Hughes 1993). It is also advantageous financially. Savings can be used to extend and improve practices and the patients of GPFHs have received priority treatment from Trusts. Because they are small compared to DHA commissioners, GPFHs can be more flexible in placing contracts or buying extra contractual referrals. For Trusts, these contracts provide useful additional income. So, despite the loss of influence at FHSA level after their representation was reduced to only one doctor, GPs have gained in other respects.

A further aspect of the health service reforms has been the stress on better information for the consumer. GPs are expected to produce practice leaflets while FHSAs are encouraged to find out what people want through surveys and consultation with local groups. This information is then used to influence their purchase of services. Although there are examples of GPs consulting with their patients about purchasing decisions in relation to preferences about hospital treatment (Glennerster, Matsaganis and Owens 1992), there is no systematic information available on how widespread this is, or how effective.

The consequences of change

The changes proposed in the new contract and *Working for Patients* were not initially welcomed by GPs. In 1989, there was bitter opposition in well-publicised media campaigns (Butler 1992). Day and Klein (1991) have argued this was in part due to the way in which the usual channels for negotiation between the profession and the state were by-passed. Changes were imposed through the Parliamentary process in a manner reminiscent of the 1946 NHS Act. However, by 1991, the overt opposition to government reforms had subsided and despite the advice of their leaders in the British Medical Association, many GPs showed themselves eager to apply for fundholding status. By 1992, about 14 per cent of the population (285 practices) was covered by fundholding practices; by 1993, this had risen to 25 per cent (Audit Commission 1993). However, the proportion of the purchasing budget controlled by GPFHs remains small at about 2 per cent. Among other GPs, many saw the financial advantages of the new contract and the greater flexibility and additional resources available through the FHSA.

There is evidence that the health reforms have increased the *pace* of change in general practice. This can be seen in a number of areas. First, practices have invested more resources in management – many practices now have full-time managers. There has also been an increase in the use of computers. This is significant as GPs' ability to monitor and control activity is dependent on the effective use of IT. In 1987, 10 per cent of practices had computers. By 1991, this had risen to more than 60 per cent and is predicted to rise to 85 per cent by 1995. Not surprisingly, a higher proportion of the larger practices are computerised (Audit Commission 1993). The size of practices, in terms of staff employed, has also increased. For example, the numbers of practice nurses alone doubled between 1988 and 1990. Many more tasks are now undertaken by other health workers under supervision from the doctor. There is also evidence of a shift of some services from the hospital. More out-patient clinics and minor surgical procedures are taking place in general practice and GPs run specialist clinics either within the practice or with the assistance of hospital consultants (Boyle and Smaje 1992). This has occurred whether GPs are fundholders or not.

Another recommendation of *Working for Patients* was the appointment of professional advisers to give clinical advice, as FHSAs themselves lacked the expertise to assess standards of medical work. The Audit Commission report (1993) indicates that professional advisers have been used sparingly as they are expensive to employ. Those who have been appointed have tended to concentrate on advice on prescribing rather than aspects of diagnosis and treatment. Reducing the costs of prescribing is a government priority and for doctors is less controversial than making judgements about practice, which is inimical to professional autonomy.

The scope of GPs' preventive work has also increased. There is evidence that government targets for screening have been met (Audit Commission 1993). However, there has been little evaluation of its effectiveness in changing health behaviour, let alone in reducing mortality rates (Haines and Iliffe 1992). The efficacy of some screening methods is questioned by doctors themselves (Allsop 1990, Hann 1993) and there is also concern about the impact of health promotion on the day-to-day work of practices. By 1993, the requirement for GPs to offer a health check to anyone on their lists between the age of 16 and 74, and the associated funding, had been withdrawn.

It is also not known how thoroughly GPs are following up their contacts with elderly people and the associated costs and benefits. The requirement to offer elderly people a home visit means that doctors can reach a section of the population that is not particularly active in seeking help. For example, one study of annual health checks for elderly people found that 43 per cent had some form of unmet need (Brown, Williams and Groom 1992).

GP fundholders in particular have gained in autonony and influence in their relationships with hospital doctors and their patients. Glennerster, Matsaganis and Owens' (1992) study of a sample of practices found a variety of innovations, with doctors taking the initiative to develop their practice and to get a better service for their patients. Further examples are given in Glennerster, Matsaganis and Hancocks (1994). Smith, Crawford and Roberts (1993) suggest how GPFHs may influence providers to meet the wishes and convenience of the practice rather than the hospital. Moreover, many GPs have made considerable savings in the first year of fundholding which could be ploughed back into their practices (Audit Commission 1993). Coulter and Bradlow (1993) in a matched sample of fundholding and non-fundholding practices in Oxford, found little difference between the two in rates of referral to hospital. This suggests that these GPFHs did not hold back on referrals to save money.

While many GPs have proved to be adept at using the opportunities the market provides, others have lagged behind. For example in 1991, a study of 2000 practices found that 60 per cent did not prepare business plans; 20 per cent did not employ practice managers; 64 per cent did not prepare budgets. Not even all GPFHs had a business plan (Quinn 1991). Leese and Bosanquet (1989) found an widening bifurcation between the larger, well-managed practice (often in a better-off area) and the small practice (in poor premises with a population ranked high on indicators of social deprivation). Market forces allowing easier movement of better-informed patients are likely to exacerbate these trends.

The recent developments in general practice have tended to favour the wealthier practices and do nothing to alleviate the already considerable variations in the way in which GPs practise (OHE 1990). For example, studies have indicated that rates of referral to hospital varied four-fold (Coulter 1992a). Patterns of prescribing varied by as much as 50 per cent. In 1990–1, practices at the lower end of the scale prescribed at a cost of £30.71 per patient and at the top end it was £62 per patient (Audit Commission 1993). Furthermore, very high levels of prescribing occurred in a small minority of practices. It has been known for some time that there are wide variations in how GPs treat quite common ailments (Acheson and Henley 1984). Moreover, GP fundholding and the advantages for patients that this brings has been more widespread in more affluent areas.

In summary, general practice continues to provide a convenient point of access to health care. With GP fundholding in particular, there appear to have been innovations and some efficiency gains.

However, there has been innovation and development in practices with or without fundholding. It is not known whether these changes are more effective in terms of patient care as there are still too few ways of measuring effective treatments. Some believe that measures to prevent ill-health have been largely ineffective. In terms of equity, the differences in what is available among practices has increased.

Changes in FHSAs

The health service reforms have extended the role of FHSAs as the lead agency for primary care development. They now have responsibility for supporting and monitoring practices. In the past, FHSAs have been hampered by weak powers, an organisational culture which stressed administration rather than management, a strong GP contract of employment and the doctor's autonomy in methods of working. There has been a conflict between their support and monitoring roles (Allsop and May 1986). For example, FHSAs have attempted to develop minimum standards for practice premises, but these have been resisted by the GPs. Also, the new arrangements have not curbed the rise of the number and costs of prescriptions which by 1994 accounted for more than 10 per cent of total NHS costs.

It is not known whether the relationships between FHSAs and their practitioners has changed significantly although there is evidence that in some areas, close cooperation is occurring with resultant benefits for primary care development (Houghton 1993, Morley 1993). It remains difficult for FHSA managers to judge the quality of medical practice in the absence of medical advice. The same applies to assessing whether health promotion clinics are indeed good value for money. And how, for example, does the FHSA deal with the inadequate practice? They cannot penalise it as this might lead to a further deterioration in services for patients.

There is also a contrary trend possible in the relations within FHSAs and their practitioners. As FHSAs take on a clearer commissioning role, and become larger as a consequence of mergers with Health Authorities, they will become distanced from GP practices. Unlike Trusts, where there is a strong management infrastructure, general practices are small and unsupported. A serious void could open between what individual practices could do and what the Department of Health wants them to do in terms of primary care. General practice requires support for the task. This could take the forms of primary care development teams with additional resources. As the Audit Commission (1993) points out, FHSAs need to draw up strategies for service development in their areas, identify priorities and undertake performance reviews to promote quality.

The effect of the reforms on GPs' opportunities and professional powers

In some respects, the developments have brought a clear increase in control over, and the surveillance of, the work of GPs. Additional data are required by the FHSA on aspects of patient activity. Annual reports must be produced and additional funds can be made contingent on providing business plans and improving practice management. Remuneration has a performance element. The FHSA's capacity for control, and that of other central bodies, has been aided by the availability of information technology. Computerised financial and patient activity systems enable the FHSA to chart the progress of practices.

At present, evidence suggests that few FHSAs have yet developed a sufficiently clear view of their role, or have the managerial capacity to control what goes on in the large number of small practices. In terms of their autonomy to control their own work and that of others, GPs with well-managed practices have more control over a range of other health workers. In relation to hospitals, GPs are able to influence the type and quality of these services for their patients. They can contribute to the process of drawing up contracts with purchasing authorities and, if they are GPFHs, they may actually place or remove contracts from particular hospital and community Trusts.

For the first time, this gives GPs power over their hospital colleagues in terms of the services they provide. The reforms have provided opportunities for the GP in a number of spheres: in relation to the scope of work; in access to resources to improve services; the span of control over others; and in their bargaining position with service providers. So far, because of the intrinsic difficulties of reviewing day-to-day practice and the weakness of FHSAs, GPs have remained relatively immune from scrutiny although their activity is now more closely monitored. Ironically, the overall effect of introducing market forces into the NHS has been to allow the central state to step back. The 'invisible hand' of the market determines the behaviour of individuals in the health arena and the visibility of government's crucial role in funding is reduced.

The consequence of this is an extension of the GPs' and other health workers' cultural authority over the well population. The purpose of screening is to detect those at risk of more serious illness so that they can be counselled about life-styles. As Armstrong argues in *The Political Economy of the Body* (1983), population medicine is an extension of the clinical gaze into those who are well and therefore is an extension of state control. Patient compliance is ensured through claims for the advantages of early detection. Doctor compliance is ensured by financial incentives.

References

Acheson, N. H. and Henley, M. (1984) 'Clinical Knowledge for General Practice', Occasional paper 27, Royal College of General Practitioners, London.

Allsop, J. (1990) *Changing Primary Care: the role of facilitators*, King's Fund Centre, London.

Allsop, J. and May, A. (1986) *The Emperor's New Clothes: Family Practitioner Committees in the 1980s*, King's Fund Publishing, London.

Armstrong, D. (1983) *The Political Economy of the Body: medical knowledge in Britain in the 20th century*, Cambridge University Press, Cambridge.

Audit Commission (1993) *Practices Make Perfect: the role of the Family Health Services Authority*, Audit Commission, Local Government Report no. 10, HMSO, London.

Bain, J. (1993) 'Budget Holding: here to stay?', *British Medical Journal*, 306, pp. 1186–88.

Boyle, S. and Smaje, C. (1992) 'Minor Surgery in General Practice: the effect of the 1990 GP contract' in Harrison, A. (ed.), *Health Care UK*, King's Fund Institute, London.

Brown, K., Williams, E. and Groom, L. (1992) 'Health Checks of Patients 75 Years and Over in Nottinghamshire after the New GP Contract', *British Medical Journal*, 305, pp. 619–21.

Butler (1992) *Patients Policies and Politics: before and after Working for Patients*, Open University Press, Milton Keynes.

Cartwright, A. (1967) *Patients and their Doctors*, Routledge & Kegan Paul, London.

Cartwright, A. and Anderson, R. (1981) 'Patients and their Doctors', Institute for Social Studies in Medical Care, Occasional Paper 8, London.

Coulter, A. (1992a) 'The Interface between Primary and Secondary Care', in Roland, M. and Coulter, A. (eds), *Hospital Referrals*, Oxford University Press, Oxford.

Coulter, A. (1992b) 'Fundholding general practices: early successes – but will they last?' *British Medical Journal*, 304, pp. 397–8.

Coulter, A. and Bradlow, J. (1993) 'The Effect of NHS Reforms on General Practitioners' Referral Patterns', *British Medical Journal*, 306, pp. 433–7.

Day, P. and Klein, R. (1991) 'Political Theory and Policy Practice: the case of general practice 1911–1991', Paper presented at the Political Studies Association Conference, University of Lancaster.

Department of Health (1989) *General Practice in the NHS: the 1990 contract*, DOH, London.

Department of Health (1992) *The Health of the Nation: strategy for health in England*, Cmnd 1986, HMSO, London.

Department of Health and Social Security (DHSS) (1981) *The Primary Health Care Team*, (Chairman: W. Harding), HMSO, London.

Department of Health and Social Security (DHSS) (1986a) *Improving Primary Health Care*, HMSO, London.

Department of Health and Social Security (1986b) *Neighbourhood Nursing: a focus for care* (Chair: Julia Cumberledge), HMSO, London.

Department of Health and Social Security (1987) *Promoting Better Health*, Cmnd 249, HMSO, London.

Glennerster, H., Matsaganis, M. and Owens, P.(1992) *A Foothold for Fundraising*, King's Fund Institute, London.

Glennerster, H., Matsaganis, M. and Hancocks, S. (1994) 'GP Fund-holding: Wild Card or Winning Hand?' in Robinson, R. and Le Grand, J., *Evaluating the NHS Reforms*, King's Fund Institute, London.

Hann, A. (1993) 'The Decision to Screen', in Mills, M. (ed.), *Prevention, Health and British Politics*, Avebury, Aldershot.

Haines, A. and Iliffe, S. (1992) 'Primary Health Care' in Beck, E., Lonsdale, S., Newman, S. and Patterson, D. (eds), *In the Best of Health? The status and future of health care in the UK*, Chapman & Hall, London.

Honigsbaum, F. (1985) 'Reconstruction of General Practice: failure of reform', *British Medical Journal*, 290, pp. 823–26.

Houghton, K. (1993) 'Peak Practices', *Health Services Journal*, 3 June, pp. 26–7.

Hughes, D. (1993) 'Letting the Market Work?' in Page, R. and Baldock, J. (eds), *Social Policy Review 5: the evolving state of welfare*, pp. 104–124, Social Policy Association, University of Kent, Canterbury.

Leese, B, and Bosanquet, N. (1989) 'High and Low Incomes in General Practice', *British Medical Journal*, 298, pp. 932–4.

London Health Planning Consortium (1981) *Primary Health Care in Inner London* (Chairman: D. Acheson), London.

Ministry of Health (1963) *The Field of Work of the Family Doctor* (Chairman: A. Gillie), HMSO, London.

Morley, V. (1993) 'Empowering GPs as Purchasers', *British Medical Journal*, 306, pp. 112–14.

Morris, R. (1993) 'Community Care and the Fundholder', *British Medical Journal*, 306, pp 635–7.

Office of Health Economics (1990) 'Variations between General Practitioners', OHE Briefing, no. 26, London.

Quinn, G. (1991) *The Management of General Practice*, Stoy Hayward Consulting and Cranfield School of Management, Cranfield.

Secretary of State for Health (1989) *Working for Patients: the Prime Minister's Review of the Health Service*, Cmnd 555, HMSO, London.

Smith, R., Crawford, M. and Roberts, H. (1993) 'Purchasing in Practice', *Health Services Journal*, 1 April, pp. 28–30.

Styles, W. (1994) 'Viol Bodies', *Health Services Journal*, 3 February, pp. 30–2.

Taylor, D. (1991) *Developing Primary Care: opportunities for the 1990s*, King's Fund Institute, London.

World Health Organisation (1985) *Health for All Targets*, WHO, Geneva.

CHAPTER 11

Policies for prevention

By 1992, the UK had developed a strategy for preventing ill-health. England, Northern Ireland, Scotland and Wales each published separate targeted proposals for improving health status. Compared with a number of other countries, the UK has been relatively slow to develop a preventive strategy which linked improvements in health staus to specific policies. For example, Canada published *A New Perspective on the Health of Canadians* in 1974 (Canada, Ministry of National Health and Welfare 1974), and the US produced *Healthy People* in 1979 with a follow up in 1990 (US Public Health Service 1979, 1990). In 1978, with the Alma-Ata declaration, the World Health Organisation launched its health promotion charter which encouraged all member states to develop plans for improving health (Document 22, page 327). This chapter examines why preventive policies have developed more strongly as part of health policy. It looks at the strategies adopted by UK governments and the factors which have shaped the decisions to follow particular health promotion paths.

The dimensions of prevention

Billis (1981) argues that, when used in relation to the physical world, the most straightforward meaning of prevention is 'to stop'. 'To prevent' means to intervene in the interaction between factors which create a result which is considered undesirable. In relation to the disease process, the causal chain of events is likely to be complex and often the links between causative agents and subsequent ill-health are unclear. Moreover, the time period between events and their manifest outcome may be considerable. In addition, a number of choices about where to intervene in the chain of events are possible. For example, there are a number of explanations of the causes of one of the most common diseases – tooth decay. Diet and environmental factors, such as type of water, may play a part in building tooth structure as well as having a later effect on vulnerability to decay. Many oppportunities for intervention occur and action could be taken by various agents. Diets may be changed; teeth protected by fluoride toothpaste; painted with fluoride; or water supplies may be treated with fluoride. Individuals, families, dentists, the local or central state could all be involved. Questions arise, therefore, about the point of intervention which is likely to be most effective in achieving the desired result.

The concept of prevention may be defined narrowly or broadly. Within medicine and epidemiology a distinction is made between primary, secondary and tertiary prevention (Document 21, page 325). Primary prevention refers to measures taken to protect health in those who are well. Examples are immunisation and vaccination and screening, to detect and reduce risk factors for disease such as high blood pressure. Secondary prevention refers to the procedures used to identify disease at a very early pre-symptomatic stage – for example, through screening for microscopic cancers in the cervix or breast, so that early treatment can be given. The term 'tertiary prevention' refers to the process of rehabilitation enabling a patient to become as fully functioning as possible after a period of illness or a disabling episode. In the medical model, responsibility for prevention is assumed to lie with the clinician.

The concepts outlined above reflect a disease-based view of prevention. Broader definitions place an emphasis on developing and maintaining healthy life-styles. As demonstrated in Chapter 6, the concept of health is variously interpreted and the basis of good health may be multi-factorial – depending on genetic factors, individual behaviour and environmental hazards. Responsibility for living a healthy life may be deemed to lie with the individual, the community or the state. Strategies to improve health by changing individual behaviour rest on the assumption that education and information on health services will encourage individuals to optimise their own health. However, policies may also involve action by health care providers, employers and the local community to promote healthy behaviour. Lastly, the central state may itself pursue public health policy through promotion and regulation. This approach is potentially so broad that social life may become redefined in terms of health.

Policies towards prevention

Principles of intervention

We already know a good deal about what makes for a healthy life. For example, Belloc and Breslaw (1972) carried out a study to relate personal behaviour to physical status. They assessed the effects on health when seven rules were followed: (a) no smoking of cigarettes; (b) sleeping for seven hours a night; (c) eating breakfast; (d) keeping weight down; (e) drinking moderately; (f) exercising daily; and (g) not eating between meals. It was concluded that health and longevity increased with the number of rules followed. For people over 75 following all the rules, health was said to be as good as for those aged 35 to 44 who followed less than three; and life expectancy at age 45 was 11 years longer for people following six or seven rules than for those following less than four. However, such findings raise a number of questions. How widespread is this knowledge? Even if it is commonly accepted, why do people not follow these rules even if they are aware that they contribute to longevity? Finally, what do any of these factors have to do with government? Are not these issues simply matters of personal choice? Policies for prevention raise questions not only about which forms of intervention are efficacious but also questions of the boundaries between government regulation and individual action.

Perceptions of the seriousness of particular health problems, the extent of knowledge about risks and benefits, may also explain why certain areas become a focus for state intervention. Values and culture may play a part as well as rational choices based on the predicted outcome in terms of health gain. There are two main strategies towards preventing ill-health: those which rely on state intervention in matters which affect health and those which rely on informing and educating individuals so that they can make choices about how to live their lives. However, structure of services has also been shown to affect policy formation.

Mills and Saward (1993) argue that in liberal democracies there are particular problems which arise in state intervention as government action aims to regulate what is deemed to be private behaviour. Political controversy may arise over particular policies and because preventive programmes are less central to party political programmes, a wide variety of policy networks may be involved in decision-making. Paradoxically, societies which have well-developed health care systems for clinical care have varied considerably in their approach to preventing ill-health. The outcomes of the policy process are less predictable than with mainstream political programmes.

Changing individual behaviour

It has been argued that government policies which seek to control individual behaviour in the interests of good health are paternalist. That is, decisions are made by government which people should make for themselves. Thus, there is public control of private behaviour. J. S. Mill, the nineteenth-century liberal political philosopher, suggested that the avoidance of harm to others was the only legitimate reason for legally compelling someone to do something they would not otherwise do. Self-regarding actions and actions where others had given their consent should fall outside the law. On these grounds, there have been objections to public health measures which require the wearing of seat belts, the screening of populations for pre-symptomatic indicators, the prevention of smoking in public places, and the addition of fluoride to the water supply.

The libertarian view is based on objections to paternalism in principle and in practice. It may be taken as a principle that people are the best judges of their own welfare. Only they are in a position to decide how high a value to put on health and the risks they are prepared to run. People have the right to decide what they do with their own bodies and the decisions they make. In more practical terms, one line of argument is that the evidence is often lacking on the relationship between a hazard and the alleged effect. For example, the evidence of the link between diet and ill-health is equivocal. The relationship between a fatty diet and a high cholesterol level, which is a risk factor for heart disease, has been contested. Some attribute high rates of heart disease to sucrose. There has also been dispute about the effect of nitrates on the water supply (see Weale 1981). It has been pointed out, too, that populations with a high wine consumption, such as in France, have lower levels of heart disease. Another strand to this argument is that evidence about the effect of certain hazards is based on aggregate populations. The direct causal links are thus obscured.

Another point to consider is that preventive programmes may have unintended effects. Thus, if it is supposed that smoking is addictive, then raising the price of cigarettes may have the effect of reducing expenditure on food rather than reducing smoking. Crawford (1977) has also argued that preventive programmes create a group of 'worried well'.

Regulatory strategies

The arguments for government regulation rest on a number of points. In practice, however, it is often difficult to separate self-regarding from other-regarding activity. For example, smokers pollute the environment for others as there is an element of 'secondary' or 'passive' smoking. Pregnant mothers who smoke put the foetus at greater risk as they tend to have lower birth weight babies, who in turn are more vulnerable to illness in later life. With a national health service, to which all citizens have to contribute, the costs of treating those whose illness is associated with smoking fall on the community as a whole. In relation to the principle that people have the right to decide how they behave, it can be said that people are not necessarily rational or enlightened. They may be in a position where choice is so conditioned by circumstances that it exists only in theory. People may learn from experience and from information so preferences may change over time. Studies of smoking, for example, suggest that people's habits and preferences are a product of their circumstances. There is evidence of this in the class bias in smoking behaviour and how this has changed over time. For example, Graham's (1987) work on women and smoking suggests that smoking is closely linked to attitudes, social circumstances and limited opportunities for choice. There is also the problem that, in relation to health issues, the effects of behaviour or circumstances are remote in time. Therefore, governments need to protect individuals on the basis of the information available to them at the time.

Perhaps the strongest argument for government regulation in the area of prevention is that preserving the right choice of individuals may not be the prime principle. There may be benefits to the collectivity from interventions. These may not involve conflicts with individual choices at all – for example, in the case of the fire-proofing of public buildings. And where they do, the benefits may outweigh the loss of individual choice. Vaccination and immunisation programmes against infectious disease have external benefits. Compulsory vaccination will bring group immunity. However, this creates what Rose (1981) calls the 'paradox of prevention' in terms of the relative costs and benefits to the group and the individual. For the collectivity, there are advantages in introducing compulsory measures. The small numbers who are damaged by vaccines are worth paying for. However, for the individual the reverse may be the case. The cost to them of vaccine damage, should it occur, is extremely high. In these circumstances, individuals gain the maximum advantage when everyone else except themselves is vaccinated.

Warner (1979) suggests that a classification can be made of different preventive health measures along a continuum which distinguishes between alternative strategies by the extent to which they depend upon active, passive or no involvement by individuals. He declares that the more individual decision-making is involved the less likely is the the success of the programme. General environmental programmes which need little or no effort on the part of the individual – such as clean air legislation; the addition of vitamin D to milk; the removal of sugar from paediatric medicines; the addition of fluoride to water supplies – can all be extremely effective. These are regulatory activities and can only be carried out by government. Thus, it can also be argued that government legislation making behaviour compulsory is more effective – for example, seat belt legislation has led to more people travelling safely in cars. But programmes which demand more individual active public involvement become less effective and have an increasing class bias in take-up.

Weale (1981) argues that in areas where there is a doubt about efficacy, there is a case for liberal paternalism. Where a link between a health hazard has been established beyond reasonable doubt, then there is an argument for state regulation. Where an association appears to be strong, evaluative trials could be introduced. He also suggests that where a choice of strategies is possible, then, rather than having a total ban on an activity which means policing of some kind, the use of the price mechanism is preferable. This allows individual choices to be made. The price mechanism could also be used in reverse – that is, to promote activities which are health-enhancing. For example, employers who provided sports facilities for their staff could receive a subsidy towards the cost of amenities.

Government policies on prevention – the 1970s

Although the stated aims of the NHS included the prevention of ill-health, in practice, public health medicine was limited to the activities of Medical Officers of Health (MOHs) in the local authorities. In 1948 the public health function was separated from hospital and GP care. At neither national nor local level was there a forum concerned with good health. The weak position of public health has inhibited the development of policies for prevention in Britain.

Until 1974, MOHs were responsible for public health and the coordination and delivery of community health services. In a study of community medicine, Lewis (1986) argues that, compared to their predecessors in the late nineteenth century, MOHs were not able to monitor and respond to the causes of ill-health in their area and nor did they have sufficient control over community services to affect policy. In relation to the latter, the social work profession within local authorities and the GPs outside them had an autonomy beyond the remit of the MOH.

In 1974, responsibility for environmental health remained with local government, while District Community Physicians (DCPs) became integrated within the structure of management of curative services in the health districts, under the general administration of the Area Medical Officer. DCPs could be used in a consultative capacity by local authorities on environmental health matters. In its evidence to the Royal Commission of the NHS (1979: 47) the Society of Community Medicine felt that this change had brought disadvantages:

> Despite many advances and improvements in environmental control, especially in the more traditional sectors of water and air, there is little evidence that the physical environment continues to improve; rather the reverse, with the environment being continually and subtly degraded.

It went on to argue that, with the lack of centrality for the community physician, some of the impetus for the development of services had been lost.

So the 1974 reorganisation further reduced the public health role of the community physicians. Their main task was to manage and integrate clinical services in the hospital and community. However, they lacked the power and authority to achieve this. Local authorities on the other hand lost a medical input in public health. As a consequence, community medicine became an unpopular specialism among doctors. On the local authority side, reorganisation served to downgrade prevention and rob it of medical leadership just as it was beginning to rise up the policy agenda. Within health districts it placed the community physician in a difficult role. The specialism ranked low in the medical hierarchy and community physicians themselves lacked both the authority and the power to manage other clinicians, while post-holders often had insufficient training in management for the task. This led to problems in recruitment to the sub-specialty and a vacuum in local health policy persisted.

At the local level, a number of individual health workers had responsibilities for promoting better health; health visitors, for example, had a statutory responsibilities to visit mothers with new babies and in relation to the health of young children. District nurses had an important role in educating informal carers; however, their work was often poorly coordinated with that of GPs. Health education officers were employed by Health Authorities to educate and inform the public. Clinical medical officers looked after the health of schoolchildren. All these workers are likely to use different information systems and ways of operating.

At the national level, there was (and still is) an extraordinarily complicated network of government departments whose activities relate to health. For example, Morris (1982) comments that 12 central government departments and agencies are concerned with the control of pesticides – although this is hardly a priority area. To take another example, occupational health is the responsibility of the Health and Safety Executive of the Health and Safety Commission. Its remit is 'the reactions of work people to their working environment and the prevention of ill-health arising from working conditions'. The Department of the Environment is responsible for the aspects of environmental health which come under local government while the DHSS is concerned with community health services. The lack of clear responsibilities for health at both central and local level made it easy for professional commitment to be diffused among the plethora of agencies. Political lobbying could be targeted to particular MPs – as it was with the tobacco lobby (Read 1993) – while policies at the level of the Executive remained piecemeal and largely ineffective.

However, the approach taken in the 1970s was limited in terms of direct government intervention. The Health Education Council, an independent but publicly funded body, founded in 1968, was seen as the major organ for publicising factors associated with ill-health. Otherwise, it was expected that health providers, particularly GPs, nurses and health education officers, would promote the cause locally.

The increasing concern for prevention

In the mid-1970s, the possibility of preventing ill-health again came onto the policy agenda. Two themes emerged from government statements on the issue. The first was a concern about the rising costs of treating illness and the second was the high rate of mortality and morbidity from heart disease and the cancers. As Chapter 6 indicated, the leading causes of illness had changed and there was also greater scepticism about the benefits of clinical medicine. During the next decade, evidence accumulated that death rates in the UK from heart disease and some of the cancers were particularly high compared to other European countries (NAO 1989). This helped to keep the issue on the agenda although governments were slow to intervene. In general, policies were left to local-level authorities to determine. When they did receive attention from Westminster, the emphasis was on education so as to allow people to make up their own minds. Relevant information was taken to be that provided by health professionals.

In 1976, the Labour government published two consultative documents on health, *Prevention and Health: Everybody's Business* (DHSS 1976a) and *Priorities for the Health and Personal Social Services in England* (DHSS 1976b). The immediate purpose was to stimulate discussion. Three elements were of particular importance. First, the focus was on individual behaviour change. Although, historically, the evidence suggested that the most effective measures for the prevention of disease were those policies implemented at the level of populations, the document declares that:

> Much ill-health in Britain today arises from over-indulgence and unwise behaviour . . . the greatest potential and perhaps the greatest problems for preventive medicine now lies in changing behaviour and attitudes to ensure health. The individual can do much to help himself, his family and the community by accepting more direct responsibility for his own health and well-being. . . . Prevention today is everybody's business.
>
> (DHSS 1976a: 7)

Second, all discussion was prefaced by a warning about the limited availability of resources. Third, emphasis was placed on the relationship between prevention and health planning. (DHSS 1978, DHSS 1981a, DHSS 1981b)

In 1977, a White Paper, *Prevention and Health*, was published (DHSS 1977a). This reiterated the message:

> . . . to ensure that people are encouraged to take more responsibility for their own health . . . and to enable them to do so, there should be a greater flow of reliable information and advice.
>
> (DHSS 1977a: 1)

An example of this policy was the approach to smoking. In 1971, the link between smoking and cancer had been established by a report by the Royal College of Physicians. Despite this, governments were reluctant to legislate. Policies were a combination of using the price deterrent through taxation, education programmes and voluntary agreements on advertising with the tobacco industry. For example, since 1970, cigarette packets have carried health warnings. However, advertising has not been banned completely and an annual increase in taxes has been rejected. Governments were unwilling to take strong regulatory action:

> . . . because cigarette smoking is a long standing habit practised by nearly half the population, it would be totally unfair to expect smokers to give up the habit.
>
> (DHSS 1977a)

Prevention and Health declared that tax increases raised the cost of smoking for those least able to afford it and, given their dependence on tobacco, some smokers might forgo necessities. Even so, governments eschewed regulation on the grounds of individual preferences.

Prevention and health – the 1980s

In the early 1980s, the policies pursued by Conservative governments continued to be based on the notions of individual responsibility. Indeed this fitted well with the values of the New Right. Although the Black Report (DHSS 1979a) had produced good evidence of the link between inequalities in income and resources and health, the issue was not on the government's agenda. The priority was economic growth.

Calnan (1991) comments that government policy continued to focus on personal behaviour:

> Government policy in relation to the control of smoking, diet, alcohol and the encouragement of exercise has been characterised by a non-interventionist approach with the emphasis on persuasion and industrial self-regulation . . . it is a paternalistic policy which has been based on authoritative knowledge and is inclined towards a more individualist orientation.
>
> (Calnan 1991: 83)

This reluctance to intervene has been attributed to a number of factors: the strength of vested interests and the weakness of those opposing them; the governments' electoral interest; and competing departmental interests. Both the tobacco and alcohol industries in the UK wield considerable economic muscle: the drinks industry accounted for 2 per cent of all employment and 5 per cent of Gross Domestic Product (GDP) in 1984 (Baggott, 1986). Both lobbies are represented in Parliament through the business and constituency interests of MPs (Calnan 1984, Baggott 1986). The voluntary self-regulation of these industries reflects British policy-making style: it creates stability for business; and for government, tax revenues are secured through a moderate approach (Baggott 1987).

Nonetheless, other pressure groups exerted a measure of influence on policy-making. Government action on smoking was prompted by a series of reports on *Smoking and Health* produced by the Royal College of Physicians between 1964 and 1983, and by the pressure group ASH (Action on Smoking and Health) established under its auspices in 1971 (Calnan 1984). The Royal College of Psychiatrists published the similarly influential *Alcohol and Alcoholism* in 1979.

While this suggests that the prestige and scientific authority of the medical professions have proved influential enough to turn smoking and, to a lesser extent, alcohol consumption into health policy issues, they seem not to have been strong enough to make the profession's recommendations effective (Calnan 1984). The weak regulation of the production and distribution of food, similarly, can be attributed to inconclusive research findings and a diversity of views within the medical profession (Calnan 1991). In turn, this suggests that pressure groups which address issues of this kind invariably face an uphill task. Their achievement lies in forcing prevention on to the political agenda, while industrial lobbies, by contrast, need only to wait and then resist change (Popham 1981). In addition, in some areas, pressure groups have lacked cohesion: the anti-alcohol lobby, for example, has been weakened by conflict between voluntary organisations (Allsop and Freeman 1993).

The effect of health education campaigns

Health education campaigns and other fiscal measures have been successful to the extent that the numbers of people smoking has fallen over the last 20 years. One out of every two adults now smoke as opposed to two out of every three previously. Figure 11.1 shows the trends.

Furthermore, there has been a shift into less 'dangerous', low-tar cigarettes. However, the recent decline is less apparent for women and the overall figures indicate marked class differences. The decrease in cigarette smoking has been most rapid among professional as compared to manual social classes. Doctors have

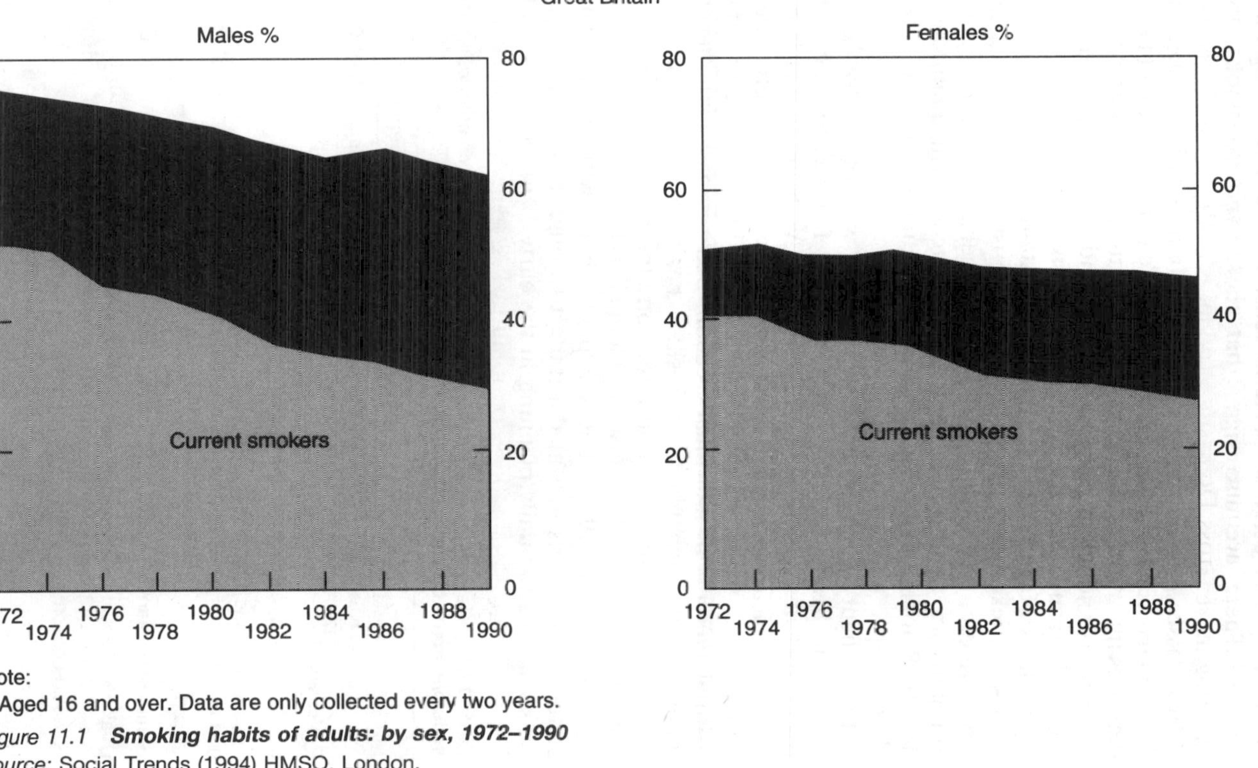

Note:
1 Aged 16 and over. Data are only collected every two years.

Figure 11.1 ***Smoking habits of adults: by sex, 1972–1990***

Source: Social Trends (1994) HMSO, London.

been the group showing the steepest reduction while the incidence of smoking has actually been increasing among working-class women. There are also signs that those who do smoke are smoking more.

In an assessment of the evidence in relation to the prevention of coronary heart disease, the Office of Health Economics (1992) indicates that there is a need to search for more effective methods. An understanding of particular living and working patterns of high-risk groups and the role which smoking and alcohol play in the lives of individuals at risk is important. Where behaviour is closely linked to custom or culture it is difficult to change. Furthermore, one of the paradoxes of a behavioural rather than a regulatory approach is that it may *increase* inequalities in health. Smoking rates have fallen more rapidly among middle-class groups.

In the light of the difficulties associated with other strategies, a resort to health education represented a fall-back position for preventive health policy. It accorded well with an emphasis on policies which were relatively inexpensive, immediately practicable, and which accorded with prevailing ideological and cultural precepts of individual freedom and responsibility. Nevertheless, efforts towards more positive health promotion became an area of significant political tension, the brunt of which was borne by the Health Education Council (HEC). The HEC had been founded in 1968. It was a public body with independent status and made its first media impact through poster campaigns on smoking and family planning in the early 1970s. In 1987, with

Table 11.1 ***Heavy cigarette smoking and consumption of alcohol above sensible limits: by socio-economic group, 1990***

	Males %		*Females %*	
	Smoking	*Alcohol*	*Smoking*	*Alcohol*
Professional	5	26	6	14
Employers and managers	12	30	7	14
Intermediate and junior non-manual	8	26	7	11
Skilled manual	17	28	11	9
Semi-skilled manual	18	26	12	9
Unskilled manual	22	26	13	6
All socio-economic groups[3]	14	27	9	11

Notes:
1 20 or more per day.
2 22 units or more for males, and 15 units or more for females, per week.
3 Adults aged 16 and over.

Source: Social Trends (1994) HMSO, London.

support from the DOH, it made use of television advertising with the *Look After Your Heart* campaign.

In the early 1980s, the HEC took an independent line. It championed the findings of the Black Report (DHSS 1979a) on inequalities in health and lobbied against the tobacco, alcohol and food industries. The Council's Canterbury Report (HEC 1984) took up the issue of coronary heart disease, calling in particular for increased government regulation of food production and distribution. In this endeavour, it was resisted by the DHSS. The 'emergency topics' of drugs and AIDS then served to heighten the public and political profile of health education (Baggott 1991). In a move designed to make health education work more responsive to the needs of the NHS, the HEC was reconstituted in April 1987 as the Health Education Authority (HEA), responsible directly to Ministers. The government's influence was soon made apparent by the ending of support for community development projects, a number of which had seemed to offer a focus for local health promotion in the 1980s (Beattie 1991). The Professional and Community Development Division which had been established at the HEA in 1988 was closed in 1989.

Thus, despite the efforts of the HEA an individualistic, *laissez-faire* model of health education supported by government has dominated its work. It has also been criticised for its ambivalent relationship with medicine. Rodmell and Watt (1986) comment that health education has relied heavily on the medical model of disease:

> Health educators constantly seek affirmation of their activities from medical practitioners who retain the power to confer the necessary status, but at the same time seek to resist the medicalisation which this conferment of status imposes.
>
> (Rodmell and Watt 1986: 3)

It is suggested that much health education thinking is based on a middle-class professional assumption that working-class people are best reached through short and simple messages. This was despite evidence that working-class people wanted more information covering a wider range of evidence which they might then be able to evaluate for themselves (Farrant and Russell 1985).

The HEA has been constrained to the same extent as the HEC by government's concerns for protecting interests in the business and industrial sector. Despite, or perhaps even because of, their attempt to widen the agenda for prevention, the work of both bodies has been limited by their dependence on government funding. In this context, government action on health education could be taken as symbolic. George sums up its weaknesses by suggesting that:

> Government ministers from both sides of the House, along with their civil servant advisers, have consistently used the HEC as an instant,

highly visible, relatively cheap and superficially plausible means of responding to pressure to 'do something' about a particular health problem . . . the quango image and the illusion of independence of the HEC allow programmes initiated for political reasons to be carried out behind a smokescreen of professional and scientific justification.

(George 1981: 51)

A change of direction: prevention in primary care and the public health

By the mid-1980s, both general practice and the public health role of community physicians were becoming a focus of policy-makers' attention. The Department of Health began to show a new interest in prevention (Klein 1989). This was supported by a growing concern for the poor health status of the UK population compared to many of its European neighbours and other developed nations (Smith and Jacobson 1988, NAO 1989). Three issues had emerged as a concern for public health. The strategies adopted to deal with these varied but together they contributed different elements to a policy shift towards prevention. The issues were the rising incidence of coronary heart disease (CHD), cervical and breast cancer, and a 'new disease', HIV/AIDS.

CHD was perceived as a problem because death rates in the UK are among the highest in the world. In 1986, Northern Ireland and Scotland had the highest CHD death rate at 298 per 100,000. This compared to 243 in England and Wales, 230 in the USA, 79 in Spain and 45 in Japan. In the UK, it was the largest single cause of death, accounting for 27 per cent of the total. Although no sector of society is immune, CHD rates are highest for men and women in the manual classes and for men and women of Asian origin. The costs of treating it are high – in 1984, hospital care for CHD was estimated to be about £300 million.

Policies in relation to preventing coronary heart disease have been focused on the risk factors in individuals. There is a broad consensus that the disease is strongly linked with cigarette smoking, high serum cholesterol levels and raised blood pressure. Taken together, these can increase by eight-fold the chances of a coronary event. There is also evidence from the United States and Australia to suggest that where active prevention policies are introduced death rates have been almost halved (NAHAT Briefing, 1989).

In relation to cancer – a term which covers a spectrum of diseases each with a particular set of causative factors – there is also a strong link with smoking. In relation to lung cancer, up to one-third of deaths have been attributed to smoking. Other factors such as alcohol consumption, occupational hazards, environmental pollutants, sexual activity and diet factors have been implicated in the incidence of particular kinds of cancer. In 1981, Peto (reporting on work carried out with Doll) argued that 80 to 90 per cent of cancers were theoretically avoidable. Table 11.2 shows the practicable ways of reducing the risk of contracting this disease. The strong association between a number of illnesses and smoking made this activity an ideal target for prevention policies. In 1989, it was estimated that smoking was responsible for 17 per cent of all deaths. Seventeen per cent of all women and 27 per cent of all men who smoke will die before the age of 65, compared to 13 per cent of the population as a whole (DOH 1989).

Table 11.2 **Reliably established (as of 1981), practicable ways of avoiding the onset of life-threatening cancer**

	Per cent of all US cancer deaths known to be thus avoidable
Avoidance of tobacco smoke	30
Avoidance of alcoholic drinks or mouthwash	3
Avoidance of obesity	2
Regular cervical screening and genital hygiene	1
Avoidance of inessential medical use of hormones or radiology	<1
Avoidance of unusual exposure to sunlight	<1
Avoidance of current levels of exposure to currently known carcinogens (for which there is good epidemiological evidence of human hazard) in i. occupational ii. food, water or urban air	

Note:
1 Excluding ways such as prophylatic protatectomy, mastectomy, hysterectomy, oophorectomy, artifical menopause or pregnancy.

Source: Peto (1981).

The first recorded death from AIDS in Britain was in 1982. By 1990, about 4100 people had contracted AIDS and about half of these had died (Social Trends 1993). However, although the size of the AIDS problem was small, the absence of cure, the high incidence of the disease in young people and the main mode of transmission through unprotected sexual intercourse made the disease a focus of media and government attention from the mid-1980s.

A role for local government in health promotion?

In the 1980s there was also a surge of interest in preventive health at local level within local government (Moran 1986) and in individual cities which participated in the WHO-sponsored Healthy Cities programme (Ashton and Seymour 1988). The then Chief Medical Officer, Donald (now Sir Donald) Acheson also had a particular concern for public health. He chaired a Committee of Inquiry into the Future Development of the Public Health Function which reported in 1988 (DHSS 1988). Interestingly, the Committee had been instructed to exclude aspects of public health which were shared by the health department with other government departments: it was told to concentrate narrowly on the role of community physicians and on arrangements for the control of communicable disease. The Committee recommended that Directors of Public Health (DsPH) should be appointed in each district, to be 'named leaders of the public health function'. These were to be accountable to the DHA general manager. While the results of the Acheson Inquiry were accepted in full by the government, the extensive report represented a restatement of problems of divided responsibilities for public health as much as it did a plausible solution.

A further factor in promoting interest in the prevention of ill-health was the interest shown by the media – both newspapers and television. In the second half of the 1980s, a number of public health problems occurred which commanded media attention. AIDS remained the most prominent of these, but others included meningitis, salmonella, Legionnaire's disease and the food scares of 1989 and 1990 (Baggott 1991). Street (1993), in a discussion of the media in relation to AIDS, suggests that its importance lay not just in the way it publicised that problem but in the way it became part of the solution. In 1986, the Department of Health used the media, and particularly television, extensively in providing information on the disease and how to avoid it.

An enhanced role for primary care

In 1981, the Royal College of General Practitioners (RCGP) argued that three areas of preventive activity were important in the general practice setting (RCGP 1981). The individual patient consultation provided an opportunity for screening and health education; systems could be developed for surveying the practice population and groups at risk; and GPs could maintain contacts with other community groups. Some were sceptical of the ability of doctors to carry out this wide variety of roles (Calnan, Boulton and Williams 1986). There were a number of obstacles to the use of general practice as the focus for illness prevention. First, there was considerable variation between practices in their structure and their capacity for health promotion. Second, the interest shown in health education by the leaders of the profession was not always shared by the ordinary GP. Third, not all GPs were convinced about the benefits of population screening and health education as the most effective means of prevention (Allsop 1990).

In 1987, the government published *Promoting Better Health* (DHSS 1987) which outlined its policies for primary care. It saw health professionals as being the main mediators of health education. They were held to be:

> . . . very well placed to persuade individuals of the importance of protecting their health; of the simple steps needed to do so; and of accepting that prevention is indeed better than cure.
>
> (DHSS 1987: para 1.12)

General practice and the primary health care team were to be the main focus for health education and the screening of practice populations for illness. In 1989, a new contract with GPs was agreed (DOH 1989). General practitioners' terms of service now included requirements to include health promotion and disease prevention (see Chapter 10). At the same time, however, the government placed new restrictions on the preventive services hitherto provided by paramedical professions. It ended free sight-testing and introduced charges for dental examination.

It is probably too early to assess the effects of these changes. The outcomes of preventive health programmes are difficult to quantify given the numbers of intervening variables; their effects may only be demonstrated in the long term. McCarthy (1992) demonstrates that the take-up of cancer screening, health checks and immunisation, and vaccination for most childhood diseases has increased. However, it must be said that, apart from childhood immunisation both the efficacy of screening in general and its place in the GP's surgery have been questioned.

The 1990 health service reforms and The Health of the Nation

In 1990, the NHS and Community Care Act brought major changes in the organisation of the NHS through the introduction of the internal market. The implications for public health and the prevention of illness are that it is now the purchasing authorities who assess the health needs of their populations and who determine the importance given to health promotion. The 1992 White Paper, *The Health of the Nation* (DOH 1992), provides for the first time a health strategy for England which complements those already published for other parts of the UK. In the context of comparative data on the health status of English regions and between different groups and classes, it identifies the major causes of illness and early deaths and sets priorities and targets. Five key areas for action are identifed: heart disease and strokes; cancers; mental illness; sexual health; and accidents. Targets are set for percentage decreases in morbidity and mortality for these areas. Health Authorities and other agencies are expected to adopt policies to achieve these targets within a given timescale.

In the context of the consultations which preceded *The Health of the Nation*, two major stategies were identified as important in achieving the goals set by government. The concept of 'health gain' has emerged as a useful tool for agencies to assess which policy or programme to pursue (Welsh Health Planning Forum 1989). It poses the question of priorities in cost-benefit terms: what sorts of investment will produce the greatest benefit in terms of 'adding years to life and life to years'? Looked at in this way, 'health gain' has parallels with the use of QALYs (quality adjusted life years) to compare the costs and benefits of interventions in the hospital sector. Like QALYS, too, notions of 'health gain' appear rational when applied to determining priorities for populations but raise ethical and political problems because they affect individuals.

A second strategy puts emphasis on 'healthy alliances'. In central government, this has taken the form of a Cabinet-level committee to coordinate the work of different departments. Within the NHS, the Management Executive has promoted joint working with outside agencies, on the basis that the strategy for health cannot be delivered by the health service alone (NHSME 1992).

The publication of *The Health of the Nation* can be seen as a step forward. The report sets targets which are a spur to endeavour and provide a comparative indicator of progress. Moreover, the White Paper underlines the importance of health education, primary care and collaboration between agencies. The 1990 reforms have also strengthened managerial accountability for the health of populations; such aims have become part of the mission statements of many commissioning Authorities and Regions. Some areas, such as Wales, have demonstrated that progress can be made. However, the approach has been criticised for being too narrowly focused on particular diseases with little recognition of the social circumstances which lead to ill health.

Critiques of UK policies

Despite the importance of *The Health of the Nation* in providing a strategic framework, the weaknesses of UK policies for prevention remain much as they have always been. First, they are too focused on individual behaviour change, and second, they are locked into the structure and culture of the NHS. Administrative structures remain fragmented and policy networks are fluid; there is a continuing lack of emphasis on health inequalities; the provision of information is emphasised but there is a lack of regulation and of a community-level political system committed to healthy alliances. The fluoridation of water supplies in order to prevent dental decay is perhaps the only area where governments and health professionals have consistently urged structural intervention on health grounds, albeit in a way which does not interfere with markets. Proposals have been resisted by citizens' rights groups and now perhaps finally eclipsed by the privatisation of water boards. In short, the responsibility for health remains with individuals.

Crawford (1977) argues that self-responsibility, self-reliance and self-discipline reflect the capitalist ethic of bourgeois individualism. It rests on a victim-blaming ideology:

> It instructs people to be individually responsible at a time when they are becoming less capable as individuals of controlling their health environment.
>
> (1977: 665)

Critics of health prevention in the general practice setting argue that it focuses on individual pathology. It creates a population of 'worried well' and has high costs with uncertain benefits (Crawford 1977; McCormick 1989; Wilkinson, Jones and McBride 1990; Cribb and Haran 1991). There is as yet little clear evidence, for example, that screening reduces deaths for either cancers or coronary heart disease (CHD). While a recent National Audit Office report on CHD suggests that rates are beginning to fall (NAO 1989), the rate of decline is significantly less than those achieved in North America with their more encompassing health promotion programmes. Difficulties remain in running efficient screening systems in general practice, particularly given the small scale and lack of managerial capacity in many of them. Errors in reading test results of cervical smears, for example, affecting thousands of women, continue to occur.

Graham (1979), in a critique of the effects of preventive work with mothers and young children, suggests that a strategy which seeks to underline individual responsibility in the area is misguided. She argues that mothers already take their responsibilities for their children seriously and that health education may increase uncertainty. The problem for many parents, and particularly women – as they still do most of the childcare – is the network of conflicting roles in which they find themselves. Admonitions to do this or that may be irreconcilable with demands already being placed on the mother. As family patterns become more complicated, with more single-parent families and serial marriages, this may become even more of a problem. Graham suggests that health education can only really become effective if it is more holistic. It must include an understanding of vulnerability to health risks due to social and emotional circumstances and an awareness on the part of health educators of the culture and the home circumstances of the families they are attempting to reach.

The lack of a proper framework for prevention

Despite Cabinet-level committees and a strategy for health, the NHS remains predominantly a service for curative care. The structure of the NHS and of ministerial government tends to fragment initiatives for collaborative working at both national and local levels. As Rudolf Klein has observed, Britain has 'a health policy but no policy for health' (Klein 1989, Baggott 1991: 192). The Department of Health, for example, effectively functions as the Department of the NHS – rather than as a department of health more broadly conceived. At the local level, Trusts now have a narrow remit to remain within budget. Purchasing authorities which have responsibility for the health of their populations cannot identify closely with particular communities as they continue to merge and split. In these circumstances, building healthy alliances is well-nigh impossible. As Klein agreed before the reforms:

> The NHS has, by the very fact of its existence, a political constituency: those whose income derives from working in it and those who, as patients, derive some direct benefits from its services. Prevention has no such constituency. Those who will benefit cannot be identified; moreover, the benefit itself is uncertain. For prevention is about the reduction of statistical risk, not about the delivery of certain benefits to specific individuals.
>
> (Klein 1989: 173)

Cunningham (1991), in a study of policies for prevention in North America, identified a number of factors contributing to a collective commitment to preventing ill-health. First, strong public health associations included health professionals, academics and lay people in a shared forum for raising public consciousness, while alliances were forged between voluntary organisations in the health field. In Cunningham's view, these associations informed public opinion and allowed government to adopt a radical anti-tobacco policy, for example, in the late 1980s. Second, the personal contribution of politicians and public health leaders in government was important. Third, and perhaps most important of all, there has been extensive community participation at the local level.

In the UK, the approach to health promotion has been diluted in a number of ways. First, the New Right ideologies which have dominated the governments of the 1980s stress a libertarian individualism and the importance of individual choice above all else. The emphasis has been on informing and educating the individual and these values sit uneasily with the collectivist approach necessary for many aspects of effective health promotion. The dislike of regulation may have populist roots. For example, in a study of the reasons for the failure to implement fluoridation programmes in a number of Scottish authorities, Brand (1969) found that there were two major reasons for the failure to implement this cheap and effective way of preventing tooth decay, one related to administrative structure, the second to politics. Administrative arrangements in relation to water are complex as the agreement of a number of local authorities which share a common water supply under a particular Water Board is needed. This creates difficulties. Second, the fluoridation of water was frequently left to a free vote in local councils rather than being a party issue. Councillors were thus often without leadership or sufficient information on which to make a judgement. In the absence of clear guidance they fell back on 'folk' knowledge and resisted attempts to interfere with the 'purity' of the water supply.

This case study may have a wider applicability to health issues which have not on the whole been seen as major party themes. The politics of health are not clearly developed and this may reflect the existence of a national health service and the consensus which has surrounded it. UK governments, irrespective of party, have found regulation in health matters politically difficult and have resorted to providing information and relying on health education as the main methods of health promotion.

Some would interpret this reluctance as due to political interests rather than political culture. Other countries have adopted more or less explicit health promotion strategies. Norway introduced differential food subsidies in the 1970s to encourage healthy eating (Ringen 1977, Ziglio 1986), and Finland has a highly developed primary care system which, it is suggested, has helped to reduce mortality rates. Although British governments have been willing to shift the emphasis to primary care, they have been unable or unwilling to give it priority in resource terms or to direct or control the activities of GPs.

They have also ignored the social and environmental determinants of ill-health. Their ideology tends to obscure the reality of disease and the impact of social inequality on health. The emphasis on personal responsibility thus plays down the wider economic and environmental influences on health and assumes that the individual has all the power and autonomy necessary to carry out decisions which affect life-style. It also tends to draw attention away from inequalities in access to life chances, goods and services and the way in which they contribute to health – disease rates are higher in the lower social classes. Furthermore, governments have been unwilling to acknowledge the relationship between low income, unequal income distribution, unemployment, poor environment and ill-health and have chosen to focus instead on the relationship between life-style and health status (Delamothe 1992, Wilkinson 1992), as is witnessed by the fate of the Black Report (DHSS 1980) and its recommendations.

References

Allsop, J. (1990) *Changing Primary Care: the role of facilitators*, King's Fund Centre, London.

Allsop, J. and Freeman, R. (1993) 'Policies for Prevention in Health Policy in the UK and the NHS', in Mills, M. (ed.), *Prevention, Health and British Politics*, Avebury, Aldershot, pp. 18–40.

Ashton, J. and Seymour, H. (1988) *The New Public Health,* Open University Press, Milton Keynes.

Avoiding Heart Attacks (1981) HMSO, London.

Baggott, R. (1986) 'Alcohol, Politics and Social Policy', *Journal of Social Policy*, 15, 4, pp. 467–80.

Baggott, R. (1987) 'Government-industry Relations in Britain: the regulation of the tobacco industry', *Policy and Politics,* 15, 3, pp. 137–46.

Baggott, R. (1990) *Alcohol, Politics and Social Policy,* Gower, Aldershot.

Baggott, R. (1991) 'Looking Forward to the Past? The politics of public health', *Journal of Social Policy,* 20, 2, pp. 191–213.

Beattie, A. (1991) 'Knowledge and Control in Health Promotion: a test case for social policy and social theory', in J. Gabe, M. Calnan and M. Bury (eds), *The Sociology of the Health Service,* Routledge, London.

Belloc, N. and Breslaw, L. (1972) 'Relationship of Physical Health Status and Health Practices', *Prevention Medicine,* pp. 409–21.

Billis, D. (1981) 'At Risk of Prevention', *Journal of Social Policy*, pp. 367–79.

Brand, J. A. (1969) 'The Politics of Fluoridation: a community conflict', *Political Studies,* XIX, 4, pp. 430–9.

Calnan, M. (1984) 'The Politics of Health: the case of smoking control', *Journal of Social Policy,* 13, 3, pp. 279–96.

Calnan, M. (1989) 'The Politics of Preventive Medicine: UK government policy and the prevention of coronary heart disease', Paper presented to the conference of the Political Studies Association, Warwick.

Calnan, M. (1991) *Preventing Coronary Heart Disease: prospects, policies and politics,* Routledge, London.

Calnan, M., Boulton, M. and Williams, A. (1986) 'The Role of the General Practitioner in Health Education: a critical appraisal', in S. Rodmell and A. Watt (eds), *The Politics of Health Education. Raising the Issues*, Routledge & Kegan Paul, London.

Canada, Ministry of National Health and Welfare (1974) *A New Perspective on the Health of Canadians* (The Lalonde Report), Government of Canada, Ottawa.

Crawford, R. (1977) 'You are Dangerous to your Health: the politics and ideology of victim blaming', *International Journal of Health Services,* 7, 4, pp. 663–80.

Cribb, A. and Haran, D. (1991) 'The Benefits and Ethics of Screening for Breast Cancer', *Journal of the Society of Public Health*, 195, pp. 63–7.

Cunningham, R. (1991) 'Promoting Better Health in Canada and the USA: a political perspective', Mimeo, Department of Politics, University of Glasgow.

Delamothe, T. (1992) 'Poor Britain' (editorial), *British Medical Journal*, 305, pp. 263–4.

Department of Health (1989) *General Practice in the NHS: the 1990 contract*, DOH, London.

Department of Health (1992) *The Health of the Nation. A Strategy for Health in England*, Cmnd 1986, HMSO, London.

Department of Health and Social Security (1976a) *Prevention and Health: everybody's business. A Reassessment of Public and Personal Health*, HMSO, London.

Department of Health and Social Security (1976b) *Priorities for Health and Personal Social Services*, HMSO, London.

Department of Health and Social Security (1977a) *Prevention and Health*, Cmnd 7047, HMSO, London.

Department of Health and Social Security (1977b) *Reducing the Risk: Safer Pregnancy and Childbirth*, HMSO, London.

Department of Health and Social Security (1978) *Eating for Health*, HMSO, London.

Department of Health and Social Security (1979) *Eating for Health: a discussion booklet,* HMSO, London.

Department of Health and Social Services (1980) *Inequalities in Health*, DHSS, London.

Department of Health and Social Security (1981a) *Care in Action: a handbook of policies and priorities of the health and personal social services in England*, HMSO, London.

Department of Health and Social Security (1981b) *Avoiding Heart Attacks,* HMSO, London.

Department of Health and Social Security (1981c) *Drinking Sensibly: a discussion document,* HMSO, London.

Department of Health and Social Security (1987) *Promoting Better Health: the government's programme for improving primary health care*, Cmnd 249, HMSO, London.

Department of Health and Social Security (1988) *Public Health in England, The Report of the Committee of Inquiry into the Future Development of the Public Health Function* (Chairman: Sir Donald Acheson), Cmnd 289, HMSO, London.

Farrant, W. and Russell, J. (1985) *A Case Study in the Production, Distribution and Use of Health Information*, Final Report, Health Education Council, HEC Publications, London.

George, D. (1981) 'Who Pulls the Strings at the HEC?', *World Medicine,* 28 Nov., pp. 51–4.

Graham, H. (1979) 'Prevention and Health: every mother's business, comment on child health policies in the 1970s', in *The Sociology of the Family: new directions for Britain*, Sociological Review Monograph 28, University of Keele.

Graham, H. (1987) 'Women's smoking and family health', *Social Science and Medicine*, 25, 1, pp. 47–56.

Harrison, L. and Tether, P. (1987) 'The Co-ordination of UK Policy on Alcohol and Tobacco: the significance of organisational networks', *Policy and Politics*, 15, 2, pp. 77–90.

Health Education Council (1984) *Coronary Heart Disease Prevention: Plans for Action*, a report based on an interdisciplinary workshop conference held at Canterbury on 28–30 September 1983, Pitman/HEC, London.

Klein, R. (1989) *The Politics of the NHS*, 2nd edn, Longman, Harlow.

Lewis, J. (1986) *What Price Community Medicine?,* Wheatsheaf, Brighton.

Maynard, A. and Tether, P. (eds) (1990) *Preventing Alcohol and Tobacco Problems*, vol 1, Avebury, Aldershot.

McCarthy, M. (1992) 'Preventive Medicine and Health Promotion', in Beck, E., Lonsdale, S., Newman, S. and Patterson, D. (eds), *In the Best of Health? The status and future of health care in the UK*, Chapman & Hall, London.

McCormick, J. (1989) 'Cervical Smears: a questionable practice', *The Lancet*, 22, p. 207.

McKeown, T. (1979) *The Role of Medicine: dream, mirage or nemesis?*, Blackwell, Oxford.

Mills, M. and Saward, M. (1993) 'Liberalism, Democracy and Prevention', in Mills, M. (ed.), *Prevention, Health and British Policy*, Avebury, Aldershot.

Moran, G. (1986) 'Health Promotion in Local Government: a British experience', *Health Promotion*, 1, 2, pp. 191–200.

Morris, J. (1982) 'Epidemiology and prevention', *Milbank Memorial Fund Quarterly*, 60, 1, pp. 1–16.

NAHAT (1989) *Coronary Heart Disease*, Briefing Paper, 17.

Naidoo, J. (1986) 'Limits to Individualism', in Rodmell, S. and Watt, A. (eds), *The Politics of Health Education: raising the issues*, Routledge & Kegan Paul, London.

National Audit Office (NAO) (1989) *Report of the Comptroller and Auditor General: NHS coronary health*, HMSO, London.

NHSME (National Health Service Management Executive) (1992) *The Health of the Nation: healthy alliances, working together*, NHSME, Leeds.

Office of Health Economics (1982) *Coronary Heart Disease: the scope for prevention*, Paper 73, Office of Health Economics, London.

Peto, R. (1981), 'Why Cancer? the causes of cancer in developed countries', reporting on work for United States Congress by Doll, R. and Peto, R. *The Times Health Supplement*, 6 Nov.

Popham, G. (1981) 'Government and Smoking: policy making and pressure groups', *Policy and Politics*, 9, 3, pp. 331–47.

Report of the Royal Commission on the National Health Service (1979) (Chairman: Sir Alec Merrison), Cmnd 7615, HMSO, London.

Read. M. (1993) 'The Failure to Implement an Anti-smoking Policy', in Mills, M. (ed.), *Prevention, Health and British Politics*, Avebury, Aldershot.

Ringen, K. (1977) 'The Case of Norway's Nutrition and Food Policy', *Social Science and Medicine*, 13, 3, pp. 31–41.

Rodmell, S. and Watt, A. (eds) (1986) *The Politics of Health Education: raising the issues*, Routledge & Kegan Paul, London.

Rose, G. (1981) 'Strategy of Prevention: lessons from cardio-vascular disease', *British Medical Journal*, 282, pp. 1847–51.

Royal College of General Practitioners (RCGP) (1981) *Health and Prevention in Primary Care*, Royal College of General Practitioners, London.

Royal College of Physicians (1980) *A Recommendation for the Prevention of Alcohol-related Disorders*, Royal College of Physicians, London.

Royal College of Psychiatrists (1979) *Alcohol and Alcoholism*, Tavistock, London.

Smith, A. and Jacobson, B. (1988) *The Nation's Health: a strategy for the 1990s*, Report of an independent steering committee, King's Fund Centre, London.

Social Trends (1993) Central Statistical Office, HMSO, London.

Stone, D. (1986) 'The Resistible Rise of Preventive Medicine', *Journal of Health, Politics, Policy and Law*, 11, 2, pp. 671–96.

Street, J. (1993) 'Teaching New Habits: the case of AIDS', in Mills, M. (ed.), *Prevention, Health and British Politics*, Avebury, Aldershot.

US Public Health Service (1979) *Healthy People: the Surgeon General's report on health promotion and disease prevention*, US Department of Health and Human Services, Washington, DC.

US Public Health Service (1990) *Healthy People 2000*, US Department of Health and Human Services, Washington, DC.

Warner, K. E. (1979) 'The Economic Implications of Prevention Health Care', *Social Science and Medicine*, 13c, pp. 227–37.

Welsh Health Planning Forum (1989) *Strategic Intent and Directions for the NHS in Wales*, NHS Directorate, Welsh Office, Cardiff.

Weale, A. (1981) 'Invisible Hand or Fatherly Hand?', *Journal of Health, Politics, Policy and Law*, 74, pp. 784–807.

Wilkinson, C., Jones, C. and McBride, J. (1990) 'Anxiety Caused by Abnormal Results of a Cervical Smear Test: a controlled trial', *British Medical Journal*, 300, p. 440.

Wilkinson, R. (1992) 'Income Distribution and Life Expectancy', *British Medical Journal*, 304, pp. 165–8.

Ziglio, E. (1986) 'Uncertainty in Health Promotion: nutrition policy in two countries', *Health Promotion*, 1, 3, pp. 257–68.

CHAPTER 12

The NHS and its users

Almost everyone in Britain is affected by the NHS. The vast majority are registered with NHS GPs and most use its hospital services. In 1991, the proportion of the population covered by private insurance was about 12 per cent (Office of Health Economics 1993) although this did not always mean they would use private care. All those who are earning contribute to the NHS as taxpayers. So what do people think of the NHS? What opportunities do they have to exercise their voice? How are their individual and collective interests expressed and protected?

Models of health care delivery

If medical care were taken as a good like any other, then market forces would simply determine what was provided for whom. The consumer would be sovereign. Assuming a particular number of suppliers of health care, and demand from users, the price mechanism would ensure that consumer preferences were met. However, since the rise of medical science, two other models for determining how medical and health care is distributed have developed. The professional model is based on the expert knowledge of the doctor or health worker and is essentially paternalist. Professionals acquire the competence to practise and are deemed to be the best judges of what is in the interest of the patient. They make choices for the patient. In the bureaucratic model, the judgement is that medical care is too important to be left to either the market or the professional. Governments set up institutional structures to ensure the delivery of medical services to the whole population and in so doing, determine what is available, often according to criteria of equity and need. The democratic process insures that this is achieved.

In the case of UK health care, a combination of the professional and bureaucratic model has left the health care user with restricted choice and a limited ability to exercise both exit and voice (Hirschman 1970). In relation to exit, the NHS is a monopoly service, as only a minority of people can afford private care. Moreover, there are only two points of entry to the NHS – through the GP or the hospital Accident and Emergency Department.

Once a person has presented themselves for treatment, then the use of resources is determined by the professional.

The possibilities for the exercise of voice are also limited. Those who use health services are in a weak position to question the strategies or choices involved in diagnosis and treatment because the provider has expert knowledge. This is the case whether the service is paid for or not. Abel-Smith comments:

> There are few fields of consumer expenditure where the consumer is as ill-equipped to exercise this theoretical sovereignty as in the health services.
>
> (1976: ch. 4)

He might also have added that there are few fields of work where the decision-making concerns matters which are so intimate or the consequences potentially so momentous.

There are also limitations in the exercise of voice on a collective level. The NHS, compared to other institutional structures providing social services, lacks democratic accountability. There is no locally elected tier and therefore, theoretically, the Secretary of State for Health and Social Services is accountable to Parliament for money spent in the NHS, for policies pursued and for mistakes made. The very scope of this task and the unwieldy nature of parliamentary scrutiny weakens accountability and sensitivity to individuals. Successive Ministers of Health have been well aware of these issues. Those on the left have tended to focus on increasing local democracy while those on the right have emphasised the importance of choice within a more market or business-orientated system.

There have been two other forces at work. First, active consumerism developed in the 1970s with the emergence of a number of campaigning groups concerned to promote the interests of the user. One such group, the National Consumer Council (NCC), established in 1975, has defined the dimensions of consumerism as concerned with 'access, information, equity, choice, redress and representation' (NCC 1986). Second, there has been the notion of 'participation', that is, an involvement of the patient in the health work of getting well and in taking part in the process of health service development. If patients are considered part of the process of health work then they are more likely to cooperate in their own treatment. Equally, those who were concerned with health service development argued that healthy ways of living and the development of appropriate health programmes, depend upon the active participation of communities and cooperation between a number of lay and professional health workers (WHO 1986). This chapter aims to explore the different approaches to involving the health care user in the development and provision of that care.

Democratic accountability

In theory, Ministers of Health have been accountable to Parliament for all aspects of the NHS. However, since the early 1980s and the establishment of the NHSME, and in 1990 of Trusts, this accountability has diminished. Nevertheless, Health Ministers deal with many thousands of issues through written and verbal questions both in the House of Commons and outside it, every year. There are *ad hoc* committees and commissions of inquiry into a variety of specific issues, many of which have been referred to in earlier chapters in this book. Standing Advisory Committees within the Department of Health keep particular aspects of the NHS under review. Within the House of Commons, the Public Accounts Committee examines how public money has been spent. Recent inquiries have been made into expenditure on information technology. The National Audit Office also periodically undertakes reviews to ensure value for money in public spending. The Select Committee on the Social Services and, since 1990, the Health Committee have investigated and commented upon a range of policy issues. The Audit Commission has a remit which covers health as well as local authorities in terms of investigating whether budgets are wisely used. It carries out assessments of particular areas to promote good practice in general.

Despite these mechanisms for ensuring accountability at a national level, the lack of an elected tier at a local level is a weakness. Health policy has largely been the concern of a few interested and involved national politicians; higher civil servants at the DHSS and DOH; the representatives and advisers of professional bodies; and, on occasions, the unions representing workers in health care. Although there is little doubt that chairs, members and officers of health authorities lobby the DOH, the political process of decision-making is largely hidden from public view. The public have therefore had little chance to participate in the formulation of regional health policy and, although there has been considerable pressure-group activity at a national level, at local level the community interest is very weakly represented.

Local accountability

In Britain, many social services are provided through elected local authorities. Health is an exception. The actions of the local authorities gain legitimacy through the election of representatives who claim to pursue the interests of the local community and those who elected them. The importance of local government is its potential to respond to needs within the limits of national policies using the resources available. In the 1940s, the substitute for locally elected health authorities was the representation of interest groups, particularly those involved in producing the service. Thus Aneurin Bevan appointed lay people to represent the community interest and health professionals (mainly doctors) to his new health service bodies, the Hospital Management Committees (HMCs) and Regional Hospital Boards (RHBs). Doctors were in this way given 'full participation in the administration' of the service. This was syndicalist rather than representative democracy. However, time was to show that local lay interests were weakly reflected in the activities of the boards and committees. Crossman (1972) later called these 'self-perpetuating oligarchies' in his impatience with the failures of the health authorities to respond to inadequacies in the service. The phrase may owe more to political rhetoric than analysis, although research studies had shown that members of health authorities were predominantly middle class, elderly and male (Royal Commission on Local Government 1969).

Bevan's solution to managing the health services was based on the assumption that running them was uncontroversial. There was an implicit acceptance that health care was about providing professionally determined, predominantly medical services. In the 1960s and 1970s, it became increasingly apparent that the health service was failing to adapt itself to changing needs and priorities and reforms were sought. One of the aims of the 1974 reorganisation was to increase democratic participation. The assumption was that this would help to implement national priorities and make the service more sensitive to local needs. Greater democracy was to be introduced in two ways – though both were within the tradition of interest group rather than of elected democracy. The first aimed to increase lay and professional representation within the health authorities, the second to create a new institution, the Community Health Council (CHC), to represent the public.

In Chapter 3, the increased staff and lay representation introduced in 1974 was described. From the evidence of research studies it was apparent that the impact of members on the running of the authorities was small. This was not due to members' lack of experience and expertise, but to their lack of power. In contrast to local government, in Health Authorities there was no party programme to create cohesion between members. Thus, they had no coherent approach to policy; nor did they have a power base as members acted as individuals. In 1982, a further reorganisation designed to increase the responsiveness of the health authorities to local needs took place. A closer relationship between those planning and those managing services was envisaged. However, District Health Authority (DHA) membership was reduced to between 16 and 18 members although the principles of appointment with local authority, trade-union and generalist representation remained. One report on DHAs by the National Association of Health Authorities (NAHA 1986) suggested that they had 'a complex balancing and mediating responsibility' between the various pressures applied by the DHSS, the NHS Management Board, the Regional Health Authority (RHA) managers and professionals within the district and the local community. The report claimed that DHAs, because of their membership, had 'some legitimacy to challenge the demands or pressures emanating from any one of these sources'. They had a particular responsibility to the local community. However, with the strengthening of health service management after the 1983 Griffiths Report, the introduction of the top-down review process and the cost-cutting exercises of the mid-1980s, the role of members was weakened further.

Finally, with the 1990 NHS Act, any pretence that appointed members represented local communities was dropped. The business model prevailed. Generalist members are now appointed by the Secretary of State and receive payment for their work. They have become non-executive Board members of Trusts and purchasing authorities working alongside managers. Recent research has shown that the majority of Board members are white male businessmen from private sector backgrounds (Cairncross and Ashburner 1992). The main function of Trusts is to attract sufficient contracts to remain financially viable. Purchasing authorities draw up contracts based on their assessment of the service needs of their population. Although contracting should involve consultation with local interest groups, there is no requirement to do so. In general, individuals as consumers and citizens have few ways of influencing the process. As was argued in the previous chapter, accountability through formal means, always weak in the NHS, has been reduced by the health service reforms.

Community Health Councils (CHCs)

In 1974, CHCs were established by Richard Crossman, the then Minister of Health, to increase democracy in the NHS through the 'representation of interests'. This notion was, however, ambiguous. It was proposed that appointees to CHCs should include both people with special knowledge to speak for the interests of vulnerable groups – who were more frequent users of the NHS – as well as those representing the public in general. There was a potential conflict between these interests which was left to the Councils themselves to resolve. Moreover, what was meant by 'representation' was never spelt out.

In 1974, CHCs were set up in each of the 229 districts in England and Wales. They were, and still are, funded by the regions who also appoint the members – drawing one-third of them from voluntary organisations, one-half from local authorities, while one-sixth are generalists. CHCs have between 18 and 24 members depending on the population and are serviced by a small secretariat. They have two major roles. The first is to keep under review the operation of the health service in the district and make recommendations for improvement. They have a right to visit NHS premises (but not GP surgeries) and to access to information. They must be consulted on planning proposals. They may also oppose a hospital closure, in which case the matter may be referred to the Secretary of State for a final decision. The second main function of the CHC is to be a source of information and advice to the public, particularly for those with special needs.

Studies of CHCs suggest that they have faced a number of problems (Klein and Lewis 1976, Maxwell and Weaver 1984). First, they have an ambiguous relationship to Health Authorities. Is their role of cooperation with NHS management simply providing a consumer input or should they oppose changes which they believe are against the user interest? The DHSS stated that the CHCs were given a special role in relation to the planning process, that they should be consulted and help to determine the setting of priorities and in so doing encourage the better use of resources. On the other hand the Association of Community Health Councils in its evidence to the Royal Commission on the NHS (1979) argued that CHCs' ability to represent the consumer was strongest when they were not seen as part of the process of management. One aspect of the problem lay in the lack of precision with which the terms 'participation' and 'consultation' have been used. Ham (1980) quotes a national survey in which 68 per cent of CHCs were shown to have had disputes with the Health Authorities on the meaning of these terms.

Ham (1980) goes on to suggest that the efficacy of CHCs, despite their good intentions, has been affected by the dominant political culture of the NHS. Members of Health Authorities (whose own legitimacy is in any case weak), and their officers, have tended to see CHCs as speaking only as individuals or speaking for narrow sectional interests. Health Authority members see *themselves* as representing the true public interest and regard the time spent in their dealings with CHCs as giving little payoff.

Winkler (1987) writes a first-hand account of the difficulties which CHC members face as lone representatives on health service planning committees.

> . . . [they] frequently get overwhelmed and feel unable to contribute. They can also become co-opted into the professional orbit and become supporters of the status quo. 'Your representative was present when a decision was taken,' is the standard excuse by authorities to stop comment by a group at a later discussion.
>
> (quoted in Seale 1993: 75)

In order to support its members, this particular CHC treated them as its own representatives and asked them to report back to a specialist group of the Council.

Second, CHCs have a low level of funding in relation to the roles they are expected to play. Hogg (1987) has estimated that in 1983–4, the funding for CHCs amounted to 8 pence per head of population. Their full-time staff members are small in number – this creates a reliance on voluntary commitment from Council members. Conversely, the role of CHCs is also limited by their lack of resources.

Third, CHCs have varied considerably in the way they have operated. Some have carried out surveys to investigate shortcomings in health care. For example, in the late 1970s, Kensington and Chelsea CHC undertook a survey on access to primary health care in inner London. In some areas, a high proportion of people were unable to register with a doctor due to the lack of NHS GPs and a high number of single-handed practices. Others, such as Hackney CHC, have campaigned to shape services in the interests of local groups (see Seale 1993 for further examples).

Exercising voice

What do people think of the NHS?

From the 1970s, surveys began to be used to establish what people thought of the NHS. These have found that users do support it and also have a high level of satisfaction. For example, the Royal Commission on the NHS commissioned two surveys, of users and patients. Both found the level of general consumer satisfaction with health services was high (Gregory 1978). In the study on patient's attitudes to the hospital service more than 80 per cent of inpatients thought that the service they received was good or very good. Simpson's (1979) study of primary care services for old people and children in a rural and an inner-city area concluded that on the whole, the NHS did provide care which was generally appreciated by its users.

Gregory's study showed that although the *general* level of professed satisfaction was high, there was in fact a large number of specific complaints. Among outpatients, for example, more than 25 per cent complained about difficulties in getting information about their progress. This rose to 31 per cent for inpatients. One in four adult inpatients complained that doctors had discussed their condition as if they were not there. Waiting times also caused dissatisfaction. Sixteen per cent of patients at outpatient clinics waited an hour after their appointment time and another 8 per cent for 45 minutes. There were also complaints about lack of privacy and early rising times for patients in hospital. Nearly half

Table 12.1 ***Causes of dissatisfaction with in-patient hospital care in the UK 1976–77***

	Percentage of respondents
Woken too early	43
Information about progress	31
Emergencies: waiting for attention	26
Food	21
Waiting for admission	20

Source: Gregory (1978) HMSO, London.

of those surveyed complained of being woken too early. In fact 44 per cent were being woken before 6.00 am and 76 per cent before 6.30 am. Table 12.1 gives a complete set of figures.

The Royal Commission (Report of the Royal Commission 1979: 133) comments:

> This seems to us a prime example of the hospital being run for the convenience of its staff rather than the patient. We do not believe that the in-patients' day cannot be so organised so that the majority of patients are able to wake up at roughly their usual time.

What is surprising is that such a high level of grumbles and grievances should be seen as compatible with a very high level of reported satisfaction. As far as the NHS is concerned, consumers do appear to be passive. Perhaps Cartwright is right when she suggested that 'behind the satisfaction of most patients there lies an uncritical acceptance and lack of discrimination which is conducive to stagnation and apathy' (Cartwright 1967: 216). This brings us full circle to Abel-Smith's point that, concerning much medical practice, users lack the knowledge and will to assess critically the treatment they receive (1976). They are patients rather than consumers, they complain about the 'hotel' aspects of care rather than treatment, the quality of which they cannot judge. To look at the question another way around, there seems to be a high capacity for health systems to generate loyalty among their recipients. On the whole, patients tend to accept what they are offered. Payer (1990) suggests that this reflects cultural attitudes; people in Britain are less critical than North Americans in relation to health care.

Since 1983, the British Social Attitudes Survey (BSAS) has provided an annual snapshot of opinions on the NHS. The most recent report indicates a number of trends. Support for an NHS funded out of taxation remains high and so does general satisfaction, but the proportion of the population who remain very satisfied has declined while the proportion who are very dissatisfied has increased. In 1983, 11 per cent were very satisfied with the NHS and 7 per cent dissatisfied while in 1987, 7 per cent were very satisfied and 15 per cent very dissatisfied. This may reflect either that services are deteriorating or that health service

Table 12.2 **Satisfaction with selected aspects of the NHS in Britain: 1983 and 1987**

	Percentage of respondents					
	Satisfied		*Neither*		*Dissatisfied*	
	1983	*1987*	*1983*	*1987*	*1983*	*1987*
Local doctors/GPs	80	79	7	8	12	13
Health visitors/district nurses	54	51	41	43	4	6
Being in hospital as an in-patient	74	67	19	19	6	13
Attending hospital as an out-patient	61	54	18	18	21	29

Source: Adapted from Bosanquet (1988) and Taylor Gooby (1987).

users are becoming more discriminating. In answer to more specific questions about the NHS, more people were dissatisfied with aspects of hospital care than with primary care (Table 12.2). Women and younger people tended to be more critical than other groups in the population.

Many studies found that NHS staff were unresponsive to patient needs. In the 1980s, local consumer surveys tended to confirm these findings although there has been no national study to replicate Gregory's work. Rather, investigations have focused on the adequacy, or otherwise, of NHS resourcing. Thus, the fifth BSAS survey asked respondents whether they thought there was a need for improvement in the quantity of certain services. The results are given in Table 12.3.

Dissatisfaction with the NHS may be one reason why more people have exercised the other consumer option of exit to choose private health care, particularly for alleviative surgery (see Chapter 8). But it is worth noting that there are even fewer avenues for exercising voice in the private sector. Perhaps it is believed that the operation of the price mechanism will keep standards high. However, patients are in no stronger a position to judge the quality of care than they are in the NHS and there are fewer ways of obtaining redress.

Surveys aimed to test consumer opinion or experiences have been used increasingly by local providers. In the 1970s, the typical

Table 12.3 **Percentage of respondents thinking there was need for improvement in certain areas in Britain: 1988**

Hospital waiting lists for non-emergency operations	87
Waiting time before getting appointments with consultants	83
Staffing levels of nurses/doctors in hospitals	73

Source: Adapted from Bosanquet (1988).

survey was carried out by a national organisation, an academic researcher, or a CHC. Usually, the aim was to investigate attitudes to services and so influence policy. Jones *et al.* (1987) review more than two hundred such surveys. In the 1980s, these were mainly carried out by Health Authorities, occasionally with assistance from CHCs. They tended to concentrate on the acceptability of a particular ward, hospital or local service rather than actively trying to find out what people wanted or the types of care to which they would give high priority. However, sometimes population-based surveys have made a valuable contribution to service development (Prescott-Clarke *et al.* 1988, Exeter and District CHC 1982, Tower Hamlets DHA 1984, Carr-Hill *et al.* 1989).

Mechamisms to protect the individual

Voicing a grievance

There are a number of mechanisms through which people can make complaint and seek redress. Family Health Service Authorities (FHSAs), previously Family Practitioner Committees, have statutory committees and a quasi-judicial procedure to hear complaints against family doctors, dentists and pharmacists for breaching their terms of contract. DHAs are obliged to maintain systems to receive and monitor patient complaints, in the hospital and community services, and mechanisms to carry out investigations if necessary. There are also elaborate procedures to investigate complaints about clinical treatment and to discipline staff employed in the NHS. For doctors, their use is relatively rare.

In 1979, the Royal Commission on the NHS criticised the plethora of complaint systems and commented:

> There needs, therefore, to be a simple and well understood mechanism through which people who use the National Health Service can suggest how it can be improved and complain when things go wrong.
>
> (para. 11.13)

However, consumer groups have continued to argue that complaints procedures are insufficiently publicised; unnecessarily complex; subject to long delays; and sometimes lack impartiality. Although there have been a number of changes (referred to below), these have been relatively limited in scope.

In 1973, the Davies Committee (DHSS 1973) recommended a national code for dealing with hospital complaints, including the introduction of an independent review. These suggestions have not been introduced but the 1985 Hospital Complaints Act obliged health authorities to establish complaint procedures. However, in 1994, a review of NHS complaints recommended a thorough overhaul of complaints systems (DOH 1994).

In addition to NHS procedures, there are professional institutions which maintain registers of the qualified. The most important of these are the General Medical Council and the United Kingdom Central Council for Nursing. Members of the public may make complaints to these bodies. However, the courts are the ultimate source of redress for those seeking to gain compensation for injury. Negligence on the part of a health care professional in authority has to be established. There is, as yet, no form of 'no fault' compensation in the UK (Ham *et al.* 1988).

Another forum for voicing a complaint is by requesting an investigation by the Parliamentary Commissioner for the Health Service. If this proceeds, complainants must give an undertaking not to seek legal redress. The Commissioner, first appointed in 1977, is empowered to investigate cases of maladministration and misadministration but matters involving clinical judgement are specifically excluded. The procedure is thorough but slow.

Since 1983, under the Mental Health Act, it has also been possible for patients who are being treated for mental illness to appeal to the Mental Health Commission against decisions about their treatment. This provides a further safeguard for those who are receiving compulsory treatment of some sort (Pilgrim and Rogers 1988).

A number of criticisms have been made of these avenues for exercising voice. Access tends to be inhibited through lack of knowledge; there is insufficient publicity; systems are complex and time consuming and often intimidating for users. A review of the problems is provided in Mulcahy, *Redress in the Public* Sector (1995).

As well as mechanisms which give voice to those who wish to complain, there are agencies which inspect services to ensure quality. The Health Advisory Service (HAS) aims to maintain the quality of care received by groups of patients who may not be able to protect themselves: for example, elderly, mentally ill people and those with learning difficulties. The HAS was established following revelations of poor patient care in a number of long-stay institutions in the late 1960s and early 1970s. Panels of specialists now visit health districts, advise on standards and policies and make recommendations. However, the implementation of these is not obligatory and a recent report has criticised the HAS's failure to develop national standards and performance indicators (Klein and Day 1990).

Trends in the use of voice

In the 1980s, data sources indicate that members of the public were increasingly likely to make use of advice services and to join organisations which represented their interests. Table 12.4 shows the trends.

Table 12.4 **Use of, and membership of, selected advisory services: UK**

	1971	*1981*	*1988*	*1991*
Citizens Advice Bureaux[1]:				
Total number of enquiries	1 500 000	4 007 000	7 015 000	8 278 000
Enquiries on health matters		148 000	197 000	160 600
Leukaemia Care Society[2]: branches	1	21	NA	75
Arthritis Care[2]: branches	64	230	431	550
National Membership	NA	NA	50 000	65 000
National Childbirth Trust: branches	37	240	353	350

Notes:
1 *Social Trends 20* (Central Statistical Office 1990) Table 11.18, p. 171.
2 Personal communication.

Making a complaint

With the exception of the General Medical Council and the courts, the mechanisms for the redress of grievances relate only to NHS, and not private sector, health care. It is worth noting that the size of awards in claims for negligence has risen steadily (Ham

Table 12.5 **Complaints from members of the public received by statutory bodies: England**

	1977/78	*1981/82*	*1985/86*	*1991/92*
Complaints received by the Health Service Commissioner UK[1]	494	586	807	972
Service Committee Hearings involving GPs (England)[2]	596	706	1287	1608
General Medical Council (UK) letters received on the conduct of doctors[3]		646	748	1301
Claims raised against 2 regional health authorities per 100 000[4]				
Region C	1.0	2.0	3.5	NA
Region E[5]	4.0	5.5	16.5	NA
Hospital complaints: England	NA	16 218	25 336	44 680

Sources:
1. The Health Service Commissioner Annual Report 1986–9.
2. Health and Personal Social Service Statistics, 1982 and 1986.
3. General Medical Council Annual Reports for 1982 and 1986.
4. Ham, *et al.* (1988).
5. Health and Personal Social Service Statistics: Hospital Complaints.

et al. 1988). Ironically, this may reflect the ability of modern hospitals to maintain the lives of severely damaged people. In 1990, the Health Authorities were given the full responsibility for claims raised against their medical employees rather than simply paying a proportion of contributions to the doctors' defence union. The Association of Victims of Medical Accidents (AVMA), a consumer group, has argued that those with complaints may lose by this as Health Authorities more vigorously defend actions to avoid additional costs (*Guardian*, 7 May 1990: 3).

Table 12.5 indicates that service users are increasingly making complaints about aspects of their health care to a variety of bodies.

Health Service users as activists

In the 1970s, the critiques of health care developed from, and assisted, the growth of a more active consumerism in health care. Social scientists became more interested in studying illness and health behaviour and how health care was viewed from the patient's perspective. There was a development of groups concerned with both self-help and active campaigning associated with specific health issues. In addition, national institutions reflecting consumer interests and concerns were strengthened.

Studies have indicated that the model of illness behaviour based on the passive consumer or patient and active doctor was an over-simplification. People may be active in relation to their health. Those with symptoms do not automatically declare themselves ill and take to their beds, nor do they necessarily consult a doctor. As Robinson (1971) showed in his study of families in South Wales, decision-making about whether to acknowledge, let alone report, illness was determined by a wide range of perceptions and evaluations which were influenced by social structure, class, family roles and work demands. In this study, women tended to under-report illness because they wished to continue to maintain their family role.

The first line of defence in illness is often self-medication. For example, Dunnell and Cartwright in *Medicine Takers, Prescribers and Hoarders* (1972) found that 41 per cent of their national sample had taken painkillers during the previous fortnight, 14 per cent indigestion remedies, 14 per cent skin ointments and antiseptics, 13 per cent throat and cough remedies – all without recourse to a doctor. People also consult others within their social network about signs and symptoms and choose to consult practitioners other than those provided through the NHS. This may be as a substitute for, or complementary to, the NHS; it may be a precursor to conventional treatment or used when this has failed.

Hughes (1958) and later Stacey (1976) argued that the patient is part of the process of health care. The patient brings conditions to the doctor in the first place and is actively involved in the process of 'producing' effective treatment. The patient does not consume a product but *is* part of the production of recovery or health. Treatment is interactive and negotiated. Analyses which made a rigid distinction between work to people and work for people excluded the patient and encouraged the objectification of the person. This could lead, suggested Illich (1976), to medical procedures which:

> . . . often turn into a kind of black magic, when instead of mobilising his healing powers, they transform the sick man into a limp and mystified voyeur of his own treatment.
>
> (1976: 53)

The interactionist perspective led to a number of studies of health care from this standpoint: Roth's account of long-stay hospitals (1963) and Stimson and Webb's study of the patient's view of general practice, *Going to the Doctor* (1975). These emphasise the ongoing drama of an illness episode of which the consultation is a small part of a longer process of management. The consultation is anticipated and made sense of by the patient afterwards and may or may not result in their following advice given. These studies and others suggest that the patient is very much part of the production of health care. The rejection of the term 'consumer' can thus be seen as part of the process of attempting to reconceptualise roles in health care so that the medical expert is only one element. This is particularly important in understanding those areas of health and medical care which do not fit the acute illness, passive patient/authoritative doctor model. Much health care is concerned with the management of chronic illness, with the discomforts of disability and old age, with coping mechanisms of self-limiting and trivial illness, where a variety of people may be involved in health care work.

Davies (1977) argued that health care can be seen as a field of work in which there are participants of various kinds providing health care within or outside the institutional setting. It is an arena in which occupational identities are forged and status is established; where some work is paid and similar work unpaid. Health policies and organisational structures aid or discourage a particular division of labour as they establish boundaries between different health care roles. Health workers and the organisational arrangements for the delivery of care may serve to socialise individuals into health roles, thus reinforcing them. Davies herself found that in a study of new mothers and health workers, the latter sought to socialise the mother into appropriate behaviour in the division of labour. This indicated where help should be sought and which health problems could be considered as trivial.

Individuals could be said to be health workers, therefore, in two dimensions. They perceive, define, make choices and cope with all stages of illness in themselves and they perform a similar role in the health care of others. There is no simple divide between health on the one side and professionally defined illness on the other. Neither is there a clear distinction between lay people on the one hand and professionals on the other. Attempts to break down barriers organisationally are occurring as there is greater recognition of the social aspects of illness and the importance of empowering patients. Parents may stay in hospital with their children. There have been experiments with patients' organisations in primary care. Community health workers have been employed to encourage groups to design their own services. Winn describes a variety of experiments in *Power to the People* (1990).

Self-help and campaigning groups

Self-help groups who may rely on either conventional or alternative therapies have become increasingly active. Lock (1986) goes so far as to call them the fourth estate in medicine. Pressure groups, particularly those concerned with disabled and chronically ill people, black people, those with HIV/AIDS and those concerned with women's health, have been active in voicing their discontents. They have been active in areas where conventional allopathic medicine has little to offer and where the experience of users provides valued knowledge and support (see, for example, Locker 1983, Brent Community Health Council 1981, Stanworth 1987).

Specialist consumer organisations concerned with health issues have maintained a high profile. For example, the Association of Community Health Councils, The Patients Association, Health Rights, the Association of Victims of Medical Accidents and the College of Health have campaigned on a variety of issues to safeguard patients' rights and can claim to have achieved some shifts in policy. For example, since 1987 the General Medical Council has increased the number of ways in which it can deal with professional conduct and misconduct (Robinson 1989, Stacey 1992). Lay representation has been strengthened on a variety of committees, such as the GMC research ethics committees, and is part of new bodies such as the licensing body which deals with embryo research (Phillips and Dawson 1982, DOH 1990).

The women's health movement has been particularly active in spreading information about self-care and 'holistic medicine'. Roberts's *Women, Health and Reproduction* (1981) is a collection of essays in which the general argument is that the disease model of illness is inappropriate to the handling of many aspects of women's health care. Bart, in an account of a self-help abortion clinic, demands the handing over of 'medical technologies', arguing that these should not remain the property of the medical profession in a hospital setting. The working of a Well Woman Clinic is also described: this is concerned with counselling and support, the sharing of health problems and treatments to develop ways of coping among women. Pressures from a variety of sources have led the Department of Health to support radical changes in handling childbirth. An indication of the shift in emphasis are the following quotations from the *Changing Childbirth* report (DOH 1993):

> In 1984, Maternity in Action gave the following guidance to health authorities. 'As unforseen complications can occur in any birth, every mother should be encouraged to have her baby in a maternity unit where emergency facilities are available'.
>
> (quoted in DOH 1993: 1)

In 1992, the Health Committee commented:

> On the basis of what we have heard, this committee must draw the conclusion that the policy of encouraging all women to give birth in hospitals cannot be justified on the grounds of safety.
>
> (quoted in DOH 1993:1)

For both women and particular ethnic groups there has sometimes been a failure of the NHS to understand sufficiently the cultural and emotional dimensions of illness which may make the NHS unacceptable. Brent Community Health Council explores these issues in its booklet, *Black People and the Health Service* (1981). Donovan (1986) and Ahmad (1993) provide reviews of the shortcomings of care for ethnic minority groups and ways of overcoming them. Further signs of active consumerism can be found in the growth and development of organised self-care around particular illnesses and disabilities. Mutual self-care groups exist for many specific conditions and Henry and Robinson's (1979) study has provided an account of the mutual support derived

Table 12.6 **Use of alternative medicine, 1989**

	Percentages	
	Seriously consider	*Personally used*
Homeopathy	37	11
Osteopathy	32	10
Faith or spiritual healing	12	5
Acupuncture	33	4
Hypnosis	19	3
Chiropractic	13	3

Source: Social Trends (1994) HMSO, London.

from the experience of sharing and learning among those with similar difficulties. Self-help groups may offer an understanding of pain, disability and dying in a supportive and non-stigmatising environment.

In addition to increasing self-help, there is also evidence of a more widespread use of alternative medicine. *Social Trends* (1994) provides data for the first time on the use of various therapies, reproduced in Table 12.6.

Health care users as active consumers

The business model

By 1990, the NHS and Community Care Act had introduced the market model into health care, bringing competition between agencies within the NHS. This has meant Trusts competing for contracts to treat patients. In theory, a Trust which does not gain sufficient patients will cease to trade. The Act is the culmination of a trend in government policy apparent in the 1980s, which aimed to strengthen control over services. An aspect of this is by encouraging the individual consumer to become more active. As Gordon argues:

> . . . the liberal idea of government consists – over and above the economic market in commodities and services, whose existence forms the classical attribution of an autonomous rationality to the processes of civil society – in the form of something like a second order market of governmental goods and services. It becomes the ambition of neo-liberalism to implicate the individual citizen, as player and partner, into this market game
>
> (1991: 36)

Managers as consumer champions

In 1983, the Griffiths Report (DHSS 1983) emphasised the concept of the consumer rather than the patient. Griffiths declared that the interests of the consumer should be central to every health care decision. Managers should go directly to the user to find out their views, through surveys and the like. Patients should have more information, be consulted about and have more involvement in decisions about health care. Griffiths saw the process of consulting CHCs to obtain community views as labyrinthine, and often unproductive.

Following the Griffiths Report, directors of quality assurance were appointed in Health Authorities to ascertain patients' views. Surveying patients and communities was encouraged as a method of establishing opinions and preferences to inform management action. From the mid-1980s, the use of these methods became relatively widespread. These took a variety of forms, from routine monitoring, such as that developed by the CASPE project and used by the Bloomsbury Health Authority (see Seale 1993), to specific surveys to target services for improvement. In 1992, the NHS Management Executive published *Listening to Local Voices* (NHSME 1992), which urged purchasing authorities to consult with local people about which services should be given priority. Layzell (1994) provides an example of how this has been done in one area, Derbyshire.

Currently, the internal market is one where GPs and purchasing authorities act as proxy consumers. Plamping and Delamothe have suggested that they can therefore become people's advocates, arguing:

> A new group of professionals will act as discriminating purchasers of services by becoming expert in assessing health needs and monitoring the quality and effectiveness of health care.
>
> (1991: 737)

However, there is currently a lack of techniques to support this kind of development. Expectations may be raised by offering participation which may then be disappointed. Furthermore, conflicts may be equally likely to be the result of a consultation process as of agreement.

Charters and the consumer

The Citizen's Charter and the raft of specific charters which followed also aimed to use the consumer to improve the service. The Charter initiative, led by the Cabinet Office Citizen's Charter Unit, was one of John Major's key policies in the early years of his premiership. The initiative was seen as a 10-year programme for transforming the management of public services. In 1992, William Waldegrave, the Minister then responsible, declared that the programme:

> . . . is part of the wider transformation of the way public services are run moving away from the old command structure to more open responsive management by clear published contracts which empower managers with the authority to run their organisations in the way that best suits the needs of those who actually use the services.
>
> (quoted in Tritter 1994)

The role of users as allies of managers in improving public services is expressed in *The Citizen's Charter First Report* thus:

> The principles of the Charter, simple but tough, are increasingly accepted. They give the citizen published standards and results; choice and competition as a spur to quality improvement; responsiveness; and

value for money to get the best possible service within the resources the nation can afford. They give more power to the citizen to choose.

(Citizen's Charter Unit 1992: i)

The means adopted to ensure that these aims are achieved was left to public services to develop in their individual charters. In general, rights are outlined and performance standards or targets given. However, there is more emphasis on the latter than the former (Tritter 1994). There is the proviso that although the government is introducing National Charter Standards:

These are not legal rights but major and specific standards which the Government looks to the NHS to achieve, as circumstances and resources allow.

(DOH 1991: 6)

NHS patients already have a number of rights – for example, to treatment, to change doctors, or to a second opinion. However, the exercise of these rights may depend on availability; on the knowledge of the patient; or on a professional decision. For example, in 1991 a Consumer's Association survey found that one in 10 patients who asked for a second opinion from their family doctor was refused (quoted in Seale 1993). *The Citizen's Charter First Report* proclaimed six principles of public service: standards, information and openness, choice and consultation, courtesy and helpfulness, putting things right and value for money. But again the emphasis is put on better management of public services in order to achieve change. This is through the privatisation of the supply of services, market testing for contracts, performance-related pay for managers and the removal of protection from competition.

In the NHS, the Patient's Charter outlined seven existing rights; three new rights and nine charter standards. In relation to the latter, specifications were either general: such as, 'all health authorities should ensure that the services they arrange can be used by everyone including children and people with special needs such as those with physical and mental disabilities . . .' (p. 13); or they were exact, '. . . you will be given a specific appointment time and be seen within thirty minutes of that time' (p. 14). From April 1992, local-level authorities, including GPs, were expected to produce local charter standards. By setting standards, the aim was to commit managers to targets against which their performance could be measured in subsequent reviews.

Complaints and redress

In 1993, the Charter Unit set up a Complaints Task Force to examine how complaints should be handled in public sector services in line with Charter principles. Later in the year, the

Task Force published a list of principles with a checklist for managers to assess how well their organisation was performing. The principles said that systems should be accessible and well publicised; simple to understand and use; allow speedy handling with time limits; ensure a full and fair investigation; respect people's desire for confidentiality; address all the points at issue; provide an effective response and appropriate redress; and supply information to management so that services can be improved. Again managers are encouraged to review their performance in the light of user views of the service.

More information for patients

Another strand to current policy is to make more information available to patients so that they can exercise more control and choice over their own treatment. An example is the approach taken by the Audit Commission's report on communication between hospitals and patients – *What Seems to be the Matter?* (Audit Commission 1993). Document 27 (page 342) shows the ways in which a lack of communication can arise. It is argued that managers should work with senior clinical staff to obtain a thorough understanding of patient's experiences and viewpoints, and actively manage the communication process through planning and costing. The review is interesting because it begins to isolate particular components of the work involved in communicating both general and clinical information. In so doing, it provides a way of setting certain standards in relation to detailed aspects of service delivery. Such standards can then be used to cost and monitor outcomes. Again, once such standards are known, this may raise patient expectations and lead to their beoming more active consumers.

Under the banner of consumerism, the Citizen's Charter initiative has taken important steps in opening up health care to greater scrutiny: providing information; comparative data on performance standards and the rest; giving ways of setting standards and improving quality; and possibly giving greater autonomy to the user. Some, like Le Grand (1992) and Davies (1993), argue that the introduction of market forces has not gone far enough. Davies, for example, would like a systematic analysis of the options open to consumers, the identification of local monopolies and the design of strategies to overcome them. Others are more critical of the reliance on competition and charters. Winkler (1987) refers to the government's approach as being a supermarket model of consumerism. Charters are only useful if people are already well informed and have money in their pockets. Pollitt (1993) concludes from a study of quality audits that, although patients are being consulted more than in the past, consultations are made usually on management terms. They may be asked what they think of the services already on offer but are rarely asked what other services they would like or how they themselves would define and assess quality.

Conclusion

This chapter has aimed to review government policy towards those who use health services. While all governments have attempted to provide some form of counterweight to the experts who provide care, the method of intervention has varied according to political ideology. The efforts to increase the democratic element favoured by Labour ministers have had little impact. Conservative policies aim to encourage the individual user to employ both voice and exit as a means of improving the service. However, because those supplying services at a local level remain in a monopoly position, this method may only be as successful as managers allow it to be. There is also a problem of balancing the needs of some individuals, those who are more active and articulate, against others who are less so. Knowledge of charter rights and methods of complaining remain limited.

There are many charters, all with different standards, principles and measures of performance. This can be confusing for users looking for the means to assess entitlement. And inevitably, there will be those who find it easier than others to understand what these entitlements are. Moreover, the stress on service standards for individuals may take attention away from the resources allocated to a service. If the standards of service are already adequate, mechanisms for redress may function well, but if they are generally poor, then there the managerial response is also likely to be poor. At the end of the day, individual consumers have little power.

There are signs that groups of health care users are becoming more active. If this can be harnessed in the purchasing process, then the NHS could develop more participative processes. However, the size of purchasing authorities is increasing – the competition between Trusts could exclude users – and they no longer serve local populations. The challenge of developing methods for involving communities, so that they have a sense of ownership over their local health care, remains.

References

Abel-Smith, B. (1976) *Value for Money in Health Services*, Heinemann, London, ch. 4.

Allsop, J. (1992) 'The Voice of the User in Health Care', in Beck, E., Lonsdale, S., Newman, S. and Patterson, D., *In the Best of Health?*

the status and future of health care in the UK, Chapman & Hall, London.

Ahmad, W. (ed.) (1993) *Race and Health in Contemporary Britain*, Open University Press, Milton Keynes.

Audit Commission (1993) *What Seems to be the Matter? communication between hospitals and patients*, HMSO, London.

Bosanquet, N. (1988) 'The Ailing State of the National Health', in Jowell, R., Witherspoon, S. and Brook, L. (eds), *British Social Attitudes*, 5th Report, Gower, Aldershot.

Brent Community Health Council (1981) *Black People and the Health Service.*

Cabinet Office and the Central Office of Information (1993) Citizen's Charter Complaints Task Force, *Effective Complaint Systems, Principles and Checklist*, HMSO, London.

Cairncross, I. and Ashburner, L. (1992) *NHS Trust Boards: the first wave – the first year*, Centre for Corporate Strategy and Change, University of Warwick.

Carr-Hill, R., Dixon, P. and McIver, S. (1989) *The NHS and its Customers I, II, III & IV*, Centre for Health Economics, York.

Cartwright, A. (1967) *Patients and their Doctors*, Routledge & Kegan Paul, London.

Citizen's Charter Unit (1992) *The Citizen's Charter First Report*, Cmnd 2101, HMSO, London.

Crossman, R. (1972) *A Politician's View of Health Service Planning*, University of Glasgow.

Davies, C. (1977) 'Comparative Occupational Roles in Health Care', *Social Science and Medicine*, 13a, 19.

Davies, H. (1993) 'The NHS Reforms: making a social market work', *Times Health Supplement*, April, pp. 7–10.

Department of Health (1990) 'Embryology Authority Membership: press release', July.

Department of Health (1991), *The Patient's Charter*, DOH, London.

Department of Health (1993) *Changing Childbirth, Report of the Expert Maternity Group* (Chair: Baroness Cumberledge), HMSO, London.

Department of Health (1994), *NHS Complaints Review*, DOH, HMSO, London.

Department of Health and Social Security (1983) *The Griffiths Management Inquiry*, DHSS, London.

Department of Health and Social Security and the Welsh Office (1973) *Report of the Committee on Hospital Complaints Procedures* (Chair: Sir Michael Davies), HMSO, London.

Donovan, J. (1986) *You Can't Buck Sickness, it Just Comes: health, illness and health care in the lives of black people in London*, Gower, Aldershot.

Dunnell, K. and Cartwright, A. (1972) *Medicine Takers, Prescribers and Hoarders*, Routledge & Kegan Paul, London.

Exeter and District CHC (1982), *Medical Services in Rural Areas*, Exeter and District CHC, Exeter.

Gordon, C. (1991) 'Government Rationality: an introduction', in Burchell, G., Gordon, C. and Miller, P. (eds) *The Foucault Effect: studies in governmentality*, Harvester Wheatsheaf, London.

Gregory, J. (1978) *Patients' Attitudes to the Hospital Service*, Royal

Commission on the National Health Service Research Paper No. 5, HMSO, London.

Ham, C. (1980) 'Community Health Council Participation in the NHS Planning System', *Social Policy and Administration*, 14, 3, Autumn, pp. 221–31.

Ham, C., Dingwall, R., Fenn, P. and Harris, D. (1988) *Medical Negligence: compensation and accountability*, Briefing paper 6, King's Fund Institute, London.

Henry, S. and Robinson, D. (1979) 'The Self Help Way to Health' in Atkinson, P., Dingwall, R. and Murcott, A. (eds) *Prospects for the National Health Service*, Croom Helm, London.

Hirschman, A. (1970) *Exit, Voice and Loyalty*, Harvard University Press, Cambridge, Mass.

HM Treasury (1991) *Competing for Quality: buying better public services*, Cmnd 1730, HMSO, London.

Hogg, C. (1987) *Good Practices in CHCs*, ACHCEW, London.

Hughes, E. C. (1958) *Men and their Work*, Free Press, Glencoe, Ill.

Illich, I. (1976) *Limits to Medicine: medical nemesis, the expropriation of health*, Marion Boyars, London.

Jones, L., Leneman, L. and MacLean, U. (1987) *Consumer Feedback for the NHS*, King's Fund Institute, London.

Klein, R. and Day, P. (1990) *Inspecting the Inspectorates*, Joseph Rowntree Memorial Trust, York.

Klein, R. and Lewis, J. (1976) *The Politics of Consumer Representation: a study of CHCs*, Centre for Studies in Social Policy, London.

Layzell, A. (1994) 'Local and Vocal', *Health Services Journal*, 20, pp. 20–30.

Le Grand, J. (1992) 'Paying for or Providing Welfare', Paper presented to the Annual Conference of the Social Policy Association, University of Nottingham, July.

Lock, S. (1986) 'Self Help Groups – the Fourth Estate in Medicine', *British Medical Journal*, 293, pp. 159–60.

Locker, D. (1983) *Disability and Disadvantage*, Tavistock Publications, London.

Maxwell, R. and Weaver, N. (eds) (1984) *Public Participation in Health*, King Edward's Hospital Fund for London, London.

Mulcahy, L. (1995) *Redress in the Public Sector*, National Consumer Council, London.

National Association of Health Authorities (NAHA) (1986) *Acting with Authority: a consultative paper*, NAHA, Birmingham.

National Consumer Council (NCC) (1986) *Measuring Up: consumer assessment of local authority services, a guideline study*, NCC, London.

NHS Management Executive (NHSME) (1992) *Listening to Local Voices*, NHSME, Leeds.

Office of Health Economics (1993) *Compendium of Statistics*, OHE, London.

Payer, L. (1990) *Medicine and Culture*, Gollancz, London.

Phillips, M. and Dawson, J. (1982) *Doctors' Dilemmas, Medical Ethics and Contemporary Sciences*, Harvester Press, Brighton.

Pilgrim, D. and Rogers, A. (1988) 'The Mental Health Act Commission, 4 years on', *The Psychologist*, 3, pp. 104–6.

Plamping, D. and Delamothe, T. (1991) 'The Citizen's Charter and the NHS', *British Medical Journal*, 26 July, p. 203.

Pollitt, C. (1993) 'The Struggle for Quality: the case of the National Health Service', *Policy and Politics*, 21, 3, pp. 161–70.

Prescott-Clarke, B., Brooks, T. and Machray, C. (1988) *Focus on Health Care, Social and Community Planning Research*, Royal Institute of Public Administration, London.

Report of the Royal Commission on the National Health Service (1979) (Chairman: Sir Alec Merrison), Cmnd 7615, HMSO, London.

Roberts, H. (ed.) (1981) *Women, Health and Reproduction*, Routledge & Kegan Paul, London.

Robinson, D. (1984) *The Process of Becoming Ill*, Routledge & Kegan Paul, London.

Robinson, J. (1989) 'The Patient's Voice at the GMC', *Health Rights*, London.

Roth, J. (1963) *Timetables, Structuring the Passage of Time in Hospital and other Careers*, Bobbs Merrill, Indianapolis.

Royal Commission on Local Government (1969) *Representation and Community*, Appendix 7, vol. III, Research Appendices, Cmnd 4040, HMSO, London.

Seale, C. (1993) 'The Consumer Voice', in B. Davey and J. Popay (eds), *Dilemmas in Health Care*, Open University Press, Milton Keynes.

Simpson, R. (1979) *Access to Primary Health Care*, Royal Commission on the National Health Service Research Paper No. 6, HMSO, London.

Social Trends (1994) Central Statistical Office, 24, HMSO, London.

Stacey, M. (1976) 'The Health Service Consumer: a sociological misconception', in Stacey, M. (ed.), *The Sociology of the National Health Service*, Sociological Review Monograph 22, University of Keele.

Stacey, M. (1992) *Regulating British Medicine: the General Medical Council*, Wiley, Chichester.

Stanworth, M. (ed.) (1987) *Reproductive Technologies*, Polity Press, Cambridge.

Stimson, G. and Webb, B. (1975) *Going to the Doctor: the consultation process in general practice*, Routledge & Kegan Paul, London.

Taylor-Gooby, P. (1987) *Citizenship and Welfare in British Social Attitudes: the 1987 Report*, Jowell, R., Witherspoon, S. and Brook, L. (eds), Gower Publishing Company, Aldershot.

Tower Hamlets DHA Department of Community Medicine (1984) *The Spitalfields Health Survey*.

Tritter, J. (1994) 'The Citizen's Charters: from users' perspectives', *Political Quarterly*, July, pp. 397–414.

Winkler, F. (1987) 'Consumerism in Health Care: beyond the supermarket model', *Policy and Politics*, 15, 1, pp. 1–8.

Winn, L. (ed.) (1990) *Power to the People*, King's Fund Centre, London.

World Health Organisation (WHO) (1986) *Targets for Health*, WHO, Geneva.

CHAPTER 13

Health policy in Britain: towards the twenty-first century

In this concluding chapter, I first aim to review the main issues which emerged from the study of substantive areas of policy covered in this book. I first look at the concerns which are likely to continue to be on policy agendas in the 1990s in the wake of the 1990 reforms – the management of health services, resource use and cost containment, community care and general practice and the prevention of ill-health. I make the assumption that the reforms are unlikely to be reversed although the direction they take might be affected by a change of government. Conservative governments are likely to continue to encourage competition and a mixed economy while alternative governments may seek greater equity and central planning. But whichever party is in power, there are certain to be continuing policy adjustments and changes.

I look next at the issues untouched by the health reforms such as the effect of poverty and the distribution of income on health, and which remain as tensions or dilemmas for government. Finally, I turn to the question of whether health care politics have shifted as managed competition has replaced the command and control model. Do corporatist politics continue at the national level? Does the cultural and social authority of medicine prevail? Is there continuing medical dominance or has 'proletarianisation' of the profession occurred? At local level, have managers emerged as another profession to challenge medicine and doctors? Will the centre dominate over the authorities at the periphery? Are there changes in the pattern of health care delivery which will alter the pattern of care into the twenty-first century? Given the limited information available, only partial and speculative answers can be given.

Key policy issues in the NHS in the wake of the 1990 reforms

Chapter 2 outlined the principles on which the NHS was based – it aimed to cover the whole population; to provide equal access to people in need of health care; it was free at the point of use; it was comprehensive in cover; it provided services of a good standard to everyone. Implicitly, it was based on notions of public service:

that is, it aimed to be egalitarian in ethos and to treat patients with respect as persons in the collective interest. These issues will be returned to in an assessment of the effects of the 1990 NHS and Community Care Act below.

Problems of management

Chapter 3 discussed problems of managing the NHS as they were approached in the 1960s and 70s. Changes in the structure of the service were seen as a solution to the problems of delivering good-quality services over the country as a whole. Through the Resource Allocation Working Party's (RAWP) reallocation policy and structures which introduced a planning system and set priorities, the NHS became a more unified service although, for government and managers, there remained considerable problems of control, particularly over policy and activity within the districts and hospitals. There were wide variations in services provided, clinical practice and costs.

The NHS reforms brought a new set of controls and incentives which were described in Chapter 9. To date the limited evidence suggests that, even prior to the reforms, managers were taking a more positive lead in their organisations (Harrison, Hunter, Marnock and Pollitt 1992, Ranade 1994). NHS management has become a more complex task with the health reforms. Moreover, the roles of managers in Trusts require different skills from those involved in commissioning. As a consequence of the reforms, the number of administrative and managerial staff has increased, particularly at senior level. In 1994 this growth was checked. Levels of staff were reviewed and a new series of reforms to incorporate the regions within the NHS Management Executive were initiated. The desire of the centre to control the health authorities at the periphery and the drive towards competition will be areas of tension in policy through the 1990s.

Problems of resources, cost containment and value for money

Chapter 4 discussed policies for resource allocation. Through the period from the 1940s, a continuous theme has been the importance of cost containment of public spending on health care. The issue is likely to remain at the top of the policy agenda although pressures on government to spend more in a tax-funded service will continue to come from those who work in health care, from those who supply the providers, particularly the pharmaceutical industry, and from the public.

British governments have been remarkably successful in keeping costs low. Culyer (1989) carried an econometric analysis of the determinants of health care across countries. He concluded that health care expenditure and the proportion of income spent on health are both greater the higher the level of GDP per capita. The UK is an exception. An analysis of seven OECD countries found that the UK spent less than would have been predicted in terms of its GDP per capita and its growth rates during the 1980s (OECD 1992). The UK also has a lower number of acute hospital beds and a lower number of doctors than other comparable countries. However, pressure to find lower-cost ways of treating people will continue in the UK. For example, day surgery is now 21 per cent of all surgery. Document 30 (page 347) shows the day surgery rates achieved by the top 25 per cent of HAs in 1991–2.

Despite these comparisons which suggest that health care in the UK is relatively underfunded, it is likely that policy will continue to focus on cost containment. This could occur in three ways – encouraging private spending, seeking cheaper treatments and establishing methods for assessing effective care. While governments will restrict public expenditure to what they believe they can afford, similar constraints may not apply to private expenditure on health care. This could expand in a number of directions through private investment in the NHS and through increasing the household share of health care costs. In the latter case, this could be led by either limiting state services and thus creating incentives to seek private insurance or private treatment or through increasing the charges for NHS services. Household expenditure on health care may therefore rise over the next decade. Either of these developments would increase the variation in the type and quality of health care for patients in different areas of the country, although the effects could be softened through regulation to achieve national aid subsidies for those on low incomes.

Health care cost, quality and outcomes

It is now widely believed that the creation of competition between those supplying health services is an effective method of financial control because it limits expenditure within fixed budgets and pushes down costs within them. Therefore a second way to contain costs is through making the commissioning/contracting process sharper and more effective. The approach is supported in a 1993 World Bank Report on *Investing in Health* where it is seen as a way of curbing expenditure on acute hospital services. Abel-Smith (1992), in a survey of European health systems, reports that a number of countries now use the contracting method, which can be adopted with a variety of funding mechanisms. Commissioning encourages the development of administrative systems to cost activity in provider agencies. In theory, the cost, quality and outcomes of services can be compared between providers and good practice encouraged.

Chapter 9 addressed the issue of whether the purchaser/provider split had increased value for money. The limited research has not produced clear findings. Bartlett and Le Grand (1994) found that first- and second-wave Trusts had lower costs than non-Trusts but this could not be attributed to being in a more competitive environment. Glennerster *et al.* (1994) found that the administrative costs of GP purchasing were greater than district purchasing, but their evidence was limited.

Three years after the NHS reforms the benefits of competition in cost terms remain theoretical due to inadequate information, local circumstances which inhibit a market structure, the high costs of the commissioning process itself and the reluctance of those working in the service to be motivated by financial incentives (Robinson and Le Grand 1994). Under Conservative governments, the emphasis on market testing is likely to increase. This involves comparing practices and outcomes within the public sector and testing these against the private sector.

In the UK, costing, pricing and financial controls were weakly developed until the internal market was introduced. And although this has put up administrative expenditure, revealing costs sharpens consideration of priorities and the management of clinical budgets. This is even more apparent when resource inputs can be related to outcomes of treatment or health gains. For example, once the costs of providing different forms of kidney dialysis are compared, or, more emotively, the cost of an intensive care cot for a premature new-born baby, decisions can be made about resource use in the light of both demand for a particular type of service and what other opportunities are being forgone. Assessing choices in relation to health gains provides a further dimension to comparing treatment interventions.

The policy focus is now on assessing the costs and benefits of specific health care practices. Only a small proportion of medical interventions have been subject to random controlled trials. One estimate is 20 per cent (Brook and Lohr 1985). The 1993 World Bank report concludes that there could be significant gains in health throughout the world for the same input in expenditure if there was a concentration on treatments which were known to effective. It states:

> Only a small share of the thousands of known medical procedures has been analyzed, but approximately fifty studied would be able to deal with more than half of the world's disease burden. Just implementing the twenty most cost effective interventions could eliminate more than 40 per cent of the total burden and three quarters of the health loss among children.
>
> (World Bank 1993: 6

In the UK, the Research and Development strategy of the DOH is focused on establishing cost-effective care which brings health gains. Methods for calculating trade-offs such as QALYs and DALYs were referred to in Chapters 4 and 6. All these methods aim to make better use of resources. They reflect an emphasis on technical/rational criteria for resource allocation rather than a reliance on professional judgement.

There is little indication yet that Health Authorities (HAs) which commission services have the information to assess health gains in relation to the services they buy, although they may use the rhetoric (Whitehead 1994). In the provider units, although there is more monitoring and evaluation, Kerrison, Packwood and Buxton (1994), who studied medical audit, found that it remained focused on peer group assessment as part of the educational process. In other words, technical/rational criteria are not yet applied. Decision-making about what procedures to follow remains the preserve of doctors. This may change in the future as information improves, but will raise moral issues.

Policies for community care and general practice

Chapters 5 and 10 considered policies for community care and general practice. From the 1970s, care in the community for those who are frail and vulnerable has been a focus for policy. This is not surprising given the socio-demographic trends. In this field, there has been a significant gap between policies and their realisation.

As the discussion on community care in Chapter 5 indicated, some have argued that the NHS no longer provides comprehensive service for the frail and vulnerable. Particular criticisms have been made of lack of funding for groups who need support following inpatient treatment. Henwood (1992) argues that services for frail elderly people have been eroded and there are inadequate facilities. The same can be said in relation to supervision and support for mentally ill people.

Government policy has been inconsistent and created perverse incentives. At local level, in both health and social services, there has been a wide variation in practice and governments have sought to contain costs but have not yet found a satisfactory way of delivering care.

With the 1990 reforms, the emphasis is on managing a package of care for people rather than fitting people to services. Local authority social services departments have been designated as the lead agency in community care and social workers given the role of care managers. People seeking social services are now obliged to contribute depending on their income level. However, questions about methods of coordination between health and social services have yet to be addressed in most areas. HA purchasing provides one arena where cross-agency discussions can occur but there are enormous information gaps in tracking and costing social care. Moreover, long-term funding issues have still to be resolved. As the community care reforms only became operational on 1 April 1993 there is little evidence available on progress.

It was argued in Chapter 10 that general practice has emerged as an important policy area. The vision for the future is of a strong system of general practice which will provide a range of services for practice populations, taking on some of the services previously provided by the hospital. The intention is to extend fundholding to enable GPs to buy facilities from the community and the hospital, thus making the practice both purchasers of services and care managers. The problems are three-fold: the lack of managerial capacity in general practice and its small scale; the variations between practices in almost every respect; and the tension between HA and general practice purchasing. At present, financial incentives are available for GPs to expand their provision of services. Overall, the differences between the quality of care between different practices remains wide (Leese and Bosanquet 1988). The future of fundholders and of their role in commissioning remains uncertain in the light of the proposals to merge HAs and FHSAs.

Currently, the pressure to evaluate interventions and outcomes is not applied to general practice with the same rigour as it is in hospital care. This may be because the former is less technical. The Chief Medical Officer's report for 1993 (DOH 1993) suggests that clinical audit is now carried out in 90 per cent of practices. It is likely that this refers to the audit of prescribing rather than looking at the efficacy of other interventions.

The prevention of ill-health

Chapter 11 examined policies for the prevention of ill-health. The UK already has an infrastructure of public health services which is based on the skills of population medicine. Until the late 1980s, these services focused on screening populations, particularly children, for illness and protecting against disease. Powers in the area of environmental health were, and remain, poorly developed. Health education has tended to be sidelined and filtered through health professionals. The approach to the prevention of ill-health has been relatively ineffective in dealing with the heart disease and the cancers. In 1992, *The Nation's Health* (DOH 1992) provided a policy framework which focused attention on particular targets for health improvements. This was a significant development, and for health authorities at least, provides a unifying framework of priorities. Nevertheless, community development remains essential.

However, the policy arena of preventive health remains diffuse.

It involves a range of agencies and pressure groups which configured differently around particular issues. The government does not, or has chosen not, to dominate. This may be for a number of reasons. Preventive health is an area where there are conflicting viewpoints about issues of personal freedom and the collective interest and about the relationship between the individual and the state. For example, if the same kind of technical/rational attitude which is being applied to medical interventions were applied in areas of prevention, then decisive action would be taken over smoking – the greatest single cause of premature death. But governments have avoided any major change to the status quo, preferring marginal price changes. In other contentious areas the resolution of issues has been left to Parliament, or government have offloaded the problem on to the local-level agencies to decide on policy as well as strategy. Because of the centrist tendency in British health policy and the divisions of responsibility, local initiatives have, with notable exceptions, been limited in effect.

In Wales, the Welsh heart programme provides an example of a more comprehensive approach to the evaluation of health gains from particular interventions. This has been linked to an active health campaign which involves communities in healthy alliances. This strategy has proved successful in North America in reducing the incidence of serious illness, particularly among the better informed. However, Whitehead (1994) concludes, on the limited evidence available, that there are few signs that health authorities are commissioning on the basis of a strategy for preventing ill-health or promoting health gain.

The new NHS: the broader questions

This section began by restating the principles of the NHS. In introducing the reforms, the government claimed a continuing commitment – the service remains tax based and therefore open to all on the basis of need. These are general principles which are difficult to operationalise and against which the NHS has arguably always fallen short. Robinson and Le Grand's (1994) edited collection, *Evaluating the NHS Reforms*, uses the criteria of quality, efficiency, choice and responsiveness, and equity. Their findings are limited and have been referred to above.

Taking a different approach, it appears that the NHS reforms so far have done little to address some major problems of delivery and policy, and have in fact created new ones. There are problems about the quantity and quality of service which relate ultimately to problems of funding. For example, waiting lists remain long in many areas although they are being managed differently. In the UK, waiting lists to see hospital consultants and to have inpatient treatment tend to be longer than in other countries (OECD 1992), and communication with patients is often poor in the NHS (Audit Commission 1993). There are few comparative data on quality compared to other systems, although in other, neighbouring European countries, payment systems favour greater patient choice and more frequent and longer patient consultations (OECD 1992).

There is now some evidence that people in the UK are less satisfied with their health care than people in other countries, but have few ways of expressing this. As well as national studies which indicate increasing dissatisfaction and complaints, an international study of 10 countries (Blendon *et al.* 1990) showed that levels of satisfaction tended to be related to the level of investment in health care. Canada, with the second highest expenditure, had the highest satisfaction rating. In answer to the statement: 'On the whole, the health system works pretty well, and only minor changes are needed to make it work better', lower levels of satisfaction were recorded in the UK and Italy, 27 to 12 per cent, which have lower levels of spending than Canada, the Netherlands, Germany and France, 56 to 41 per cent.

In relation to equity, one of the main tenets of the NHS, the service remains relatively equitable in terms of access to care and outcomes measured by mortality rates. For example, study of five European Union countries (Van Doorslaer, Wagstaff and Rutten 1993), looked at the UK in terms of equity measured by the ability to pay and treatment according to need. Financing was 'mildly progressive' in the UK compared to other countries. In terms of health status measured by life expectancy, the UK does slightly better than many countries which have higher levels of per capita spending (Le Grand 1987). Document 29 provides comparative data. However, it is not known what contribution is made by health services and what is due to other material and behavioural factors in relation to these findings. The health service reforms may have increased inequity simply because they have created greater diversity.

The health reforms have not provided more money for health care but they have revealed more clearly the ways in which care is, and always has been, rationed. Health authorities must fit commissioning within budgets. This makes priority setting explicit. The health reforms have done little to ensure that health authorities making these decisions are accountable to local populations, however. Mechanisms may be in place for involving local people but there are many possible definitions of consultation and participation. In practice a number of tensions may arise over power to influence or determine decisions. Current practice has not been assessed and monitored. Trusts are also not accountable to anyone other than their Boards. Critics of the Conservative government's policy in creating 'Next Steps' agencies to run public services have pointed to a general 'democratic deficit' in the 'market-testing' process. This is especially so in health care where there is a weak tradition of public involvement.

Poverty and ill-health: off the policy agenda?

The issue which remained off the policy agenda is the relationship between poverty and ill-health. The World Bank Report (1993) highlights two issues which, it argues, are fundamental to improving health status. The first is the importance of maintaining household income and the second is maintaining the health of children. The Report states:

> What people do with their lives and those of their children affects their health far more than anything that governments can do. But what they can do is determined, to a great extent, by income and knowledge – factors which are not completely within their control. In every society the capabilities, income and status of women extend a powerful influence on health.
>
> (World Bank 1993: 37)

The Report goes on to demonstrate, on the basis of an analysis of 70 countries, that both the level of schooling of women and per capita income have a strong effect on health status. The higher the national income and the better the level of education, the more likely its people are to live long and healthy lives. Furthermore, the distribution of income and the numbers of people suffering from poverty are also significant in affecting health status.

A matter for concern is that the legacy of 1980s' policies have bequeathed growing disparity between incomes in the UK along class and geographical lines. On the basis of research evidence, Davey-Smith and Egger (1993) demonstrate that mortality differentials increased between those living in deprived neighbourhoods and the inhabitants of affluent districts in the North of England and in Glasgow in the 1980s. They also argue that social policies have redistributed income in favour of the better-off. Hills (1993), in a detailed evaluation of incomes and benefits, shows that the numbers in poverty have increased, and argues that:

> . . . whatever the definition: the numbers of people with low incomes increased over the 1980s – substantially so if any kind of relative measuring rod is used.
>
> (Hills 1993: 3)

Income differentials have also increased and although the effect has been blunted by welfare benefits, these have not compensated entirely for the widening gap. There has therefore been a rise in inequality (Hills 1993). The World Bank Report comments on the flattening of the rise in life expectancy in the UK as compared to Japan and attributes this to income distribution. It says:

> Japan and the UK had similar income distributions and life expectancies in 1970, but they have diverged since then. Japan now has the highest life expectancy in the world and a highly egalitarian income distribution. In the UK, where income distribution has widened since the mid-1980s, life expectancy is now more than three years shorter than in Japan.
>
> (World Bank 1993: 40)

Given the importance given of women's income to family health, it is also a matter of concern that lone parents and their families, most of whom are women, are a growing proportion of the population. The numbers increased from 8 per cent to 19 per cent between 1971 and 1991, giving the UK the highest number of lone parents among OECD countries. In 1986, 59 per cent of lone-parent families were receiving Income Support, the only official measure of 'poverty' in the UK (Hills 1993). Judge and Benzeval (1993), in a discussion of the available evidence, suggest that there is strong evidence of a high risk of mortality (and associated morbidity) among the children of lone parents.

Unlike the other areas of health care where there are few party political differences, the issue of inequalities and how far they should be tolerated brings out differences in social policy approach between the major political parties. How far inequalities continue to widen will depend on both economic growth and which government is in power over the next decade.

The politics of the new NHS

In Chapter 1 of this book, it was argued that the 'command and control' model of health care was both a product of, and a support to, the configuration of political interests. Government established the NHS as a result of democratic pressure and a Parliamentary mandate, the form was based on the provision of personal illness services within an organisational hierarchy. Professional interest groups, particularly the medical profession, were involved in negotiations throughout and subsequently, the pattern of politics at national level was corporate. At the local level, the lack of central and managerial control allowed considerable professional autonomy. In Elston's terms, the profession enjoyed cultural and social authority as well as professional autonomy (Elston 1991).

Have the NHS reforms, with their emphasis on managed competition, altered the balance of interests? A number of US commentators argue that in the US health care system, there has been a 'deprofessionalisation', and a 'proletarianisation' of medicine (McKinlay 1988, Morone 1993), although a contrary view is also expressed (Mechanic 1991). There are two aspects to this process. First, it involves a loss in the power to make decisions and second, a routinisation of work. In the US, it is argued that as health insurance companies own hospitals and clinics, they have become the dominant interest group. Within health organisations, decision-making is curtailed by cost considerations and work is routinised by applying approved procedures and protocols which provide technical, formula-driven answers to medical interventions. Moreover, computerised records allow greater surveillance of medical work carried out.

In relation to UK health care, there are two questions. The first is whether politics remains corporatist at the national level and whether there is discussion and agreement with the medical profession over policy developments. The second is whether the system of commissioning has reduced professional autonomy and social authority within the Trusts. The third is whether there are broader changes which will affect the cultural authority of medicine more generally. Answers to these questions can only be speculative as there is a dearth of empirical studies.

Butler demonstrates that the health care reforms were introduced with little consultation and against considerable opposition (Butler 1992). Klein and Day (1991) argue that a distinction should be made between normal and exceptional politics. Major legislative change in 1946 and again in 1989–90 brought a breakdown of the usual process of bargaining and negotiation. Government exerted its sovereignty in Parliament. However, little is known of current political processes at central level. Organisation at the centre is divided between the Department of Health in London and the NHS Management Executive in Leeds[1]. The profession has a token presence on the Boards at the centre and at commissioning level. Currently, the power of HAs over Trusts is unclear. In some areas, purchasers call the tune, in others the reverse may occur. If HAs are to become larger and fewer in number, they may have greater influence on the activity of Trusts but have little effect on the day-to-day work. The extent of influence will depend on how information systems develop to ensure effective purchasing and on whether there is a range of local competitors.

At the local level, where most doctors work, the politics of hospital work differs from that of general practice. In Chapter 9, the evidence suggested that managers had become a more dominant force in terms of leading their organisations strategically as well as numerically. Trusts must now remain financially viable and this suggests that managers could increasingly dominate the agenda. However, in many hospitals, changes have brought doctors and managers into a more effective partnership rather than increasing the power of one over the other. Ranade (1994) suggests that in many Trusts, doctors are becoming the managers of clinical services while managers deal with external relationships. At this level, there is little sign of a reduction of social authority in the division of labour of doctors as a whole. However, there may be less individual autonomy for individual clinicians. Hunter

(1993) considers that although there is currently the element of a partnership between doctors and managers, in the longer run, managers are likely to capture the agenda as they will be able to control the organisational parameters of medical work.

In relation to the routinisation of medical work through the use of rational/technical criteria, the evidence is that as yet, costing systems and clinical protocols are too poorly developed to pose a threat to professional autonomy. While it is likely that these will develop and alter the micro-politics of health care, current trends suggest that clinicians will endeavour to control their use. Also, as Payer (1990) points out, the UK has had a tradition of embracing the evidence from random-controlled trials. On the whole, the profession has been concerned to use treatments which are known to be effective. This may mean assessing medical work but this does not mean that doctors lose control of the process.

Within general practice, the health reforms have enhanced the power of GPs in relation to their hospital colleagues, although many GPs appear reluctant to take advantage of the opportunities offered. It is more difficult for managers to keep GPs' clinical practice under surveillance. This is partly because their work is intrinsically less technical and partly because their mode of working is more akin to that of a small business (Allsop 1994). Within general practice the social authority of the doctor remains unchallenged although GPs are becoming primarily managers of care.

In relation to the balance between the centre and the peripheral authorities in health care, the NHS remains a very centralised service. Regulatory mechanisms continue to remain strong. The absorption of the NHS Management Executive into the Department of Health, and of regions into the NHS Management Executive, together with market-testing and centrally validated protocols and guidelines, suggest that tight controls over money and activity will be maintained. What is less clear is whether the centre will also drive policy priorities where these do not relate to value for money. Will it be left to the purchasing authorities to implement *Health of the Nation* targets and the health side of community care? Currently, there is no clear policy at the centre on these issues.

Finally, it can be concluded that managed competition has introduced a new dynamic into health care politics in the UK. The consequences, however, are complex: they may reduce the medical mandate in some ways but enhance it in others. It could be that, in the longer run, the cultural authority which has been accorded to medical knowledge will reduce. If this were to happen, this would fundamentally change the position of the profession as its area of monopoly would be narrowed. In the twenty-first century changes already under way or under consideration could develop further. Primary and community care will continue to expand and the role of the hospital reduce.

This is likely to be accompanied by an increase in the range of specialist health care workers and the scope for self care by people themselves. If local authorities were to take over the role of purchasers of health care as well as of social services, an element of democratic control would be introduced into health care. The consequences of this could be profound.

Note

1. From mid-1994, this became known as the NHSE, the NHS Executive. This may indicate a weakening of central management of the service.

References

Abel-Smith, B. (1992) 'Cost Containment and New Priorities in the EC', *The Milbank Quarterly*, 70, 3, pp. 393–416.

Allsop, J. (1994) 'Shifting Spheres of Opportunity: GPs and the health service reforms', in Johnson, T., Larkin, G. and Saks, M. (eds), *The Professions in Transition*, Routledge, London.

Audit Commission (1993) *What Seems to be the Matter?* Audit Commission, London.

Barlett, W. and Le Grand, J. (1994) 'The Performance of Trusts', in Robinson, R. and Le Grand, J. (eds), *Evaluating the NHS Reforms*, King's Fund Institute, London.

Blendon, R., Leitman, R., Morrison, I. and Donclan, K. (1990) 'Satisfaction with Health Systems in their Nations', *Health Affairs*, Summer.

Brook, R. and Lohr, K. (1985) 'Efficiency, effectiveness, variations and quality', *Medical Care*, 23, pp. 710–22.

Butler, J. (1992) *Patients, Policies and Politics*, Open University Press, Milton Keynes.

Culyer, A. (1989) 'Cost-containment in Europe', *Health Care Financing Review*, Annual Supplement.

Davey-Smith, G. and Egger, M. (1993) 'Socioeconomic Differentials in Wealth and Health', *British Medical Journal*, 307, pp. 1085–6.

Day, P. and Klein, R. (1991) 'Political Theory and Policy Practice: the case of general practice 1911–1991', Paper presented at the Political Studies Association Conference, Lancaster, 15–17 April.

Department of Health (1992) *The Nation's Health, in England*, HMSO, London.

Department of Health (1993) Report of Chief Medical Officer, 1993, HMSO, London.

Elston, M. (1991) 'The Politics of Professional Power: medicine in a changing health service', in Gabe, J., Calnan, M. and Bury, M. (eds), *Sociology of the Health Service*, Routledge, London.

Glennerster, H., Matsaganis, M., Owens, P. and Hancock, S. (1994) 'GP fundholding: wild card or winning hand?', in Robinson, R. and Le Grand, J., *Evaluating the NHS Reforms*, King's Fund Institute, London.

Harrison, S., Hunter, D. J., Marnock, G. and Pollitt, C. J. (1992) *Just Managing: Power and culture in the National Health Service*, Macmillan, London.

Henwood, M. (1992) 'Through a Glass Darkly: community care and elderly people', Research Report 14, King's Fund Institute, London.

Hills, J. (1993) *The Future of Welfare: a guide to the debate*, Joseph Rowntree Foundation, York.

Hunter, D. (1993) 'Doctors as Managers: poachers turned gamekeepers?', *Social Science and Medicine*, 35, 4, pp. 557–66.

Judge, K. and Benzeval, M. (1993) 'Health Inequalities: new concerns about the children of single mothers', *British Medical Journal*, 306, pp. 677–80.

Kerrison, S., Packwood, T. and Buxton, M. (1994) 'Monitoring Medical Audit' in Robinson, R. and Le Grand, J., *Evaluating the NHS Reforms*, King's Fund Institute, London.

Klein, R. and Day, P. (1991) 'Britain's Health Care Experiment', *Health Affairs*, 10, pp. 39–59.

Leese, B. and Bosanquet, N. (1988) 'High and Low Incomes in General Practice', *British Medical Journal*, 298, pp. 932–4.

Le Grand, J. (1987) 'Inequalities in Health: some International comparisons', *European Economic Review*, 31, pp. 182–91.

McKinlay, J. (ed.) (1988) 'The Changing Character of the Medical Profession', *The Milbank Quarterly*, 66 (supp. 2).

Mechanic, D. (1991) 'Sources of Countervailing Power in Medicine', *Journal of Health Politics, Policy and Law*, 15, pp. 129–43.

Morone, J. (1993) 'The Health Care Bureaucracy: small changes, big consequences', *Journal of Health Politics, Policy and Law*, 18, 3, pp. 723–39.

OECD (1992) *The Reform of Health Care: a comparative analysis of seven OECD countries*, OECD, Paris.

Payer, L. (1990) *Medicine and Culture*, Gollancz, London.

Porter, A. and Porter, J. (1980) 'Anglo-French Contrasts in Medical Practice', *British Medical Journal*, 26 April.

Ranade, W. (1994) *A Future for the NHS? Health care in the 1990s*, Longman, Harlow.

Robinson, R. and Le Grand, J. (1994) *Evaluating the NHS Reforms*, King's Fund Institute, London.

Van Doorslaer, E., Wagstaff, A. and Rutten, F. (1993) *Equity in the Finance and Delivery of Health Care*, European Community, Brussels.

Welsh Health Planning Forum (1989) *Local Strategies for Health: a new approach to strategic planning*, Welsh Office, Cardiff.

Whitehead, M. (1994) 'Is it Fair? Evaluating the equity implications of the NHS reforms', in Robinson, R. and Le Grand, J., *Evaluating the NHS Reforms*, King's Fund Institute, London.

World Bank (1993) *Investing in Health*, World Bank, Geneva.

PART FIVE

Documents

List of Documents

Document 1
THE CHADWICK PRESCRIPTION FOR PUBLIC HEALTH

ON THE COSTS OF PREVENTIBLE ILL-HEALTH

It appears that fever, after its ravages amongst the infant population, falls with the greatest intensity on the adult population in the vigour of life. The periods at which the ravages of other diseases, consumption, smallpox, and measles take place, are sufficiently well known. The proportions in which the diseases have prevailed in the several counties will be found deserving of peculiar attention.

A conception may be formed of the aggregate effects of the several causes of mortality from the fact, that of the deaths caused during one year in England and Wales by epidemic, endemic, and contagious diseases, including fever, typhus, and scarlatina, amounting to 56,461, the great proportion of which are proved to be preventible, it may be said that the effect is as if the whole county of Westmorland, now containing 56,469 souls, or the whole county of Huntingdonshire, or any other equivalent district, were entirely de-populated annually, and were only occupied again by the growth of new and feeble population living under the fears of a similar visitation. The annual slaughter in England and Wales, from preventible causes of typhus which attacks persons in the vigour of life, appears to be double the amount of what was suffered by the Allied Armies in the battle of Waterloo . . .

ON THE CAUSES OF ILL-HEALTH

First, as to the extent and operation of the evils which are the subject of the inquiry: That the various forms of epidemic, endemic, and other disease caused, or aggravated, or propagated chiefly amongst the labouring classes by atmospheric impurities produced by decomposing animal and vegetable substances, by damp and filth, and close and overcrowded dwellings prevail amongst the population in every part of the kingdom, whether dwelling in separate houses, in rural villages, in small towns, in the larger towns – as they have been found to prevail in the lowest districts of the metropolis.

That such disease, wherever its attacks are frequent, is always found in connexion with the physical circumstances above specified, and that where those circumstances are removed by drainage, proper cleansing, better ventilation, and other means of diminishing atmospheric impurities, the frequency and intensity of such disease is abated; and where the removal of the noxious agencies appears to be complete, such disease almost entirely disappears . . .

Secondly. As to the means by which the present sanitary conditions of the labouring classes may be improved:
The primary most important measures, and at the same time the most practicable, and within the recognized province of public administration, are drainage, the removal of all refuse of habitations, streets, and roads, and the improvement of the supplies of water . . .

That for the protection of the labouring classes and of the ratepayers against inefficiency and waste in all new structural arrangements for the protection of the public health, and to ensure public confidence that the expenditure will be beneficial, securities should be taken that all new local public works are devised and conducted by responsible officers qualified by the possession of the science and skill of civil engineers . . .

The advantages of uniformity in legislation and in the executive machinery, and of doing the same things in the same way (choosing the best), and calling the same officers, proceedings, and things by the same names, will only be appreciated by those who have observed the extensive public loss occasioned by the legislation for towns which makes them independent of beneficent, as of what perhaps might have been deemed formerly aggressive legislation.

From: Edwin Chadwick, *Report on the Sanitary Conditions of the Labouring Population of Great Britain* (1842), 1965 edn by M. W. Flinn, Edinburgh University Press, p. 78

Document 2
THE HEALTH OF THE POPULATION, 1901

Increase in numbers is commonly regarded as a sign of national progress, and as evidence of the soundness of the State. Recent growth of population in the United Kingdom, however, is actually a symptom of political decline. A vast population has been created by the factory and industrial systems, the majority of which is incapable of bearing arms.

Spectacled school-children hungry, strumous and epileptic, grow into consumptive bridegrooms and scrofulous brides, and are assured beforehand of the blessing of the Church, the aid of the compassionate, and such solace as hospitals provided wholesale by unknown donors can supply. If a voice be raised in protest against the unhealthy perversion of the command, 'Be ye fruitful and multiply' it is drowned in a chorus of sickly emotion . . .

In the Manchester district 11,000 men offered themselves for war service between the outbreak of hostilities in October 1899 and July 1990. Of this number 8000 were found to be physically unfit to carry a rifle and stand the fatigues of discipline. Of the 3000 who were accepted only 1200 attained the moderate standard of muscular power and chest measurement required by the military authorities. In other words, two out of every three men willing to bear arms in Manchester district are virtually invalids.

From: Arnold White, *Efficiency and Empire*, Methuen (1901), pp. 100–3

Document 3
HEALTH AND HEALTH SERVICES IN THE 1930s: THE REPORT FROM POLITICAL AND ECONOMIC PLANNING

WHAT IS HEALTH?

Health means more than not being ill. A new attitude is needed, involving not so much a departure from the old as a more thorough grasp of the different elements in health policy. Many people are at any given moment suffering from defects, injuries or sickness so pronounced as to make them unable to carry on ordinary occupations and leisure activities. These are the 'cases' with which a large part of the organised health services mainly deal. But in addition there are far larger numbers of people suffering temporarily or permanently from less acute defects, injuries or inadequacies which are not sufficient to unfit them for work or play, and may not even be noticed at all, but nevertheless suffice to place them in an unnecessarily weak position for creating and maintaining good physique, energy, happiness or resistance to disease. Provided that the argument is not pushed too far it is useful to bear in mind a distinction between the mass of socially and economically incapacitating disabilities usually treated as cases of ill-health and the even larger mass of deficiencies and disabilities which do not incapacitate and are often unrecognised or not thought serious. No contemporary health policy can be considered adequate which does not deal with the second group as well as the first.

Until recently medicine was inevitably confined largely to work of a salvage nature. Neither knowledge, nor imagination, nor physical resources were adequate to pass the stage of patching up ill-health and to create boldly and consciously the conditions in which a healthy population could grow and flourish. While efforts at effecting the cure of diseases cannot be relaxed, efforts at prevention of ill-health can and must be increased. The aspect of raising standards of nutrition and of fitness should be given much more prominence. Health must come first: the mere state of not being ill must be recognised as an inacceptable substitute, too often tolerated or even regarded as normal. We must, moreover, face the fact that while immense study has been lavished on disease no one has intensively studied and analysed health, and our ignorance of the subject is still so deep that we can hardly claim scientifically to know what health is. To the extent that health is a positive element mere negative attempts to palliate or even to cure specific diseases cannot be regarded as a solution to the problem.

In the first and most important range of health-creating services come those activities which provide more and better food, housing, recreation, and social and economic security, and which stimulate the knowledge and will to make use of these facilities. The really essential health services of the nation are the making available of ample safe fresh milk to all who need it, the cheapening of other dairy products, fruit and vegetables, new accommodation to replace slums and relieve overcrowding, Green Belt schemes, playing-fields, youth hostels and physical education, social insurances which relieve the burden of anxiety on the family and advances in employment policy which improve security of tenure or conditions of work and, finally, education in healthy living through training and propaganda. Health problems are frequently the result of social and industrial conditions, and the attempt to deal with these problems piecemeal results in a lopsided development of the health services. It is necessary to remember that there are often two alternative policies for dealing with ill-health – either to treat the cases or to deal with the social and economic conditions producing the cases.

Personal health services, whether preventive or curative, can only deal effectively with limited numbers of persons, and they can hardly be made satisfactory so long as the numerical burden of cases thrown upon them is excessively inflated by wholesale failures in education or in essential social and economic provision. The more careless about health the community is, and the more often its members need serious doctoring, the worse doctoring they are likely to get, because the cases coming up for attention will be too many and at too late a stage.

The report concludes:

What does the Report show? To sum it up, it describes how a bewildering variety of agencies, official and unofficial, have been created during the past two or three generations to work for health mainly by attacking specific diseases and disabilities as they occur, and by maintaining the sufferers. To a much more limited extent attempts have successfully been made to find out and to eradicate the social and economic causes of sickness and disability such as bad housing, sanitation and water supply, and dangerous or unhealthy working conditions.

Although all these efforts have had remarkable results they have failed to give the nation an acceptable measure of good health or to reduce the economic burden of sickness and accidents. Perhaps the most fundamental defect in the existing system is that it is overwhelmingly preoccupied with manifest and advanced diseases or disabilities and is more interested in enabling the sufferers to go on functioning in society somehow than in studying the nature of health and the means of producing and maintaining it. From this it naturally follows that millions of pounds are spent in looking after and trying to cure the victims of accidents and illnesses which need never have occurred if a fraction of this amount of intelligence and money had been devoted to tracing the social and economic causes of the trouble and making the necessary readjustments. While everyone knows that cholera, bubonic plague, malaria, scurvy and other scourges have been eliminated by the engineer or through raising the standard of living rather than by medical treatment, we are all too apt to think of health in terms of curing and treating disease, and to ignore or underrate the extent to which habits of life, the layout of our towns and buildings, labour management, transport, food manufacturing and distribution and so forth can and must be brought into the campaign for fitness. Basically health is a problem of knowledge and education. The type of survey as we have attempted should be carried out much more thoroughly as an essential and continuous function of government. There should be men and women constantly tracing back into the factory, the office, the traffic system and the home the origins of defects and diseases which are a burden on the nation. There should also be in the universities and the schools men and women evolving and conveying to the new generation an attitude of life based on healthy minds and bodies and prepared to face the implications, instead of stopping short, as we still do, at the stage of lip service.

From: *Report on the British Health Services*, Political and Economic Planning, London (1937)

Document 4
THE 1944 WHITE PAPER: AN ACCOUNT OF THE INADEQUACIES OF EXISTING HEALTH SERVICES

The record of this country in its health and medical services is a good one. The resistance of people to the wear and tear of four years of a second world war bears testimony to it. Achievements before the war – in lower mortality rates, in the gradual decline of many of the more serious diseases, in safer motherhood and healthier childhood, and generally in the prospect of a longer and healthier life – all substantiate it. There is no question of having to abandon bad services and to start afresh. Reform in this field is not a matter of making good what is bad, but of making better what is good already.

The present system has its origins deep in the history of the country's social services. Broadly, it is the product of the last hundred years, though some of its elements go much further back. But most of the impetus has been gathered in the last generation or two; and it was left to the present century to develop most of the personal health services as they are now known . . .

The main reason for change is that the Government believe that, at this stage of social development, the care of personal health should be put on a new footing and be made available to everybody as a publicly sponsored service. Just as people are accustomed to look to public organisation for essential facilities like a clean and safe water supply or good highways, accepting these as things which the community combines to provide for the benefit of the individual without distinction of section or group, so they should now be able to look for proper facilities for the care of their personal health to a publicly organised service available to all who want to use it – a service for which all would be paying as taxpayers and ratepayers and contributors to some national scheme of social insurance.

In spite of the substantial progress of many years and the many good services built up under public authority and by voluntary and private effort, it is still not true to say that everyone can get all the kinds of medical and hospital service which he or she may require. Whether people can do so still depends too much upon circumstances, upon where they happen to live or work, to what group (e.g. of age, or vocation) they happen to belong, or what happens to be the matter with them. Nor is the care of health yet wholly divorced from ability to pay for it, although great progress has already been made in eliminating the financial barrier to obtaining most of the essential services. There is not yet, in short, a comprehensive cover for health provided for all people alike. That is what it is now the Government's intention to provide.

To take one very important example, the first-line care of health for everyone requires a personal doctor or a family doctor, a general medical practitioner available for consultation on all problems of health and sickness. At present, the National Health Insurance scheme makes this provision for a large number of people; but it does not give it to the wives and the children and the dependants. For extreme need, the older Poor Law still exists. For some particular groups there are other facilities. But for something like half the population, the first-line health service of a personal medical adviser depends on what private arrangements any particular person can manage to make.

Even if a person has a regular doctor – and this is not now assured to all – there is no guaranteed link between that doctor and the rest of necessary medical help. The doctor, both in private practice and in National Health Insurance practice, has to rely on his own resources to introduce his patient to the right kinds of special treatment or clinic or hospital – a great responsibility in these days of specialised medicine and surgery – or the patient has to make his own way to whatever local authority or other organisation happens to cater for his particular need.

When a hospital's services are needed, it is far from true that everyone can get all that is required. Here it is not so much a question of people not being eligible to get the service which they need, as a matter of the practical distribution of those services. The hospital and specialist services have grown up without a national or even an area plan. In one area there may be already established a variety of hospitals. Another area, although the need is there, may be sparsely served. One hospital may have a long waiting list and be refusing admission to cases which another hospital not far away could suitably accommodate and treat at once. There is undue pressure in some areas on the hospital out-patient departments – in spite of certain experiments which some of the hospitals have tried (and which should be encouraged) in arranging a system of timed appointments to obviate long waiting. Moreover, even though most people have access to a hospital of some kind, it is not necessarily access to the right hospital. The tendency in the modern development of medicine and surgery is towards specialist centres – for radiotherapy and neurosis, for example – and no one hospital can be equally equipped and developed to suit all needs, or to specialise equally in all subjects. The time has come when the hospital services have to be thought of, and planned, as a wider whole, and the object has to be that each case should be referred not to one single hospital which happens to be 'local' but to whatever hospital concentrates specially on that kind of case and can offer it the most up-to-date technique.

Many services are also rendered by local authorities and others in special clinics and similar organisations, designed for particular groups of the population or for particular kinds of ailment or medical care. These are, for the most part, thoroughly good in themselves, and they are used with advantage by a great many people in a great many districts. But, owing to the way in which they have grown up piecemeal at different stages of history and under different statutory powers, they are usually conducted as quite separate and independent services. There is no sufficient link either between these services themselves or between them and general medical practice and the hospitals.

In short, general medical practice, consultant and specialist opinion, hospital treatment, clinic services for particular purposes, home nursing, midwifery and other branches of health care need to be related to one another and treated as many aspects of the care of one person's health. That means that there has to be somewhere a new responsibility to relate them, if a service for health is to be given in future which will be not only comprehensive and reliable but also easy to obtain.

Last, but not least, personal health still tends to be regarded as something to be treated when at fault, or perhaps to be preserved from getting at fault, but seldom as something to be positively improved and promoted and made full and robust. Much of present custom and habit still centres on the idea that the doctor and the hospital and the clinic are the means of mending ill-health rather than of increasing good health and the sense of well-being. While the health standards of the people have enormously improved, and while there are gratifying reductions in the ravages of preventable disease, the plain fact remains that there are many men and women and children who could be and ought to be enjoying a sense of health and physical well-being which they do not in fact enjoy. There is much subnormal health still, which need not be, with a corresponding cost in efficiency and personal happiness.

These are some of the chief deficiencies in the present arrangements which, in the view of the Government, a comprehensive health service should seek to make good . . .

THE SCOPE OF A 'COMPREHENSIVE' SERVICE

The proposed service must be 'comprehensive' in two senses – first, that it is available to all people and, second, that it covers all necessary forms of health care. The general aim has been stated at the beginning of this Paper. The service designed to achieve it must cover the whole field of medical advice and attention, at home, in the consulting room, in the hospital or the sanatorium, or wherever else is appropriate – from the personal or family doctor to the specialists and consultants of all kinds, from the care of minor ailments to the care of major diseases and disabilities. It must include ancillary services of nursing, of midwifery and of the other things which ought to go with medical care. It must secure first that everyone can be sure of a general medical adviser to consult as and when the need arises, and then that everyone can get access – beyond the general medical adviser – to more specialised branches of medicine or surgery. This cannot all be perfected at a stroke of the pen, on an appointed day; but nothing less than this must be the object in view, and the framing of the service from the outset must be such as to make it possible.

From: *A National Health Service*, Ministry of Health, Cmnd 6502, HMSO, London (1944), pp. 6–9

Document 5
LABOUR (ANEURIN BEVAN) AND CONSERVATIVES (RICHARD LAW) DEBATE THE INTRODUCTION OF THE NATIONAL HEALTH SERVICE

MR BEVAN: The first reason why a health scheme of this sort is necessary at all is because it has been the firm conclusion of all parties that money ought not to be permitted to stand in the way of obtaining an efficient health service. Although it is true that the national health insurance scheme provides a general practitioner service and caters for something like 21 million of the population, the rest of the population have to pay whenever they desire the services of a doctor. It is cardinal to a proper health organisation that a person ought not to be financially deterred from seeking medical assistance at the earliest possible stage. It is one of the evils of having to buy medical advice that in addition to the natural anxiety that may arise because people do not like to hear unpleasant things about themselves, and therefore tend to postpone consultation as long as possible, there is the financial anxiety caused by having to pay doctors' bills. Therefore, the first evil that we must deal with is that which exists as a consequence of the fact that the whole thing is the wrong way round. A person ought to be able to receive medical and hospital help without being involved in financial anxiety.

In the second place, the national health insurance scheme does not provide for the self-employed, nor, of course, for the families of dependants. It depends on insurance qualification, and no matter how ill you are; if you cease to be insured you cease to have free doctoring. Furthermore, it gives no backing to the doctor in the form of specialist services. The doctor has to provide himself, he has to use his own discretion and his own personal connections, in order to obtain hospital treatment for his patients and in order to get them specialists, and in very many cases, of course – in an overwhelming number of cases – the services of a specialist are not available to poor people.

Not only is this the case, but our hospital organisation has grown up with no plan, with no system; it is unevenly distributed over the country and indeed it is one of the tragedies of the situation, that very often the best hospital facilities are available where they are least needed. In the older industrial districts of Great Britain hospital facilities are inadequate. Many of the hospitals are too small – very much too small.

Furthermore – I want to be quite frank with the House – I believe it is repugnant to a civilised community for hospitals to have to rely upon private charity. I believe we ought to have left hospital flag days behind. I have always felt a shudder of repulsion when I have seen nurses and sisters who ought to be at their work, and students who ought to be at their work, going about the streets collecting money for the hospitals. I do not believe there is an hon. Member of this House who approves that system. It is repugnant, and we must leave it behind – entirely. But the implications of doing this are very considerable.

I have been forming some estimates of what might happen to voluntary hospital finance when the all-in insurance contributions fail to be paid by the people of Great Britain, when the Bill is passed and becomes an Act and they are entitled to free hospital services. The estimates I have go to show that between 80 per cent and 90 per cent of the revenues of the voluntary hospitals in these circumstances will be provided by public funds, by national or rate funds. [An. HON. MEMBER: 'By workers' contributions.'] And, of course, as the hon. Member reminds me, in very many parts of the country it is a travesty to call them voluntary hospitals. In the mining districts, in the textile districts, in the districts where there are heavy industries it is the industrial population who pay the weekly contributions for the maintenance of the hospitals. When I was a miner I used to find that situation when I was on the hospital committee. We had an annual meeting and a cordial vote of thanks was moved and passed with great enthusiasm to the managing director of the colliery company for his generosity towards the hospital; and when I looked at the balance sheet, I saw that 97½ per cent of the revenues were provided by the miners' own contributions; but nobody passed a vote of thanks to the miners . . .

MR LAW: . . . We accept the principle, and we accept the consequences that flow from it. We understand, for example, that once we are committed, as we are gladly committed, to the principle of a 100 per cent service, we require an enormous expansion and development in the health services as a whole. We understand, once we accept the principle, that we are committed to a far greater degree of coordination, or planning as it is usually called, than we have ever known before . . . if my right hon. and learned Friend the Member for North Croydon (Mr Willink) had still been Minister of Health, had the General Election results gone another way, I do not doubt that he would have introduced, before this, a Bill which would have differed from this Bill only in that my right hon. and learned Friend would not have attempted to control, own and direct the hospital services of this country or to interfere with that age-old relationship which exists, always has existed, and in our view ought to continue to exist, between a doctor and his patient. Therefore, the right hon. Gentleman is not entitled to say – he has not said it, but he might – that we will the end without the means. We will both the end and the means. We will this end, a comprehensive and efficient health service. We are willing to support any practicable means that will give us that end.

But we differ from the right hon. Gentleman on this issue. We believe that the right hon. Gentleman could have reached his end, and a better end, by other means, and by better means. We believe that he could have established a health service, equally comprehensive, better coordinated and far more efficient, if he had not been determined to sweep away the voluntary hospitals; if he had not been determined to weaken the whole structure of English local government by removing from the field of local government one of the most important and vital responsibilities of local authorities; and if he had not sought to impose upon the medical profession a form of discipline which, in our view and in theirs, is totally unsuited to the practice of medicine, an art, a vocation, however you like to call it, which depends above all else upon individual responsibility, individual devotion and individual sympathy.

From: *Hansard*, 30 April 1946

Document 6
THE BEVERIDGE REPORT AND THE ROLE OF A HEALTH SERVICE

ASSUMPTION B. COMPREHENSIVE HEALTH AND REHABILITATION SERVICES

426. The second of the three assumptions has two sides to it. It covers a national health service for prevention and for cure of disease and disability by medical treatment; it covers rehabilitation and fitting for employment by treatment which will be both medical and post-medical. Administratively, realisation of Assumption B on its two sides involves action both by the departments concerned with health and by the Ministry of Labour and National Service. Exactly where the line should be drawn between the responsibilities of these Departments cannot, and need not, be settled now. For the purpose of the present Report, the two sides are combined under one head, avoiding the need to distinguish accurately at this stage between medical and post-medical work. The case for regarding Assumption B as necessary for a satisfactory system of social security needs little emphasis. It is a logical corollary to the payment of high benefits in disability that determined efforts should be made by the State to reduce the number of cases for which benefit is needed. It is a logical corollary to the receipt of high benefits in disability that the individual should recognise the duty to be well and to co-operate in all steps which may lead to diagnosis of disease in early stages when it can be prevented. Disease and accidents must be paid for in any case, in lessened power of production and in idleness, if not directly by insurance benefits. One of the reasons why it is preferable to pay for disease and accident openly and directly in the form of insurance benefits, rather than indirectly, is that this emphasises the cost and should give a stimulus to prevention. As to the methods of realising Assumption B, the main problems naturally arise under the first head of medical treatment. Rehabilitation is a new field of remedial activity with great possibilities, but requiring expenditure of a different order of magnitude from that involved in the medical treatment of the nation.

427. The first part of Assumption B is that a comprehensive national health service will ensure that for every citizen there is available whatever medical treatment he requires, in whatever form he requires it, domiciliary or institutional, general, specialist or consultant, and will ensure also the provision of dental, ophthalmic and surgical appliances, nursing and midwifery and rehabilitation after accidents. Whether or not payment towards the cost of the health service is included in the social insurance contribution, the service itself should

(i) be organised, not only by the Ministry concerned with social insurance, but by Departments responsible for the health of the people and for positive and preventive as well as curative measures;

(ii) be provided where needed without contribution conditions in any individual case.

Restoration of a sick person to health is a duty of the State and the sick person, prior to any other consideration. The assumption made here is in accord with the definition of the objects of medical service as proposed in the Draft Interim Report of the Medical Planning Commission of the British Medical Association:

(a) to provide a system of medical service directed towards the achievement of positive health, of the prevention of disease, and the relief of sickness;
(b) to render available to every individual all necessary medical services, general and specialist, and both domiciliary and institutional.

From: *Report on Social Insurance and Allies Services* (Chairman: Sir W. Beveridge), Cmnd 6404, HMSO, London (1942), paras 426–7

Document 7
THE SHARED VERSION OF THE NHS

This common, or at least widely-shared account contained at least nine major features:

1 Health care politics are characterized as, in a broad sense, incrementalist. This means that changes in health service outputs (for example from an emphasis on acute hospital medicine to community-based forms of care) tend to be slow, and/or of narrow scope, rather than systematic or radical. This, in turn, derives from the distribution of power between the main 'actors' (ministers, civil servants, health authority members, NHS managers, doctors, other health care professionals and – occasionally – trade unions) and, institutionally, between 'centre' and 'periphery'.
2 The policy process is usually one of 'partisan mutual adjustment' (PMA), in which no one actor or institution can impose change, though several may be able to veto it.
3 Within this PMA process, the medical profession continues to wield enormous influence, at least in the 'defensive' sense of being able to frustrate those who wish to alter its training, conditions of service or patterns of practice.
4 The position of the lay health authority members is often weak relative to both clinicians and senior managers.
5 The position of consumer organizations is usually even weaker. On the other hand their increased activity and 'density' over the last two decades signifies a broadening of the *dramatis personae* in the process of partisan mutual adjustment at least for certain *types* of issue. However, these issues which are characterized by broader, pluralistic bargaining have tended not to be of the strategic type. Decisions concerning resource allocations, service priorities and the evaluation of effectiveness and efficiency remain fairly inaccessible to consumer groups. NHS management has tended to be highly 'introverted'.
6 The 'centre' possesses little direct operational control over the implementation of most national policies. It does, however, exercise considerable influence principally through (a) its control over the global sum of resources going into the NHS; (b) the allocation of this total between health authorities; (c) specific approval of large capital schemes and (d) the increasing practice (in England and Wales but less so in Scotland) of 'earmarking' revenue funds for particular purposes.
7 The role of health authority managers within this system of partisan mutual adjustment has usually been reactive. The emphasis has been on 'fire-fighting', diplomacy, conflict-avoidance and consensus-seeking, including maintenance of some notion of 'fair shares' in allocative disputes.
8 The policy inertia resulting from the distribution of power between

the health departments, health authorities and the medical profession is further exacerbated by the extreme occupational complexity of the health service as a whole.

9 The whole complex and slow-moving edifice has been underpinned by an extremely durable political consensus. This consensus has existed both internally and externally. It has existed internally in the sense that no subsequent government has directly challenged the basic deal struck between the then Labour government and the medical profession during the 'founding' period of 1946–8. Nor have either government or NHS managers tried to mount any major, frontal criticism of the 'medical model' of ill-health. It has existed externally in the high and continuing public popularity of the NHS, a popularity which has ensured it very high ratings (topped only – occasionally – by the monarchy) in numerous attitudes surveys concerning public institutions and services.

From: Harrison, S., Hunter, D.J. and Pollitt, C., *The Dynamics of British Health Policy*, 1990 pp. 6–7

Document 8
KEITH JOSEPH'S RATIONALE FOR THE PROPOSED REORGANISATION IN 1974

NATIONAL HEALTH SERVICE REORGANISATION: ENGLAND

Foreword

For two years I have been responsible for the National Health Service – and for the personal social services.

Throughout this time my respect for the achievements of the National Health Service has steadily grown. Whatever its defects we would be utterly wrong to take for granted the massive performance of this remarkable network of services and the ease of mind that it has brought to all the people of this country. I am sure that they feel a deep sense of gratitude to all those involved: to the members of the governing authorities; to the men and women who make their careers in the service, whether in direct contact with patients or in supporting services; and to the voluntary workers.

But at the same time I have come to recognise, as many others have, that while this good work will continue, nothing like its full potential can be realised without changes in the administrative organisation of the service.

Hence this White Paper. It is about administration, not about treatment and care. But the purpose behind the changes proposed is a better, more sensitive, service to the public. Administration is not of course an end in itself. But both the patients and those who provide treatment and care will gain if the administration embodies both a clear duty to improve the service and the facilities for doing so.

Let me illustrate this. Everyone is aware of gaps in our health services. Even for acute illness, where we provide at least as good a service for our whole population as any country in the world, there are some respects in which we achieve less than we could. On the non-acute side the service for the elderly, for the disabled, and for the mentally ill and the mentally handicapped have failed to attract the attention and indeed the resources which they need – and all the more credit to the staff, who have toiled so tirelessly for their patients despite the difficulties.

It is well understood now, moreover, that the domiciliary and community services are under-developed – that there is a need for far more home helps, home nurses, hostels and day centres and other services that support people outside hospital. Often what there is could achieve more if it were better co-ordinated with other services in and out of hospital. It is well understood too that there must be more emphasis on prevention – or at the least on early detection and treatment.

For the imbalances and the gaps Governments must take their share of the responsibility. Resources were and still are stretched. The acute services had a legitimate priority. But the shortcomings were not rational.

They did not result from a calculation as to the best way to deploy scarce resources. They just happened.

Why did they just happen? Because it has never been the responsibility – nor has it been within the power – of any single named authority to provide for the population of a given area of a comprehensible size the best health service that money and skills available can provide. There has been no identified authority whose task it has been, in co-operation with those responsible for complementary services, to balance needs and priorities nationally and to plan and provide the right combination of services for the benefit of the public.

It is to enable such an authority to operate in each area, with the best professional advice, that the Government proposes to reorganise the administration of the National Health Service as explained in this White Paper.

The National Health Service is one of the largest civilian organisations in the world. Its staff is growing rapidly. It contains an ever-growing multitude of skills that depend on and interact with each other. It serves an ever-growing range of health needs with ever more complex treatments and techniques. And though the Government has made substantial additions to a programme of expenditure which was already planned to grow at an above-average rate, there is never enough money – and never likely to be – for everything that ideally requires to be done. Nor, despite the great increase since 1948, are there ever enough skilled men and women.

Real needs must therefore be identified, and decisions must be taken and periodically reviewed, as to the order of priorities among them. Plans must be worked out to meet these needs and management and drive must be continually applied to put the plans into action, assess their effectiveness and modify them as needs change or as ways are found to make the plans more effective.

Effective for what? – to improve the service for the benefit of all. The plans must therefore be effective in providing what patients need: primarily, treatment and care in hospital; support at home; diagnosis and treatment in surgery, health centre or out-patient clinic; or day care.

Furthermore they must include arrangements whereby the public can express their wishes and preferences, and know that notice will be taken of them. That is why I attach great importance to the establishment of strong community health councils, and to improved methods for inquiring into complaints, including the appointment of a health ombudsman.

The health service depends crucially on the humane planning and provision of the personal social services, and therefore on effective and understanding collaboration with local government. No doubt arguments will continue about the theoretical advantages of making both health and social services the responsibility of a single agency. But the formidable practical difficulties, which have been fully argued elsewhere, rule this out as a realistic solution, and require us to concentrate instead on ensuring that the two parallel authorities – one local, one health – with their separate statutory responsibilities shall work together in partnership for the health and social care of the population. This White Paper demonstrates the Government's concern to see that arrangements are evolved under which a more coherent and smoothly interlocking range of services will develop for all the needs of the population.

The doctor and other professional workers will gain too. The organisational changes will not affect the professional workers on which the complex of health services is so largely built. The professional workers will retain their clinical freedom – governed as it is by the bounds of professional knowledge and ethics and by the resources that are available – to do as they think best for their patients. This freedom is cherished by the professions and accepted by the Government. It is a safeguard for patients today and an insurance for future improvements.

But the organisational changes will also bring positive gains to the professional worker. He – or she – will have the opportunity of organising his or her own work better and of playing a much greater part than hitherto in the management decisions that are taken in each area. At the same time the more systematic and comprehensive analysis of needs and priorities that will lie behind the planning and operations of each area will help professional workers to ensure their skills bring the greatest possible benefit to their patients.

We are issuing a White Paper and promoting legislation about the administration of the National Health Service, solely in order to improve the health care of the public. Administrative reorganisation within a unified health service that is closely linked with parallel local government services will provide a sure foundation for better services for all.

KEITH JOSEPH
Secretary of State for Social Services

From: *National Health Service Reorganisation: England*, Cmnd 5055, HMSO, London (1972), pp. v–vii

Document 9
OBJECTIVES OF THE NHS, 1979

The Merrison Commission outlined the objectives of the NHS in the following way;

ENCOURAGING AND ASSISTING INDIVIDUALS TO REMAIN HEALTHY

We consider it legitimate and positively desirable to devote public resources to the maintenance and promotion of personal as well as public health, not only by the constraints of law but also by offering exhortation, education and incentives. The NHS cannot cover the whole field. Though protracted unemployment and poor social conditions may impair the quality of life and health, it is the responsibility of other organs of government to promote employment and to care for the environment. The encouragement and advancement of good personal health is vitally important . . . It is a proper objective of the NHS to keep the individual in good health.

EQUALITY OF ENTITLEMENT

We consider, like the framers of the original legislation, that the NHS should be available without restriction by age, social class, sex, race or religion to all people living in the UK.[1] We are in no doubt that one of the most significant achievements of the NHS has been to free people from fear of being unable to afford treatment for acute or chronic illness, but we regret that they must often wait too long for such treatment.

A BROAD RANGE OF SERVICES OF A HIGH STANDARD

This is perhaps the most difficult matter we have to discuss and it is at the heart of our terms of reference. We deal with it more fully in Part II of the report, but our definition of this objective includes health promotion, disease prevention, cure, care and after care. The NHS was, from the first, designed to be a comprehensive service. The 1944 White Paper said:

> The proposed service must be 'comprehensive' in two senses – first, that it is available to all people and, second, that it covers all necessary forms of health care.

The impossibility of meeting all demands for health services was not anticipated. Medical, nursing and therapeutic techniques have been developed to levels of sophistication and expense which were not foreseen when the NHS was introduced.

Standards of cure and care within a given level of resources are in practice largely in the hands of the health professions. They are nevertheless of the greatest concern to the patient. The aim must always be to raise standards in areas where there are deficiencies, but not at the expense of places where services are already good. The NHS has achieved much. It should remain an objective of a national health service to see that it has an active role in disseminating high standards. Sir George Godber, Chief Medical Officer at the Department of Health and Social Security 1960–73, puts the point thus:

> The burden upon the NHS is that of generalization from the example of the best and the result of having such a national service should be the more rapid development of improved services available to all.

EQUALITY OF ACCESS

It is unrealistic to suppose that people in all parts of the United Kingdom can have equal ease of access to all services of an identical standard. Access to the highest standard of care will be limited by the numbers of those who can provide such care. There are parts of the country which are better or worse provided with services than others. We draw attention . . . to the special problems of rural areas and declining urban areas . . . Nonetheless, a fundamental purpose of a national service must be equality of provision so far as this can be achieved without an unacceptable sacrifice of standards . . .

A SERVICE FREE AT THE TIME OF USE

Charges for services within the NHS have always been a matter of controversy, and have led on occasion to the resignation of ministers . . . there are three points to be made here. First, the purpose of charges may be to raise revenue, or discourage the frivolous use of the service, or both. Second, charges may be made for a service which, though provided by or through the NHS, is not essential to the care of treatment of patients – for example, amenity beds in NHS hospitals. Third, in any consideration of charges, it is important to stress that 'free at the time of use' is quite different from 'free'. We do not have a free health service; we have a service to which all taxpayers, employees and employers contribute, regardless of the use they make of it. The effect of this is that those members of the community who do not require extensive use of the NHS help to pay for the care of those who do. It is worth remembering that about 60% of the total expenditure of the NHS goes on children, the old, the disabled, the mentally ill and the mentally handicapped.

SATISFYING REASONABLE EXPECTATIONS

This objective can be considered from the point of view of the individual patient, or more generally. Most patients lack the technical knowledge to make informed judgements about diagnosis and treatment. Ignorance may as easily be a reason for a patient being satisfied with his treatment as for his being dissatisfied. One aspect of care on which he will be reliable, however, is whether he has been humanely treated. While doctors are properly deferred to as experts on the technical aspects of medicine, options, when they exist, should be carefully explained and wherever feasible the choice of treatment left to the patient and his relatives. Maximum freedom of choice seems to us an important aspect of this objective although we recognise that there may sometimes be practical limitations on complete freedom of choice for patients. A patient, or potential patient, who is capable of deciding for himself, should be free to:

> consult a doctor, dentist, or other health professional;
> change his practitioner;
> choose a particular hospital or unit with the help of his general practitioner; and
> refuse treatment or advice where the health and safety of others would be endangered.

More generally, it is important for any health service to carry its users with it, given that it can never satisfy all the demands made upon it. It is misleading to pretend that the NHS can meet all expectations. Hard choices have to be made. It is a prime duty of those concerned in the provision of health care to make it clear to the rest of us what we can reasonably expect.

A NATIONAL SERVICE RESPONSIVE TO LOCAL NEEDS

Health services meet different situations in different parts of the country. The range, speed of development and pattern of service delivery will need to vary. Some services can best be provided on a national or regional basis; specialised treatment may require complicated equipment and a higher degree of expertise than can be provided in every community. But if inflexibility is to be avoided, health authorities should implement national policy in the context of their particular geographical and demographic constraints.

Note:
[1] We propose no change in policy towards providing treatment to non-residents of the UK. It is right that those who fall ill while they are in this country should continue to receive treatment under the NHS but that unless there is a reciprocal agreement with a particular country a charge should be made if treatment is specifically sought in the UK.

From: *Report of the Royal Commission on the National Health Service* (Chairman: Sir Alec Merrison), Cmnd 7615, HMSO, London (1979), pp. 9–12

Document 10
THE COURT REPORT'S VIEW OF THE 'SOCIAL DIMENSION': ILL-HEALTH AND DISABILITY IN CHILDREN

We have already had occasion to refer repeatedly to the correlation between social class and the prevalence of ill-health and disability in children. As we pass from the children of professional families to those of unskilled workers there is a significant increase in bedwetting, squint, stuttering, dental disease and non-infective seizures, and bronchitis and pneumonia and infective diarrhoea are more frequent and more severe. Disease does not occur in a bodily system but in a child, a member of a particular family living in a particular community. Illness in childhood cannot be fully understood without reference to the child's development and social circumstances. Conventional classifications fail to reveal the adverse social factors that may lie behind a diagnostic label and contribute to the form, management and outcome of the illness. Poverty, inadequate housing and unemployment are still with us; and although the majority of parents care for their children faithfully and well, many are hindered from doing so by physical or mental illness, or instability in their personal relationships.

The effect of environment can also be seen in growth. In one group of urban children at 15 children in social classes I and II were on average 4.5 cm taller and 4.4 kg heavier than children in social classes IV and V. In a national study,[1] when all adverse factors were compounded, the 'social' difference in height was nearly 14 cm. In a study[2] of all short children (below the third centile), in a northern city at the age of 10, 82% were normal in terms of freedom from disease. The majority of the families however belonged to social classes IV and V and the children had been brought up in poor conditions. In at least a third of these 'normal' children the adverse social conditions were considered the cause of their deficient growth. Short stature can be normal; it can also be a disease of the social environment and an important pointer to a group of socially deprived children. *There is now extensive evidence that an adverse family and social environment can retard physical, emotional and intellectual growth, lead to more frequent and more serious illness and adversely affect educational achievement and personal behaviour*.

Infant deaths, 1964, England and Wales, number and rate per 1,000 legitimate live births – social class

I & II		*III*		*IV & V*	
1,714	(12.8)	7,101	(17.2)	4,931	(20.8)

Children 1–14, 1959–63, England and Wales, numbers of deaths (and rates per 100,000 per year) - social class

Age	*I*	*II*	*III*	*IV*	*V*
1–4	436(69.0)	1,329(73.4)	6,147(88.7)	2,324(93.3)	1,521(154.0)
5–9	209(32.8)	818(35.1)	3,243(41.1)	1,234(41.4)	744(66.6)
10–14	173(29.6)	823(28.8)	2,771(31.3)	1,091(30.3)	555(41.4)

A special analysis of the 1959–63 child deaths shows that the death rate for children aged 1–4 and 5–9 in Social Class V was approximately twice that in Social Classes I and II and more than 50% higher than that for Social Class IV. The differences for children aged 10–14 are less striking, but nevertheless the death rate in Social Class V was a third higher than that for Social Class IV. The difference in deaths from respiratory diseases is particularly noticeable. For children aged 1–4 the death rate from pneumonia in Social Class V was 25.2 per 100,000 compared with 13.9 for Social Class IV and 10.0 for Social Class I. Children in Social Class V experienced considerably higher death rates from accidents, poisonings and violence. Although these figures relate to a period 15 years ago and the death rate from disease and accident has fallen appreciably since then it is unlikely that the large social class differences have been eliminated. They are a sad commentary on avoidable deaths in childhood.

Notes:

[1] Davis, R., Butler, N. and Goldstein, H. (1972) *From Birth to Seven*, Second Report of the National Child Development Study, Longman in association with the National Children's Bureau.

[2] Lacey, K. A. and Parkin, M. J. (1974) 'The normal short child', *Arch. Dis. Child*, 49, 417–24.

From: *Fit for the Future. Report of the Committee on Child Health Services* (Chair: Donald Court), Cmnd 6684, HMSO, London, Vol. 1, p. 50

Document 11
RESOURCE ALLOCATION – THE NATURE OF THE PROBLEM – DEFINITIONS AND DISTINCTIONS: THE 2ND RAWP REPORT OUTLINES THE BASIS FOR ALLOCATING RESOURCES

INTRODUCTION AND BACKGROUND

1.1 There is ample evidence to demonstrate that demand for health care throughout the world is rising inexorably. England has no immunity from this phenomenon. And because it can also be shown that supply of health care actually fuels further demand, it is inevitable that the supply of health care services can never keep pace with the rising demands placed upon them. Demand will always be one jump ahead. This is a problem for Government and society in general and not, fortunately, one to which the Working Party was called upon to address its mind. We mention it at the beginning of this Report, however, to emphasize two points. Firstly that the resources available to the NHS are bound to fall short of requirements as measured by demand criteria and secondly that supply of facilities has an important influence on demand in the locality in which they are provided.

1.2 Supply of health facilities is, in England as elsewhere, also variable and very much influenced by history. The methods used to distribute financial resources to the NHS have, since its inception, tended to reflect the inertia built into the system by history. They have tended to increment the historic basis for the supply of real resources (e.g. facilities and manpower); and, by responding comparatively slowly and marginally to changes in demography and morbidity, have also tended to perpetuate the historic situation.

1.3 This led us in our Interim Report to interpret the underlying objective of our terms of reference as being to secure, through resource allocation, that there would eventually be equal opportunity of access to health care for people at equal risk. We reaffirm this view. It has involved us in seeking criteria which are broadly responsive to relative need, not supply or demand, and to employ those criteria to establish and quantify in a relative way the differentials of need between different geographical locations. For practical purposes these geographic locations must correspond with those into which the NHS is organized to administer the delivery of health care, viz, Regions, Areas and Districts.

1.4 In searching for criteria which are responsive in this way, we have had perforce to consider only those criteria, the supporting statistical data for which are readily available and reliable at all three levels of disaggregation required. We have further taken as an aim the desirability of keeping the methods proposed as simple as possible, consistent with the overall objective. the degree of refinement necessary is to some extent a matter of judgment, but we have not by any means regarded perfection in this context as an aim. On the contrary, we have rejected many approaches which might have made the criteria more sensitive, but which on examination would have led to much greater complexity with little significant change in the result.

1.5 *Resource allocation is concerned with the distribution of financial resources which are used for the provision of real resources. In this sense it is concerned with the means rather than the end. We have not regarded our remit as being concerned with how the resources are deployed.* This must be a matter for the administering Authorities and is essentially part of their policy-making, planning and decision-making functions in response to central guidelines on national policies and priorities. Resource allocation will clearly have an important influence on the discharge of those functions and be the most critical guideline within which they have to be discharged. This serves, however, to emphasize the importance, as our terms of reference direct, of ensuring that the availability of the finite resource at the NHS's disposal should be determined in relation to criteria of need.

CRITERIA OF NEED

Size of Population

1.6 Health care is for people and clearly the primary determinant of need must be the size of the population. This must therefore be the basic divisor used to distribute the resources available to each level required.

Population Make-up

1.7 The make-up of the population is, however, critical. People do not have identical needs for health care. For example, the elderly (men and women aged 65 and over) form about 14% of the total population, yet they occupy more than half the non-psychiatric hospital beds (excluding maternity). Women have needs different from men, and children too are heavy users of health care facilities. Similarly, patterns of morbidity are different between the sexes at different ages. Thus the age/sex make-up of the population needs to be taken into account as well as its size.

Morbidity

1.8 Even when differences due to age and sex are fully accounted for, populations of the same size and make-up display different morbidity characteristics. The reasons are simple enough to guess but harder to quantify; environment, social circumstances, heredity, occupation etc all play a part. But a population-based measure of need which takes no account of different patterns of morbidity would ignore geographic variations which, on the data available, are significant.

Cost

1.9 The costs of providing care in response to need are also variable. Some conditions are very expensive to treat, others less so. It is not enough to use criteria which predict the likely incidence of the more expensive forms of care, unless at the same time some account is taken of the differential cost involved. Furthermore, the costs of exactly the same form of care may vary from place to place depending on local variations in market forces. A clear example of this is the weighting paid to staff employed in the London area.

Health Care Across Administrative Boundaries

1.10 The populations for which the administering Authorities are responsible for delivering health care are primarily those who reside within their geographic boundaries. In some cases these responsibilities are adjusted to take account of people residing in overlap areas – by means of formal agency or extra-territorial management arrangements. For resource allocation purposes the population needs to be that for which the Authority exercises a management responsibility.

1.11 But these arrangements do not take account of patients who receive cars outside the managed area of their particular Authority. Patient flows across boundaries result from the fact that few Areas and Districts are entirely self-sufficient in terms of the services they provide. In some cases these 'deficiencies' are planned, e.g. Regional specialties, in others they are unplanned and are often the inevitable consequence of new and arbitrary administrative boundaries not matching established patterns of health care delivery. To a large extent unplanned patient flows are also a measure of geographical disparity in health care provision. Whether patient flows are from choice or necessity, the populations used for revenue allocations need to be adjusted to take account of the movement. And such adjustment ought also to reflect the different costs of care involved.

Medical and Dental Education

1.12 The NHS has a responsibility to provide clinical facilities for the teaching of students qualifying through the University Medical Schools. Service facilities which are used for medical and dental education are more costly to provide. The incidence of these costs is, however, unrelated either to the size of the needs of the populations served by the hospitals where medical and dental education is undertaken. Means must therefore be found of identifying the additional costs necessarily involved and protecting those costs from the effects of allocation processes based upon population and service need criteria.

Capital Investment

1.13 Health services require considerable capital investment in buildings, plant and equipment. Whilst the need for capital investment may to a considerable extent be measurable by criteria similar to those used for determining need for current expenditure, there is one significant difference. As mentioned earlier in this chapter, the distribution of capital stock is still very much influenced by the historic patterns of health care delivery. There are not only geographic inequalities in the quantity of stock available but also in its age and condition. Nor do these factors of quantity and quality go hand in hand. Regions which are well provided in quantitative terms may, for the same historic reasons, have a large proportion of ageing stock. Furthermore, the effects of population movement, demographic change and the redefinition of administrative boundaries have all exacerbated the 'mislocation' problem.

From: DHSS, *Sharing Resources for Health in England*, Report of the Resource Allocation Working Party, HMSO, London (1976), pp. 7–10

Document 12
COMMUNITY CARE: AIMS FOR LOCAL LEVEL AUTHORITIES OUTLINED IN THE 1971 WHITE PAPER

(i) Ensuring that the family with a handicapped member has the same access to general social services as other families and to special additional help as required.

(ii) Preventing unnecessary segregation of mentally handicapped children or adults from other people of similar age and from the general life of the local community.

(iii) Preventing mental handicap if possible and reducing the severity of its effects.

(iv) Providing a comprehensive initial assessment and periodic reassessment of the needs of each handicapped person and his family.

(v) Providing stimulation, social training and education, and purposeful occupation or employment for each mentally handicapped person.

(vi) Enabling each mentally handicapped person to live with his own family, if this does not impose an undue burden on them or him.

(vii) Enabling the mentally handicapped person who has to leave home temporarily or permanently to maintain links with his own family.

(viii) Providing a homelike substitute home for those mentally handicapped people who need one, with sympathetic and constant human relationships.

(ix) Providing an adequate range of residential services for mentally handicapped people in every area.

(x) Fostering proper co-ordination of relevant services and in the application of relevant professional skills to individual mentally handicapped people and their families, regardless of administrative frontiers.

(xi) Developing local authority personal social services for mentally handicapped people as an integral part of services provided under the Local Authority Social Services Act 1970 (and other legislation).

(xii) Fostering close collaboration between local authority personal social services for mentally handicapped people and services provided by other local authority departments and with GPs, hospitals and other services for people who are disabled.

(xiii) Fostering partnerships in the planning and operation of hospital and local authority services.

(xiv) Encouraging voluntary help for mentally handicapped people and their families.

(xv) Encouraging understanding and help from the immediate and wider community for the mentally handicapped person and his family.

From: DHSS, Government response to the second report from the Social Services Committee, 1984–85 session, *Community Care with Special Reference to Adult Mentally Ill and Mentally Handicapped People,* Cmnd 9674, HMSO, London, p. 52

Document 13
WORKING FOR PATIENTS (1989): THE GOVERNMENT'S PROPOSALS

Key changes:
The Government is proposing seven key measures to achieve these objectives:

FIRST: to make the Health Service more responsive to the needs of patients, as much power and responsibility as possible will be delegated to local level. This includes the delegation of functions from Regions to Districts, and from Districts to hospitals. The detailed proposals are set out in the next chapter. They include greater flexibility in setting the pay and conditions of staff, and financial incentives to make the best use of a hospital's assets.

SECOND: to stimulate a better service to the patient, hospitals will be able to apply for a new self-governing status as NHS Hospital Trusts. This means that, while remaining within the NHS, they will take fuller responsibility for their own affairs, harnessing the skills and the services they provide. They will therefore have an incentive to attract patients, so they will make sure that the service they offer is what their patients want. And in turn they will stimulate other NHS Hospitals to respond to what people want locally. NHS hospital Trusts will also be able to set the rates of pay of their own staff and, within annual financing limits, to borrow money to help them respond to patient demand.

THIRD: to enable hospitals which best meet the needs and wishes of patients to get the money to do so, the money required to treat patients will be able to cross administrative boundaries. All NHS hospitals, whether run by health authorities or self-governing, will be free to offer their services to different health authorities and to the private sector. Consequently a health authority will be better able to discharge its duty to use its available funds to secure a comprehensive service, including emergency services, by obtaining the best service it can whether from its own hospitals, from another authority's hospitals, from NHS Hospital Trusts or from the private sector.

FOURTH: to reduce waiting times and improve the quality of service, to help give individual patients appointment times they can rely on, and to help cut the long hours worked by some junior doctors, 100 new consultant posts will be created over the next three years. This is in line with the number of fully trained doctors ready for consultant appointments in the relevant specialties. The new posts will be additional to the two per cent annual expansion of consultant numbers already planned.

FIFTH: to help the family doctor improve his service to patients, large GP practices will be able to apply for their own budgets to obtain a defined range of services to the patient, GPs will be encouraged to compete for patients by offering better services. And it will be easier for patients to choose (and change) their own GP as they wish.

SIXTH: to improve the effectiveness of NHS management, regional, district, and family practitioner management bodies will be reduced in size and reformed on business lines, with executive and non-executive directors. The Government believes that, in the interests of patients and staff, the era in which a £26 billion NHS is run by authorities which are neither truly representative nor fully management bodies must be ended. The confusion of roles will be replaced by a clear remit and accountability.

SEVENTH: to ensure that all concerned with delivering services to the patient make the best use of the resources available to them, quality of service and value for money will be more rigorously audited. Arrangements for what doctors call medical audits will be extended through the Health Service, helping to ensure that the best quality of medical care is given to patients. The Audit Commission will assume responsibility for auditing the accounts of health authorities and other NHS bodies, and will undertake wide-ranging value for money studies.

From: *Working for Patients* (1989), HMSO, London para 1.9

Document 14
CASES ILLUSTRATING THE DIFFICULTY OF DISTINGUISHING BETWEEN CLINICAL AND POLICY DECISIONS IN HEALTH CARE

CASE 1: OBSTETRICS

The major teaching hospital in the West Midlands Region has exceptional skills and resources to detect potential abnormalities among prospective mothers and their babies. It has a dual role: first, it serves the Region as a centre of excellence, taking referrals from other hospitals in the Region; second, it has a district general hospital maternity role with respect to the District within which it is situated. Upon examination of the way in which this latter role is actually carried out, some interesting facts emerge. Women living in the four electoral wards of the District, where there are low perinatal mortality rates have ten times the chance of having their babies in this hospital as women living in parts with high perinatal mortality rates. In the worst electoral ward in the District, the perinatal mortality rate (over a five-year period) is 35.8 per 1,000 live births. Women living there have a one in thirty chance of being delivered in the centre of excellence on their doorsteps. The best electoral ward has a perinatal mortality rate of 17.22: women living there have a one in two chance of being delivered there. Two alternative conclusions may be drawn from these figures. If perinatal mortality is regarded as principally the consequence of social and economic deprivation, as implied by the work of the National Perinatal Epidemiology Unit in Oxford, then it may be argued that the hospital ought to be directing its efforts simply to cope with the situation on a remedial and short-term basis, while leaving the causes to be dealt with elsewhere. Thus, the hospital should admit a higher proportion of women from wards with high perinatal mortality rates. If, however, it is argued that the figures show that, where the hospital does a great deal of work, perinatal mortality is lower (as a result of the hospital's effective work), then surely any *additional* resources for the hospital should be tied to increased workloads in wards where those perinatal mortality rates are at present relatively high. But this has not happened. Instead, substantial additional funds have been allocated for nurse staffing, with the aim of increasing the hospital's annual throughput by 1,000 births, without any conditions being attached. Thus funding is in no way linked to specific desired outcomes. The pattern of obstetric care, says the Authority, is a matter properly to be determined by consultant staff, although it is their booking policies which are at the root of the problem. Clinical freedom is thereby extended beyond the care of the individual patient, to the realms of resource allocation and political decision-making . . .

CASE 2: EYES

Recent development in the technology of ophthalmology have enabled consultants to perform extremely sophisticated operations which take a great deal of time. In consequence, waiting lists for relatively simple operations, such as the removal of cataracts, have built up. Sometimes the equipment that consultants are using to enable them to perform more intensive work has been obtained outside the NHS, by voluntary and public donation. This is likely to be the case especially where there is a strong industrial tradition and numbers of industrialists prepared to act philanthropically. Additionally, of course, the revenue consequences of such acquisitions or gifts are rarely met by the original donors, and thereby become a burden on the service. Now it *may* be that the public, if asked, would wish this more intensive ophthalmic work to be carried out, in preference to larger numbers of cataract operations. But the question is never put. It is not the kind of issue considered by health authorities. Prior to 1974, public discussion, too, was non-existent. Now, in a limited way, such issues are beginning to arise in local media, through the work of CHCs. Once again, the boundaries of clinical freedom have been extended to allow consultant medical staff to determine just how the Service will operate and subvert substantially the NHS planning system, and with it any sense of priorities determined in a quasi-democratic way through the health authorities' deliberations.

From: Burkeman, S., 'A Consumer's Response to Merrison and Patients First', *The Yearbook of Social Policy in Britain, 1979*, Brown, M. and Baldwin, S. (eds), Routledge & Kegan Paul, London (1980), pp. 129–30

Document 15
THE 'MEDICAL' MODEL

Probably the most important model is that which we have called the 'medical' model. It seems to have two major components: the *disease* component and the *engineering* component. Typically, the disease component holds that illness, as manifested in signs and symptoms, is due to pathological processes in the biochemical functions of the body. Specific pathogens cause specific diseases which are, as it were, 'hosted' by the patient's body. The emphasis on specific, individual etiology leads to emphasis on individual specific cures. Newer, multicausal theories of disease do not fundamentally question the basics of the disease approach which emphasises the disease rather than the patient, cure rather than prevention, and individuals rather than populations. These emphases on illness rather than health imply the engineering component by which diseases, their detection and treatment become increasingly technical. This engineering approach is summarised by McKeown thus:

> . . . Medical education begins with the study of the structure and function of the body, continues with examination of disease processes, and ends with clinical instruction on selected sick people; medical service is dominated by the image of the acute hospital where the technological resources are concentrated; and medical science reflects the mechanistic concept, for example in the attention given to the chemical basis of inheritance and the immunological response to transplanted organs. These researches are strictly in accord with the physical model, the first being thought to lead ultimately to control of gene structure and the second to replacement of diseased organs by normal ones. (T. McKeown, 'A Historical Appraisal of the Medical Task', in G. McLachlan and T. McKeown (eds), *Medical History and Medical Care*, OUP, 1971, p. 30.)

From: Illsley, R., 'Everybody's Business? Concepts of Health and Illness', in *Health and Health Policy. Priorities for Research*, Social Science Research Council, June 1977, Appendix 4, p. 3

Document 16
WORK AND HEALTH

1. Engels, who came to live in England in 1842, in his account 'The Conditions of the Working Class in England' drew attention to ill health due to working conditions. In Engels' view many disorders were a consequence of the physical demands of industrialism. He discussed curvature of the spine, deformities of the lower extremities, flat feet, varicose veins, and leg ulcers as manifestations of work demands that required long periods of time in an upright posture. Engels commented on the health effects of posture, standing and repetitive movements.

All these affections are easily explained by the nature of factory work . . . The operatives . . . must stand the whole time. And one who sits down, say upon a window-ledge or a basket, is fined, and this perpetual upright position, this constant mechanical pressure of the upper portions of the body upon spinal column, hips, and legs, inevitably produces the results mentioned. This standing is not required by the work itself . . .

He also commented on the condition in cotton mills which led to 'brown lung' or byssinosis.

In many rooms of the cotton and flax-spinning mills, the air is filled with fibrous dust, which produces chest affections, especially among workers in the carding and combing-rooms . . . The most common effects of this breathing of dust are blood-spitting, hard, noisy breathing, pains in the chest, coughs, sleeplessness - in short, all the symptoms of asthma . . .

Engels discussed pulmonary disorder among coal miners. He reported that unventilated coal dust caused both acute and chronic pulmonary inflammation that frequently progressed to death. Engels observed that 'black spittle' – the syndrome now called coal miners' pneumoconiosis, or black-lung – was associated with other gastrointestinal, cardiac, and reproductive complications. By pointing out that this lung disease was preventable, Engels illustrated the contradiction between profit and adequate health conditions in capitalist industry.

Every case of this disease ends fatally . . . in all the coal-mines which are properly ventilated this disease is unknown, while it frequently happens that miners who go from well to ill-ventilated mines are seized by it. The profit-greed of mine owners which prevents the use of ventilators is therefore responsible for the fact that this working-men's disease exists at all.

From: *The Condition of the Working Class in England*, Engels, F. (first published 1845), Progress Publishers, Moscow (1973), pp. 190–3, 279

2. Ruth Cavendish in her account of working with women on a production line also comments on work conditions and their effects on health.

The speed of the line affected your whole body. Constant physical pressure for eight hours left you tensed up. We all felt the same. I don't know whether assembly line workers suffer from stress diseases more than other types of worker, but it wouldn't surprise me. Arlene had recently started seeing 'a butterfly' in front of her eyes and the doctor said she had high blood pressure. Many women are taking Valium and Librium for 'nerve trouble'. They all looked older than their age, pale, tired and drawn. They thought I was about eight years younger than I was and I thought them years older. Even the 20-year olds had deep lines round their eyes.

My diary was full of days when I was 'bursting inside', 'gone over my physical limit', 'whirring', or had 'pains in the chest and felt faint'. It must be bad for the heart to push yourself so hard, and work at a pace much faster than is normal for the body.

It certainly took years off their lives. Apart from looking worn out, they thought fifty was old and didn't expect to live much after sixty or retirement age. That was realistic statistically, given that manual workers have a much lower life expectancy than professional workers. The two labourers who died while I was there were just under sixty, and three other men were said to have dropped dead from heart attacks on the shopfloor during the past year. On my last day, one of the progress chasers, in his mid-forties, had a heart attack. Alice thought the fact it was only men who dropped dead at work proved that 'we women are much stronger'. But the older women did look really haggard and some had difficulty keeping up with the speed.

You also suffered from various aches and pains. Sitting in the same position all day was almost unbearable – it made me feel like a stiff slug that couldn't even stretch. Backache and neckache were common, and excruciatingly painful.

From: Cavendish, R., *Women on the Line*, Routledge & Kegan Paul (1982), p. 118

Document 17
THE TUC'S COMMENT ON THE BLACK REPORT

According to the *Black Report*, health differences between classes and inequalities of life-chances can be traced through all stages of a person's life. This can effectively be illustrated if we take the case of two hypothetical families – the Jones and the Smythes.

Mr Smythe is the financial director of a large company. Mrs Smythe does not work and she is soon to give birth to her third child. They live in a pleasant suburb on the edge of the green belt with their two children, Emily aged five, and Rodney aged 10. They own their own home and the area where they live is mainly populated by professional people. There are plenty of recreational and sporting facilities, good schools and a brand new health centre in the locality.

Mr Jones is an unskilled labourer at a factory. His wife supplements the family income by working as an office cleaner. They live in a high rise block of flats in the centre of the city. The flats were built in the late fifties and are poorly serviced with play areas and parks. The Joneses also have two children, Janet aged five and John aged 10. Mrs Jones is also expecting her third child. The family is registered with a local GP whose list of patients is already oversubscribed.

These two imaginary families are at opposite ends of the social scale in terms of occupation, and income. In between there are different shades of grey, but how are these two different families likely to fare under the existing National Health Service arrangements? Based on the *Black Report* these are some of the likely outcomes.

There is a 60 per cent probability that Mrs Jones will not have consulted an obstetrician by the fifth month of her pregnancy. By that time it may be too late to diagnose congenital abnormalities like spina bifida or blood disorders in her unborn baby.

Mrs Jones's poorer living standards will probably mean her standard of nutritional diet is poor. She is nearly twice as likely as Mrs Smythe to die in childbirth, or her baby to be still-born or die within the first few months of life.

If her baby is a boy and survives birth, he is still four times more likely to die before his first birthday than Mrs Smythe's new-born son.

Like his brother John, the new-born Jones boy is ten times more likely to die, before he is 14, through an accident involving fire, a fall or drowning, than his counterpart Rodney Smythe. John is seven times more likely to be knocked down and killed in a road accident.

Similar disadvantages will follow him into adult life. In only one case – asthma – is Rodney more likely to die than John at an early age.

Though statistics show that Janet Jones is not as likely to be an accident victim as her brother, her individual health and life expectancy will tend to follow the pattern of her mother and maternal grandmother.

Mr Jones's health and life expectancy is also considerably poorer than that of Mr Smythe – and if his son also becomes a manual worker his health is likely to follow a similar pattern too.,

Although the actual health of all families has improved since the setting up of the NHS, the relative gap between professional and unskilled manual workers has actually widened.

Contrary to popular belief, Mr Jones is much more likely to die of lung cancer or duodenal ulcer than Mr Smythe. He is twice as likely to die of a disease affecting the nervous system; three times as likely to suffer and die from a parasitic disease; four times as likely to incur a mental disorder, or a respiratory disease and die.

In contrast, the Smythe family are more likely to follow a nutritionally satisfactory diet, to consult preventive services such as dentists, chiropodists and opticians. Mrs Smythe is more likely to have planned her family than Mrs Jones, or to have been screened to test if she might have treatable breast or cervical cancer. The *Black Report* comments that health facilities tend to be geared towards the middle-class consumer rather than the working class.

Also the high-density urban areas where working-class people live tend to have a lower per-capita expenditure than the suburban areas which are not so densely populated. The Smythe family are likely to have frequent medical check-ups as a matter of course – the Jones are more likely to use their GP after illness has set in, and consequently visit him more often.

The unavoidable inference from the *Black Report* is that the people whose health is at greatest risk are those with the lowest incomes, and worst living conditions. Families like the Jones are the ones most at risk – they are also getting the worst deal out of the NHS.

This evidence must lead to the inevitable conclusion that the NHS is not doing its job as well as it might, and the current run-down into a two-tier system of private care and state care envisaged by the Government will make matters worse.

But of even greater concern, the establishment of an efficient health service alone would not be enough. It is living standards rather than health-care services which determine the overall state of people's health. The living standards of many ordinary working people are so low that their health and life span are severely affected.

From: Trades Union Congress, *The Unequal Health of the Nation: A TUC Summary of the Black Report*, TUC, London (1981)

Document 18
UNEMPLOYMENT AND HEALTH IN FAMILIES

Fagin and his associates carried out a study of 22 families where the male breadwinner had been unemployed for at least 16 weeks and came to the general conclusions shown below:

Our interviews with the families revealed close associations in time between changes in health and the experience of unemployment. As we have described, health changes were not restricted to the male breadwinner; his wife and children often reported fluctuations. Health did not necessarily worsen after unemployment; some families actually reported less health problems. And often the recurrence of marked worsening of a previous illness, and not the emergence of a new illness, co-incided with the event of unemployment,

The following are summaries of what we think are the main areas of concern about health and unemployment that appeared in the families we interviewed.

1. Following the onset of unemployment, spouses with previous histories of poor health suffered relapses and an aggravation of their previous illnesses. This is usually more marked in the male breadwinner, especially if his disability or handicap had neither prevented him from keeping a job nor caused his unemployment. The deterioration in the wife's health, in particular if they were not working, could have been associated with the insecurity accompanying unemployment and the emotional and physical changes in her husband.
2. Male breadwinners with previous records of ill-health may improve following the onset of unemployment. We observed this when ill-health was a manifestation of unhappiness, instability, or high stress at the work place.
3. For men with previous poor health records, returning to work may be associated with fewer reported health problems. This could be due to the threat of losing the job through illness and further long-term unemployment.
4. The wife of a man who cannot return to work because of health problems may also report fewer health difficulties than before her husband lost his job, especially if she has to work and the family relies on her income.
5. The loss of a job can set in motion psychological changes which in some male breadwinners result in clinical depression, with feelings of sadness, hopelessness and self-blame, lethargy, lack of energy and loss of self-esteem, insomnia, withdrawal and poor communication, loss or gain of weight, suicidal thoughts, impulsive, sometimes violent outbursts, and an increased use of tobacco or alcohol. These men are often treated by their General Practitioners with medication (mild tranquillisers and anti-depressants), especially if the men's confidence and self-esteem depended to a large extent on

their jobs. If the depression occurs immediately after the loss of the job, anxiety and agitation pre-dominate; but if it occurs after many months of unsuccessful job search, it is characterised particularly by lethargy, resignation and withdrawal. The wives of these men, especially if they are not employed, may also become depressed.

6. The job loss may also be accompanied by physical symptoms of a kind usually considered to be precipitated by psychological mechanisms. These symptoms include asthmatic attack, skin lesions such as psoriasis, backaches and headaches. These occur mainly in the male breadwinners.
7. Health problems or an established illness in the unemployed male breadwinner relieves the tension he experiences when he cannot regain employment. The dictum that 'it is better to be sick and unemployed, than healthy and unemployed' seems to be true for a jobless man in our society.
8. The return to employment is not necessarily associated with fewer reports of health problems. A wife who expected her life style to change when her husband returned to work was disappointed, and developed a depression which required expert help. Health problems in the male breadwinner may be associated with the extra strain he experiences trying to avoid losing his job again. One young man in our sample had a mild coronary a few months after finding a job.
9. Unemployment can affect children's health. The younger children of men who were out of work for longer periods commonly had disturbances in feeding habits, were prone to accidents, sleeping difficulties, behaviour problems and other ailments.
10. The unemployed man's prior relationship to his job, his perception of society's attitudes to his joblessness, his chances of regaining employment, the strength of the marital and family relationships, his wife's employment status, the degree of financial stress imposed by his unemployment, the power of the sick-role in his family, and his ability to fill his empty time with other activities, interests or marginal employment: all these contribute to the final outcome of physical and mental wellbeing in the families of the unemployed.

From: Fagin, L., *Unemployment and Health in Families*, DHSS, London (1981), pp. 114–17

Document 19
HEALTH AND ILLNESS: THE IMPRINT OF TIME

(This extract is from Wadsworth's *The Imprint of Time* (1991). This reviews the work of a longitudinal study of children born in 1946 and their subsequent development to adulthood. In 1991, the subjects were 45 years old.)

There is no doubt that, as with premature death, illness at all stages in adult life is more common in the manual classes than the non-manual. It is therefore appropriate to ask in a long-term follow-up study how far back in life the origins of illness may be traced, and to see whether the risk factors for illness in later life differ between the sexes and the social classes. Answers to such questions would be useful in understanding the development of illness, as well as in planning most effective ways for health services to work.

(a) LONG-TERM ILLNESS, THE EXAMPLE OF EPILEPSY THAT BEGAN IN CHILDHOOD

The important questions of how individuals with long-term illness manage in everyday life, and how such illness affects the life chances of sufferers have both been examined in this study.

Epilepsy provides an interesting example of the problems of coping with a long-term, serious illness, since it not only brings some restrictions in choice of lifestyle and career, but also anxiety about heritability of the condition, worries about having a seizure in public, concern about what others may think, and whether or not they will treat you differently because of this illness. These last aspects have for many years been lumped together, rather unsatisfactorily, in the portmanteau term 'stigma' when, as more recent observers have pointed out, it is at least necessary to differentiate the sufferer's feelings about having epilepsy from the way that those with epilepsy are treated in daily life.

By the time they were 26 years old 9.5 per thousand study members were diagnosed as having epilepsy, two-thirds of them having uncomplicated epilepsy (6.4 per thousand) and one-third (3.1 per thousand) epilepsy complicated with other conditions, such as Down's syndrome or other congenital problems.

Teachers' reports of pupils' behaviour and chances of educational achievement were compared between those with epilepsy and those without any long-term illness, comparing with two sets of study children from similar social and family backgrounds. There were practically no differences in teachers' reports and expectations, except that rather more attention-seeking and aggressive behaviour was reported amongst those with epilepsy. There was a tendency for children with epilepsy to be more neurotic, perhaps as a result of their physical illness. There was little difference between sufferers, together with higher levels of discontent about their working lives and about the fact that life had not been good to them. It was concluded therefore that perhaps the self-concepts of sufferers had undergone a change by this age, moving away from the neurotic and attention-seeking style of adolescence to a more introspective style in adult life.

(b) LONG-TERM ILLNESS AND LIFE CHANCES

There is now a very great deal of evidence to show that ill health and premature death are disproportionately experienced by people in lower social classes, but it is not at all clear how far this is a result of known class differentials in the uptake of care and advice, or exposure to harmful substances nor yet how and when this process begins. There is evidence from this study that social class differences in illness in adult life may in part originate in childhood. This can be seen first in the study of those who were seriously ill in childhood, and then in the study of health habits.

If serious illness is taken to be that which kept a child in hospital for a minimum of twenty-eight consecutive days or away from school for three consecutive weeks or more, then 388 men (15 per cent of men whose health histories were known up to 26 years) and 311 women (13 per cent of women with known health histories) had had serious illness by the time they were 10 years old. These people who had been seriously ill as children were twice as likely as others to be seriously ill in early adult life, up to age 26 years. Their chances of educational achievement were reduced if they were male and by age 26 years men's social class position achieved through their occupation, was less likely to be higher and more likely to be lower than their father's if they had been seriously ill in childhood. This was especially marked in those from manual social class families of origin.

By 36 years it was clear that the seriously ill child who had continued to be seriously ill up to 25 years was significantly less likely than others to marry and, if a woman, less likely to have children. This group of 160 persons (31 per thousand in this cohort, and likely to be greater in later born groups as survivors of serious illness in childhood increase in number) who were seriously ill both as children and in early adult life seemed especially vulnerable at 36 years, because their comparatively high rates of renting rather than buying their homes, their relatively low chances of marriage, and their higher rates of parental death meant that they had much less fundamental social support, although they were arguably amongst those in greatest need.

From: Wadsworth, M., *The Imprint of Time*, Oxford University Press, 1991 pp. 135–6

Document 20
THE WHITEHALL STUDY: CLASS AND CORONARY HEART DISEASE

The Whitehall study is of 17,000 civil servants working in government offices in London. It shows heart disease deaths for four ranks of office workers: administrators, executives, clerical and 'other'. The death rate from heart disease is four times as high among the most junior as among the most senior staff. The shaded bands at the bottom of the columns in Fig. 1 show how much of these differences can be explained by all the major known risk factors for heart disease. If instead we marked just the amount that behaviour can influence heart disease, probably less than a quarter of the differences would be explained. This is despite the fact that heart disease has been studied in more detail than almost any other single disease. It has been suggested that, even if you observe all the behavioural do's and don'ts, your most likely cause of death is still heart disease.

Lung cancer is the only major cause of death for which known risk factors explain the bulk of the disease. Behaviour makes very much less difference to other causes of death where our ignorance of risk factors is so much greater.

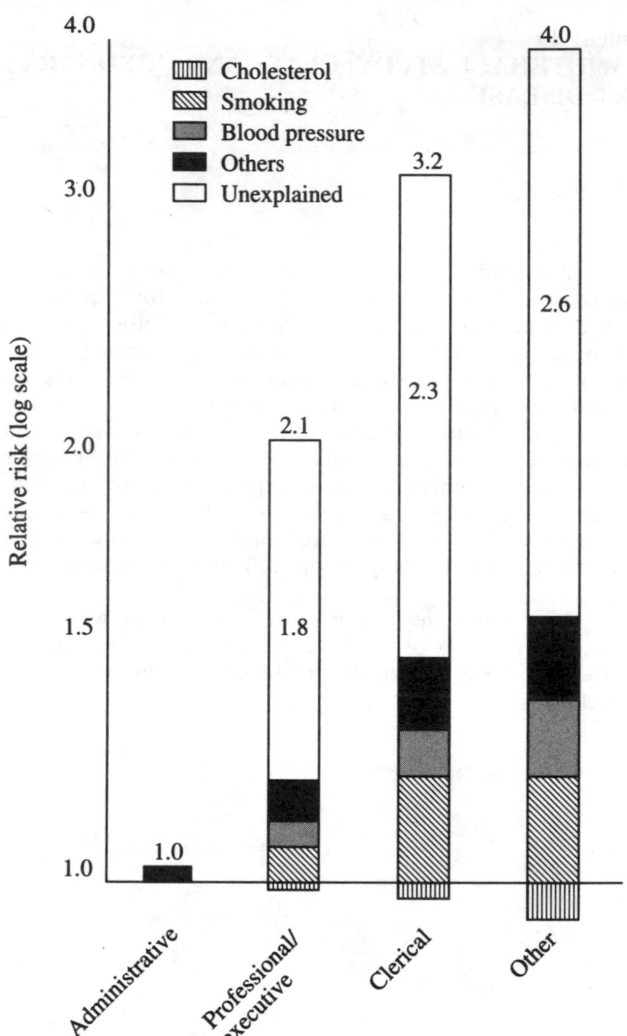

Figure 1 The relative risk of death from coronary heart disease among 17,000 civil servants working in Whitehall offices

The bars show a 4-fold difference in risk between senior and junior workers. The shaded part shows the relatively small amount of the differences explained by the major known risk-factors. ('Others' include height, body mass, exercise and glucose tolerance.)

From Rose, G. and Marmot, M., 'Social Class and Coronary Heart Disease', *British Heart Journal*, 1981, 13–19

Document 21
DEFINITION OF PREVENTION

INTRODUCTION

Prevention in relation to health is either an attempt to prevent disease or disability before it occurs (primary prevention), the early detection and treatment of conditions with a view to returning the patient to normal health (secondary prevention), or the continuing treatment of disease or disability to avoid needless progression or complications (tertiary prevention).

Prevention permeates virtually all aspects of the health services, not simply those which are normally regarded as mainly or wholly preventive. Moreover, a great deal of vital preventive activity takes place outside the National Health Service in such fields as education, housing, transport, employment, social services and environmental planning; and there are yet other fields at both national and local level which also offer important opportunities for prevention, for example, in the areas of taxation, prices and consumer protection, food hygiene and the provision of leisure and recreational facilities.

PRIMARY PREVENTION

This is action which prevents the occurrence of certain diseases or disabilities. Immunisation and vaccination are specific forms of primary prevention which have been particularly effective in recent years in helping to eradicate many of the major infectious diseases. Improved sanitation, safe water supplies, better housing and nutrition are all examples of primary prevention which have saved the lives of millions and improved the quality of life for all.

In the National Health Service, services mainly or wholly concerned with primary prevention include health education, fluoridation, immunisation and vaccination, family planning, health visiting and some aspects of ante- and post-natal care; but primary prevention is an important aspect of many other health services.

Examples of primary prevention outside the National Health Service are clean air and anti-pollution controls, motorcycle crash helmet and car seat belt legislation and much of the work of the factory inspectorate and the environmental health services.

SECONDARY PREVENTION

Secondary prevention is the early detection of a condition which, if appropriately treated, would be cured – so returning the patient to normal health. This form of preventive activity usually takes the form of screening techniques and periodic medical examinations. In general, though not invariably, a selective approach to screening has been adopted in this country, screening efforts being concentrated on 'high risk' groups for particular conditions. In child and school health especially, medical examinations are becoming increasingly selective.

Outside the National Health Service wide secondary prevention is carried out in the Employment Medical Advisory Service and the occupational health services in screening workers at risk of industrial diseases.

TERTIARY PREVENTION

This is concerned with minimising disability arising out of existing disease or injury. The continuing treatment of established disease to arrest its progress is a form of tertiary prevention. So too are those methods of treatment aimed at the rehabilitation of the patient who has recovered from an acute attack of disease or in whose case the disease process has been wholly or partially arrested. Tertiary prevention is a function of a wide range of health services and is particularly important in the case of sufferers from chronic diseases or conditions such as diabetes mellitus, epilepsy, mental disorder, spinal injury and deformities of the feet.

In addition to services provided by the NHS, educational, occupational and social services agencies frequently have important roles to play in tertiary prevention and the rehabilitation of individual patients.

From: DHSS/DES. *Prevention and Health*, HMSO, London (1977), p. 82

Document 22
SUMMARY OF THE ALMA-ATA DECLARATION

The international conference on primary health care, held in September 1978 in Alma-Ata, the capital of the Soviet Republic of Kazakstan, expressed the need for urgent action by all governments, all health and development workers, and the world community to protect and promote the health of all the people of the world. The declaration reads as follows:

1) The conference strongly reaffirms that health, which is a state of complete physical, mental and social wellbeing, and not merely the absence of disease or infirmity, is a fundamental human right and that the attainment of the highest possible level of health is a most important worldwide social goal whose realisation requires the action of many other social and economic sectors in addition to the health sector.
2) The existing gross inequality in the health status of the people particularly between developed and developing countries as well as within countries is politically, socially and economically unacceptable and is, therefore, of common concern to all countries.
3) Economic and social development, based on a new international economic order, is of basic importance to the fullest attainment of health for all and to the reduction of the gap between the health status of the developing and developed countries. The promotion and protection of health of all people is essential to sustained economic and social development and contributes to a better quality of life and to world peace.
4) The people have the right and duty to participate individually and collectively in the planning and implementation of their health care.
5) Governments have a responsibility for the health of their people which can be fulfilled only by the provision of adequate health and social measures. A main social target of governments, international organisations, and the whole world community in the coming decades should be the attainment of all peoples of the world by the year 2000 of a level of health that will permit them to lead a socially and economically productive life. Primary health care is the key to attaining this target as part of development in the spirit of social justice.
6) Primary health care is essential health care based on practical, scientifically sound and socially acceptable methods and technology, made universally accessible to individuals and families in the community through their full participation and at a cost that the community and country can afford to maintain, at every stage of their development, in the spirit of self-reliance and self-determination. It forms an integral part both of the country's health system, of which it is the central function and main focus, and of the

overall social and economic development of the community. It is the first level of contact of individuals, the family, and community with the national health system bringing health care as close as possible to where people live and work, and constitutes the first element of a continuing health care process.

7) Primary health care:
   a) reflects and evolves from the economic conditions and socio-cultural and political characteristics of the country and its communities and is based on the application of the relevant results of social, biomedical, and health services research and public health experience.
   b) addresses the main health problems in the community, providing promotive, preventive, curative, and rehabilitative services accordingly.
   c) includes at least: education concerning prevailing health problems and the methods of preventing and controlling them; promotion of food supply and proper nutrition, an adequate supply of safe water and basic sanitation; maternal and child health care, including family planning; immunisation against the major infectious diseases; prevention and control of locally endemic diseases; appropriate treatment of common diseases and injuries; and provision of essential drugs;
   d) involves, in addition to the health sector, all related sectors and aspects of national and community development, in particular agriculture, animal husbandry, food, industry, education, housing, public works, communications and other sectors; and demands the co-ordinated efforts of all those sectors;
   e) requires and promotes maximum community and individual self-reliance and participation in the planning, organisation, operation and control of primary health care, making fullest use of local, national and other available resources; and to this end develops through appropriate education the ability of communities to participate;
   f) should be sustained by integrated, functional, and mutually supportive referral systems, leading to the progressive improvement of comprehensive health care for all, and giving priority to those most in need;
   g) relies, at local and referral levels, on health workers, including physicians, nurses, midwives, auxiliaries, and community workers as applicable, as well as traditional practitioners as needed, suitably trained socially and technically to work as a health team and to respond to the expressed health needs of the community.
8) All governments should formulate national policies, strategies, and plans of action to launch and sustain primary health care as part of a comprehensive national health system and in co-ordination with other sectors. To this end, it will be necessary to exercise political will, to mobilise the country's resources and to use available external resources rationally.
9) All countries should co-operate in a spirit of partnership and service to ensure primary health care for all people since the attainment of health by people in any one country directly concerns and benefits every other country. In this context, the joint WHO/UNICEF report

on primary health care constitutes a solid basis for the further development and operation of primary health care throughout the world.

10) An acceptable level of health for all the people of the world by the year 2000 can be attained through a fuller and better use of the world's resources, a considerable part of which is now spent on armaments and military conflicts. A genuine policy of independence, peace, détente, and disarmament could and should release additional resources that could well be devoted to peaceful aims and in particular to the acceleration of social and economic development of which primary health care, as an essential part, should be allotted its proper share.

From: World Health Organisation, Geneva, 1978, *Primary health care: report of the International Conference on primary health care, Alma-Ata*, pp. 2–6

Document 23
THE COMPLEXITY OF AGENCIES INVOLVED IN THE CARE OF THE IMPAIRED

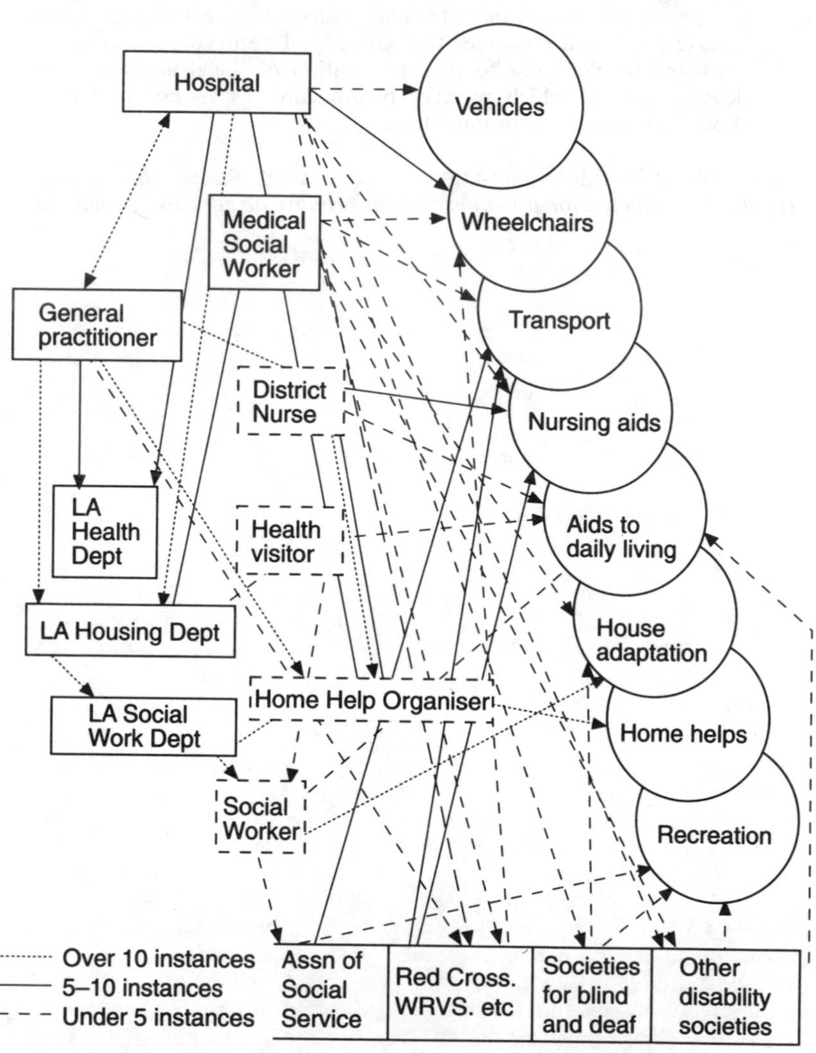

The actual weight of referrals, in one sample of 200 impaired people, for services to help with daily living in the community.

From: Blaxter, M., *Principles and Practice in Rehabilitation*, Royal Commission on the NHS, Cmnd 7615, HMSO, London (1979) p. 455

Document 24
TWO VIEWS OF THE DOCTOR

1. THE LIMITATIONS OF THE MEDICAL PROFESSION

George Bernard Shaw had some caustic things to say about the medical profession when he wrote the preface to *The Doctor's Dilemma* in 1911. Below are some extracts from the original preface.

On the character of doctors . . .

Again I hear the voices indignantly muttering old phrases about the high character of a noble profession and the honor and conscience of its members. I must reply that the medical profession has not a high character; it has an infamous character. I do not know a single thoughtful and well-informed person who does not feel that the tragedy of illness at present is that it delivers you helplessly into the hands of a profession which you deeply mistrust, because it not only advocates and practises the most revolting cruelties in the pursuit of knowledge, and justifies them on the grounds which would equally justify practising the same cruelties on yourself or your children, or burning down London to test a patent fire extinguisher, but, when it has shocked the public, tries to reassure it with lies of breath-bereaving brazenness. That is the character the medical profession has got just now. It may be deserved or it may not; there it is at all events: and the doctors who have not realised this are living in a fool's paradise. As to the honor and conscience of doctors, they have as much as any other class of men, no more and no less.

On our dependence on doctors . . .

If mankind knew the facts, and agreed with the doctors, then the doctors would be in the right; and any person who thought otherwise would be a lunatic. But mankind does not agree, and does not know the facts. All that can be said for medical popularity is that until there is a practicable alternative to blind trust in the doctor, the truth about the doctor is so terrible that we dare not face it. Moliere saw through the doctors; but he had to call them in just the same. Napoleon had no illusions about them; but he had to die under their treatment just as much as the most credulous ignoramus that ever paid sixpence for a bottle of strong medicine. In this predicament most people, to save themselves from unbearable mistrust and misery, or from being driven by their conscience into actual conflict with the law, fall back on the old rule that if you cannot have what you believe in you must believe in what you have. When your child is ill or your wife dying, and you happen to be very fond of them, or even when, if you are not fond of them, you are human enough to forget every personal grudge before the spectacle of a fellow creature in pain or peril, what you want is comfort, reassurance, something to clutch at, were it but a straw. This the doctor brings you.

You have a wildly urgent feeling that something must be done; and the doctor does something. Sometimes what he does kills the patient; but you do not know that; and the doctor assures you that all that human skill could do has been done. And nobody has the brutality to say to the newly bereft father, mother, husband, wife, brother, or sister, 'You have killed your lost darling by your credulity.'

On the difficulty of judging standards of practice . . .

Fortunately for the doctors, they very seldom find themselves in the position [of being accused of malpractice], because it is so difficult to prove anything against them. The only evidence that can decide a case of malpractice is expert evidence; that is, the evidence of other doctors; and every doctor will allow a colleague to decimate the whole countryside sooner than violate the bond of professional etiquette by giving him away. It is the nurse who gives the doctor away in private, because every nurse has some particular doctor whom she likes; and she usually assures her patients that all the others are disastrous noodles, and soothes the tedium of the sick-bed by gossip about their blunders. She will even give a doctor away for the sake of making the patient believe that she knows more than the doctor. But she dare not, for her livelihood, give the doctor away in public. And the doctors stand by one another at all costs.

Thus everything is on the side of the doctor. When men die of disease they are said to die from natural causes. When they recover (and they mostly do) the doctor gets the credit of curing them. In surgery all operations are recorded as successful if the patient can be got out of the hospital or nursing home alive, though the subsequent history of the case may be such as would make an honest surgeon vow never to recommend or perform the operation again. The large range of operations which consist of amputating limbs and extirpating organs admits of no direct verification of their necessity. There is a fashion in operations as there is in sleeves and skirts; the triumph of some surgeon who has at last found out how to make a once desperate operation fairly safe is usually followed by a rage for that operation not only among the doctors, but actually among the patients. There are men whom the operating table seems to fascinate: half-alive people who through vanity, or hypochondria, or a craving to be the constant objects of anxious attention or what not, lose such feeble sense as they ever had of the value of their own organs and ideal of a clean bill of health. He has a safe, dignified, responsible, independent position based wholly on the public health; whereas the private practitioner has a precarious, shabby-genteel, irresponsible, servile position, based wholly on the prevalence of illness.

. . . and in conclusion . . .

let me sum up my conclusion as dryly as is consistent with accurate thought and live conviction.

1. Nothing is more dangerous than a poor doctor: not even a poor employer or a poor landlord.
2. Of all the anti-social vested interests the worst is the vested interest of ill-health.
3. Remember that an illness is a misdemeanour; and treat the doctor

as an accessory unless he notifies every case to the Public Health Authority.

4. Treat every death as a possible and, under our present system, a probable murder, by making it the subject of a reasonably conducted inquest; and execute the doctor, if necessary, *as* a doctor, by striking him off the register.
5. Make up your mind how many doctors the community needs to keep it well. Do not register more or less than this number; and let registration constitute the doctor a civil servant with a dignified living wage paid out of public funds.
6. Municipalize Harley Street.
7. Treat the private operator exactly as you would treat a private executioner.
8. Treat persons who profess to be able to cure diseases as you treat fortune tellers.
9. Keep the public carefully informed, by special statistics and announcements of individual cases, of all illnesses of doctors or in their families.
10. Make it compulsory for a doctor using a brass plate to have inscribed on it, in addition to the letters indicating his qualifications, the words 'Remember too that I am mortal'.
11. In legislation and social organization, proceed on the principle that invalids, meaning persons who cannot keep themselves alive by their own activities, cannot, beyond reason, expect to be kept alive by the activity of others. There is a point at which the most energetic policeman or doctor, when called upon to deal with an apparently drowned person, gives up artificial respiration, although it is never possible to declare with certainty, at any point short of decomposition, that another five minutes of the exercise would not effect resuscitation. The theory that every individual alive is of infinite value is legislatively impracticable. No doubt the higher the life we secure to the individual by social organization, the greater his value is to the community, and the more pains we shall take to pull him through any temporary danger or disablement. But the man who costs more than he is worth is doomed by sound hygiene as inexorably as by sound economics.
12. Do not try to live for ever. You will not succeed.
13. Use your health, even to the point of wearing it out. That is what it is for. Spend all you have before you die; and do not outlive yourself.
14. Take the utmost care to get well born and brought up. This means that your mother must have a good doctor. Be careful to go to a school where there is what they call a school clinic. where your nutrition and teeth and eyesight and other matters of importance to you will be attended to. Be particularly careful to have all this done at the expense of the nation, as otherwise it will not be done at all, the chances being about forty to one against your being able to pay for it directly yourself, even if you know how to set about it. Otherwise you will be what most people are at present: an unsound citizen of an unsound nation, without sense enough to be ashamed or unhappy about it.

From: The Preface to *The Doctor's Dilemma: A Tragedy*, Bernard Shaw (first published 1911), Constable & Co Ltd, London, 1932 (standard edn), pp. 4–5, 10, 11, 12, 64, 77–8

2. THE QUALITIES OF A 'GOOD' DOCTOR

John Berger discusses a country doctor . . .

He is acknowledged as a good doctor. The organization of his practice, the facilities he offers, his diagnostic and clinical skill are probably somewhat under-rated. His patients may not realize how lucky they are. But in a sense this is inevitable. Only the most self-conscious consider it lucky to have their elementary needs met. And it is on a very basic, elementary level that he is judged a good doctor.

They would say that he was straight, not afraid of work, easy to talk to, not stand-offish, kind, understanding, a good listener, always willing to come out when needed, very thorough. They would also say that he was moody, difficult to understand when on one of his theoretical subjects like sex, capable of doing things just to shock, unusual.

How he actually answers their needs as a doctor is far more complicated than any of these epithets imply. To understand this we must first consider the special character and depth of any doctor-patient relationship.

The primitive medicine-man, who was often also priest, sorcerer and judge, was the first specialist to be released from the obligation of procuring food for his tribe. The magnitude of this privilege and of the power which it gave him is a direct reflection of the importance of the needs he served. An awareness of illness is part of the price that man first paid and still pays for his self-consciousness. This awareness increases the pain or debility. But the self-consciousness of which it is the result is a social phenomenon and so with this self-conscious arises the possibility of treatment, of medicine.

We cannot imaginatively reconstruct the subjective attitude of a tribesman to his treatment. But within our culture today what is our own attitude? How do we acquire the necessary trust to submit ourselves to the doctor?

We give the doctor access to our bodies. Apart from the doctor, we only grant such access voluntarily to lovers – and many are frightened to do even this. Yet the doctor is a comparative stranger.

The degree of intimacy implied by the relationship is emphasized by the concern of all medical ethics (not only ours) to make an absolute distinction between the roles of doctor and lover. It is usually assumed that this is because the doctor can see women naked and can touch them where he likes and that this may sorely tempt him to make love to them. It is a crude assumption, lacking imagination. The conditions under which a doctor is likely to examine his patients are always sexually discouraging.

The emphasis in medical ethics on sexual correctness is not so much to restrict the doctor as to offer a promise to the patient: a promise which is far more than a reassurance that he or she will not be taken advantage of. It is a positive promise of physical intimacy without a sexual basis. Yet what can such intimacy mean? Surely it belongs to the experiences of childhood. We submit to the doctor by quoting to ourselves a state of childhood and simultaneously extending our sense of family to include him. We imagine him as an honorary member of the family.

In cases where the patient is fixated on a parent, the doctor may become a substitute for the parent. But in such a relationship, the high degree of sexual content creates difficulties. In illness we ideally imagine the doctor as an elder brother or sister.

Something similar happens at death. The doctor is the familiar of death. When we call for a doctor, we are asking him to cure us and relieve our suffering, but, if he cannot cure us, we are also asking him to witness our dying. The values of the witness is that he has seen so many other die. (This rather than prayers and last rites, was also the real value which the priest once had.) He is the living intermediary between us and the multitudinous dead. He belongs to us and he has belonged to them. And the hard but real comfort which they offer through him is still that of fraternity.

It would be a great mistake to 'normalize' what I have just said by concluding that quite naturally the patient wants a *friendly* doctor. His hopes and demands, however contradicted by previous experience, however protected they may be by scepticism, however undeclared even to himself, are much more profound and precise.

In illness many connexions are severed. Illness separates and encourages a distorted, fragmented form of self-consciousness. The doctor, through his relationship with the invalid and by means of the special intimacy he is allowed, has to compensate for these broken connections and reaffirm the social context of the invalid's aggravated self-consciousness

When I speak of fraternal relationship – or rather of the patient's deep, unformulated expectation of fraternity – I do not of course mean that the doctor can or should behalf like an actual brother. What is required of him is that he should recognize his patient with the certainty of an ideal brother. The function of fraternity is recognition.

This individual and closely intimate recognition is required on both a physical and psychological level. On the former it constitutes the art of diagnosis. Good general diagnosticians are rare, not because most doctors lack medical knowledge, but because most are incapable of taking in all the possibly relevant facts – emotional, historical, environmental as well as physical. They are searching for specific conditions instead of the truth about a man which may then suggest various conditions. It may be that computers will soon diagnose better than doctors. But the facts fed to the computers will still have to be the result of intimate, individual recognition of the patient.

On the psychological level recognition means support. As soon as we are ill we fear that our illness is unique. We argue with ourselves and rationalize, but a ghost of the fear remains. And it remains for a very good reason. The illness, as an undefined force, is a potential threat to our very being and we are bound to be highly conscious of the uniqueness of that being. The illness, in other words, shares in our own uniqueness. By fearing its threat, we embrace it and make it specially our own. That is why patients are inordinately relieved when doctors give their complaint a name. The name may mean very little to them; they may understand nothing of what it signifies: but because it has a name, it has an independent existence from them. They can now struggle or complain *against* it. To have a complaint recognized, that is to say defined, limited and depersonalized, is to be made stronger.

The whole process, as it includes doctor and patient, is a dialectical one. The doctor in order to recognize the illness fully – I say fully because the recognition must be such as to indicate the specific treatment – must first recognize the patient as a person: but for the patient – provided that he trusts the doctors and that trust finally depends upon the efficacy of his treatment – the doctor's recognition of his illness is a help because it separates and depersonalizes that illness.

From: Berger, J., *A Fortunate Man. The Story of a Country Doctor*, Penguin, London (1967), pp. 62–74

Document 25
A MORE BUSINESS-LIKE APPROACH TO HEALTH CARE

Greater competition over the past decade has gone hand in hand with fundamental management reform of the public sector.

This means moving away from the traditional pyramid structure of public sector management. The defects of the old approach have been widely recognised: excessively long lines of management with blurred responsibility and accountability; lack of incentives to initiative and innovation; a culture that was more often concerned with procedures than performance. As a result, public services will increasingly move to a culture where relationships are contractual rather than bureaucratic.

The Government's programme of reform will continue into the 1990s with the aim of:

- making managers accountable for performance within a clear framework of objectives and resources;
- distinguishing the roles of policy formulation and service delivery;
- introducing, wherever feasible, contracts and service level agreements which define standards of performance and responsibility for meeting them.

All these changes enable managers to focus on buying the best standard of service achievable within a given budget.

In central government, the Next Steps programme, launched in 1988, is reorganising the business of government to take greater account of the needs of customers. Executive functions are being transferred to Agencies headed by Chief Executives who are set tough financial and quality targets and given the management and budgetary freedom to help them do their job more effectively. This is in itself akin to a contractual relationship: Ministers agree the terms on which the Agency Chief Executive will carry out a defined task within a defined budget. This gives Chief Executives a strong incentive to buy all the services they need from the most advantageous supplier, whether within or outside the public sector, so that they can meet both the quality and financial targets that Ministers have set.

The NHS reforms have given health authorities the strategic role of assessing the health needs of their population and purchasing care to meet them. The job of providing health care – whether in a directly managed unit or a trust – is undertaken by the management of those units. Separation of the role of customer and provider, negotiating contracts for services, makes hospital managers accountable for performance against specified standards and allows health authority managers to achieve the best value for their resources.

For local services, the Government's model of an enabling authority will promote more effective, business-like management, which pays more attention to customer requirements and value for money. The separation of service delivery from strategic responsibilities enables authorities to concentrate on the core responsibilities of setting priorities and standards and finding the best way of meeting them. We set out new approaches to achieve more business-like management methods in a consultation paper on the internal management of local authorities issued in July.

From: *Competing for Quality*, H.M. Treasury, HMSO, 1991, p. 2

Document 26
ILLICH AND THE LIMITS OF MEDICINE

Illich, in *The Limits of Medicine* presents an extreme statement of the effects of medicalisation. He argues that institutionalised medicine has become a threat to health through social, clinical and structural iatrogenesis. This has been a consequence of industrialisation, bureacratisation and professionalisation of medicine. Iatrogenesis, 'damage done by the provider', has according to Illich occurred on three levels: the clinical, the social and the structural. Clinical iatrogenesis occurs when pain, sickness and death result from the provision of medical care. Illich recounts a tale of the illness caused by the effects of drugs; and 'fashionable operations', operations which are at best effective, at worst damage the patient; irksome, painful, time-consuming diagnostic procedures. In summary, 'a professional and physician-based health must produce clinical damage which outweighs its practical benefits'.

DOCTOR-INFLICTED INJURIES OR CLINICAL IATROGENESIS

Unfortunately, the futility of medical care is the least of the torts a proliferating medical enterprise inflicts on society. The impact of medicine constitutes one of the most rapidly expanding epidemics of our time. The pain, dysfunction, disability and even anguish which result from technical medical intervention now rival the morbidity due to traffic, work and even war-related activities. Only modern malnutrition is clearly ahead.

The technical term for the new epidemic of doctor-made disease, *Iatrogenesis* is composed of the Greek words for 'physician' (*iatros*) and for 'origin' (*genesis*). Iatrogenic disease comprises only illness which would not have come about unless sound and professionally recommended treatment had been applied. Within this definition, a patient can sue his therapist if the latter, in the course of his treatment, has not applied a recommended treatment and thus risked making him sick.

In a more general and more widely accepted sense, clinical iatrogenic disease comprises all clinical conditions for which remedies, physicians or hospitals are the pathogens or 'sickening' agents. I will call this plethora of therapeutic side-effects *clinical-iatrogenesis*.

Medicines have always been potentially poisonous, but their unwanted side-effects have increased with their effectiveness and widespread use. Every 24 to 36 hours, from 50% to 80% of adults in the US and UK swallow a medically prescribed chemical. Some take a wrong drug, others get a contaminated or old batch, others a counterfeit, others take several drugs which are dangerous, or take them in dangerous combinations, others receive injections with improperly sterilized syringes or brittle needles. Some drugs are addictive, others mutilating, others mutagenic, although perhaps only in synergy with food colouring or insecticide. In some patients, antibiotics alter the normal bacterial flora and induce super-infection, permitting more resistant organisms to proliferate and invade the host. Other drugs contribute to the breeding of drug-resistant strains of bacteria. Subtle kinds of poisoning thus have spread even faster than the bewildering variety and ubiquity of nostrums. Unnecessary surgery is a standard procedure. Disabling non-diseases result from the medical treatment of non-existent diseases and are on the increase: the number of children disabled in Massachusetts from cardiac non-disease exceeds the number of children under effective treatment for cardiac disease.

Doctor-inflicted pain and infirmity have always been a part of medical practice. Professional callousness, negligence and sheer incompetence are age-old forms of malpractice. With the transformation of the doctor from an artisan exercising a skill on personally known individuals into a technician applying scientific rules to classes of patients, malpractice acquired a new anonymous, almost respectable status. What had formerly been considered an abuse of confidence and a moral fault can now be rationalized into the occasional breakdown of equipment and operators. In a complex technological hospital, negligence becomes 'random human error', callousness becomes 'scientific detachment', and incompetence becomes a 'lack of specialized equipment'. The depersonalization of diagnosis and therapy has turned malpractice from an ethical into a technical problem.

In 1971, between 12,000 and 15,000 malpractice suits were lodged in US courts. However, doctors are vulnerable in court only to the imputation of having acted against the medical code, of having been guilty of the incompetent performance of prescribed treatment, or of dereliction out of greed or laziness. Most of the damage inflicted by the modern doctor does not fall into any of these categories. It occurs in the ordinary practice of well-trained men who have learned to bow to prevailing professional judgement and procedure, even though they know (or could and should know) what damage they do.

The US Department of Health calculates that 7% of all patients suffer compensatable injuries while hospitalized, though few of them do anything about it. Moreover, the average frequency of reported accidents in hospitals was higher than in all industries but mines and high-rise construction. A national survey indicates that accidents were the major cause of death in US children, and that these accidents occurred more often in hospitals than in any other kind of place. One in 50 children admitted to a hospital suffered an accident which required specific treatment. University hospitals are relatively more pathogenic, or, in blunt language, more sickening. It has been established that one out of every five patients admitted to a typical research hospital acquires an iatrogenic disease, sometimes trivial, usually requiring special treatment, and in one case in thirty leading to death. Half of these episodes resulted from complications of drug therapy; amazingly, one in ten came from diagnostic procedures. Despite good intentions and claims to public service, with a similar record of performance a military officer would be relieved of his command, and a restaurant or amusement centre would be closed by the police . . .

SOCIAL AND STRUCTURAL IATROGENESIS

On a second level, medical practice sponsors sickness by reinforcing a morbid society that not only industrially preserves its defectives, but also exponentially breeds demand for the patient role. On the one hand defectives survive in increasing numbers and are fit only for life under institutional care, while on the other hand, medically certified symptoms exempt people from destructive wage-labour and excuse them from the struggle to reshape the society in which they live. Second level iatrogenesis finds its expression in various symptoms of social over-medicalization . . .

STRUCTURAL IATROGENESIS

On a third level, the so-called health professions have an even deeper, structurally health-denying effect insofar as they destroy the potential of people to deal with their human weakness, vulnerability and uniqueness in a personal and autonomous way. Structural iatrogenesis . . . is the ultimate backlash of hygienic progress and consists in the paralysis of healthy responses to suffering. It strikes when people accept health management designed on the engineering model, when they conspire in an attempt to produce something called 'better health' which inevitably results in the heteronomous, managed maintenance of life on high levels of sub-lethal illness. This ultimate backlash of medical 'progress' must be clearly distinguished from both clinical and social iatrogenesis.

From: Illich, I., *Limits to Medicine: Medical Nemesis*, Marion Boyars, London (1975), pp. 21–7

Document 27
PROBLEMS OF COMMUNICATION IN PATIENT CARE

The standard letter assumes patients know the consultant's name and are not referred to more than one consultant at a time.

Why is the out-patient office permanently engaged? The switchboard operators know of it, but do the managers?

CASE STUDY

Mrs Rogers had been referred to hospital by her GP and received a letter with the date and time of an out-patient appointment (1). She rang the hospital three times to find out if the consultation was for her eyes, or for her heavy periods. On each occasion the switchboard put her through to the appointments office which seemed to be permanently engaged (2). So she finally gave up, knowing she would find out on the day.

Arriving at the hospital she could see no signs for out-patients. Eventually a volunteer directed her to the Haldane Wing (3). After waiting for some time in the out-patient clinic, she overheard part of a conversation about cancer from a consulting room (4), but did not have time to feel too uncomfortable about it as a nurse called her into another room and told her to undress and wait on the couch (5).

The privacy and confidentiality of the consultation is lost, and the patient waiting outside is exposed to needless anxiety.

The out-patient department is named after a retired consultant. New patients get lost, but volunteers have no channels for influencing decisions about signposting.

The doctors arrived with Mrs Rogers' medical notes and asked her what the matter seemed to be? Not without a sense of humour, she said she assumed she was there for her periods rather than her eyesight! The doctor did an internal examination, a cervical smear and said he would like her to have a 'scrape'. She heard the words 'routine' and 'nothing to worry about', but was also remembering the talk of cancer she had overheard. Had he taken a smear because he suspected cancer, she wondered? Although he asked if she had any questions, she did not know where to begin (6). What was a 'scrape'? Did it involve cutting? When would she get the smear result? She felt uncomfortable talking while she was still undressed, and was anxious to put her clothes back on.

Ordinary rules of social conduct are broken as the patient meets someone for the first time who is dressed and standing while she is undressed and lying on a couch.

The doctor assumes that patients will be reassured by his emphasis on the routine nature of the operation, and that if they do not ask questions it is because there is nothing more they want to know.

On the day of the operation, a nurse told her off for bringing too much money and her expensive watch with her. As this was the first time she had been in hospital for an operation, she was worried about what else she had done wrong. On her bedside locker she found a booklet with all the information she needed. 'What a shame I didn't see this before,' she thought (7).

The in-patient booklet fails to fulfil its purpose because of a poor distribution system.

A doctor arrived with a consent form. He did not mention a 'scrape' but did talk about a 'D&C', the anaesthetic, and when she would get the results. Mrs Rogers was startled – after her out-patient appointment she had concluded that the operation was to treat her periods – not that the 'scrape' was an investigation and that there was any question of results (8).

The house officer does not know what patients are told in clinic and so he does not know he is passing on new information or using different words from the consultant. This is the first time anyone has referred to 'results' and the patient's worries about cancer resurface.

At home Mrs Rogers received a questionnaire asking what she felt about the level of noise on the ward, and if the toilets were clean. As she ticked the boxes she thought, this was not really what she wanted to tell them about, but the three lines for other comments were not really enough (9) (10).

If Mrs Rogers did not speak or read English, how would the hospital have communicated with her?

The design of the hospital survey did not include finding out what was important to patients.

From: *What Seems to be the Matter?*, Audit Commission, London, 1993, p. 4

Document 28

THE 'NEW CONTRACT' FOR GENERAL MEDICAL PRACTITIONERS, 1990: AN OUTLINE SUMMARY

SERVICE DELIVERY, PLANNING AND MONITORING

FHSAs will plan service development in order for the resources available to be used to best effect. LMCs should be consulted, and GPs supplied with aggregated information about health care provision and achievements in their areas. FHSAs should develop effective working relationships with DHAs and Regional outposts to ensure appropriate service provision, and analyse GP referral patterns. GPs must produce for FHSAs annual reports describing their practice services and plans. The FHSA may invite them to add further data if it is needed.

PRESCRIBING

FHSAs are required to establish rational prescribing policies for their localities, and monitor individual practice prescribing.

PRACTICE TEAMS

The new contract requires FHSAs to determine the percentage of practices' staff costs to be reimbursed, with the total spending now restricted to a cash limited amount in each area. Practice staffing is to be reviewed on a three-yearly basis. Bars on the range of professionals employable which applied under the previous 'ancillary staff scheme' have been lifted.

PREMISES: COST RENT AND IMPROVEMENT GRANTS

Standards for premises are tightened and cost rents made payable in line with regional variations in costs. FHSAs can set the level of improvement grant payable within a defined range. Cash limits now apply.

COMPUTERS

The new contract enables help to be offered towards the cost of purchasing/leasing hardware and software for GPs. Training costs may also be met.

MEDICAL MANPOWER

FHSAs have more discretionary power in relation to defining satisfactory arrangements to meet local needs. Key changes include the introduction of a retirement age of 70 as from April 1991; the use of Jarman indicators in considering manpower needs in deprived localities; GPs must be available for direct consultation for at least 26 hours over at least five days; newly appointed GPs should live within a 'reasonable' distance of the surgery and FHSAs must be notified of GPs' other professional appointments.

INFORMATION FOR CONSUMERS

More information must be supplied for consumers. For example, medical directors must give data on the sex, age/date of qualification, clinic sessions and practice staff offered by each practitioner. Special services (e.g.: child health surveillance), languages and the availability of link-workers may also be indicated. GPs should produce leaflets. Changing doctors is made easier. FHSAs should carry out consumer surveys. They must also offer an annual home visit and assessment to patients over the age of 75.

REMUNERATION SYSTEM

The new contract abolishes a considerable number of established GP payments such as seniority and childhood immunisation on a capitation basis and modifies the basic allowance and night payments system, as well as the higher capitation payment for patients over 75. New payments introduced include those for registration examinations of new patients; the achievement of defined immunisation and cervical screening targets; minor surgery; undergraduate supervision/education; child health surveillance; and health promotion clinic provision. Also, a deprived area supplement to the basic practice allowance is introduced, based on Jarman index measures.

MEDICAL EDUCATION

GPs are now entitled to a payment for each undergraduate medical student they are responsible for. As to postgraduates' medical education, they are entitled to receive a fee of a little over £2000 a year provided at least ten half day education sessions are attended. However, travel costs and session fees must be paid from this, unlike the case previously.

From: Terms of service for doctors in General Practice, Department of Health, London (1989)

Document 29

A COMPARATIVE TABLE OF HEALTH INPUTS AND OUTPUTS (1) 1991

Country	Life Expectancy at birth	Perinatal Mortality per 1000 popn.	Doctor per 1000 popn.	Hospital bed per 1000 popn.	Per Capita Health Expenditure	Health Expenditure as % of GDP		
						Total	*Public*	*Private*
Australia	77	10	2.3	5.6	1331	7.7	5.4	2.3
Canada	77	8	2.2	16.1	1945	9.1	6.8	2.4
France	77	9	2.9	9.3	1869	8.9	6.6	2.3
Italy	77	12	4.7	7.5	1426	7.5	5.8	1.7
Japan	79	6	1.6	15.9	1538	6.5	4.8	1.6
Netherlands	77	10	2.4	5.9	1500	7.9	5.7	2.2
Sweden	78	7	2.7	6.2	2343	8.8	7.9	0.9
USA	76	10	2.4	5.3	2763	12.7	5.6	7.0
Germany	78	7	2.7	8.7	1588	6.3	5.3	1.0
UK	77	10	1.4	6.3	1039	6.1	5.2	0.9

From: *Investing in Health: World Bank*, Oxford University Press, New York 1993; OECD Facts and Trends, Paris 1993

A COMPARATIVE TABLE OF HEALTH INPUTS AND OUTPUTS (2)

Country	Tobacco Consumption (Kilos per year) *1974*	*1990*	Babies with Low Birth Weight % *1985*	Years of Life Lost per 1000 popn. (1990)	% of Total Government Expenditure *1980*	*1991*
Australia	2.9	2.0	6	9	10.0	12.7
Canada	3.8	2.6	6	9	6.7	5.1
France	2.8	2.3	5	10	14.8	15.3
Italy	2.2	1.9	7	10	12.6	—
Japan	3.5	2.4	5	8	—	—
Netherlands	3.8	3.0	4	10	10.7	12.4
Sweden	1.9	1.5	4	11	2.2	0.8
USA	3.8	2.6	7	11	10.4	13.8
Germany	3.2	2.3	5	12	19.0	18.1
UK	2.6	1.9	7	12	13.5	13.3

From: *Investing in Health: World Bank*, Oxford University Press, New York, 1993

Document 30
EVALUATING HEALTH CARE INTERVENTIONS, 1993

Table A: Targets for day surgery by procedure

Treatment	Percentage of treatment
Inguinal hernia repair	11
Breast lump excision	44
Anal fissure excision	68
Varicose vein stripping/ligation	23
Cystoscopy	67
Circumcision	55
Excision of Dupuytren's contracture	28
Carpal tunnel decompression	81
Arthroscopy	59
Excision of ganglion	83
Orchidopexy	32
Cataract extraction	7
Correction of squint	12
Myringotomy	82
Sub-mucous resection	13
Reduction of nasal fracture	80
Operation of bat ears	37
Dilation and curettage	66
Laparoscopy	49
Termination of pregnancy	80

Note: Based upon Audit Commission data on the rates of day surgery achieved by the top 25 per cent of health authorities in 1991–2

Table B: Cost per QALY for various interventions

Treatment	Cost per QALY (August 1990)(£)
Cholesterol testing and treatment by diet (adults aged 40–69)	220
Neurosurgical intervention for head injury	240
Advice to stop smoking from general practitioner	270
Neurosurgical intervention for subarachnoid haemorrhage	490
Antihypertensive treatment to prevent stroke (aged 45–64)	940
Pacemaker implantation	1100
Hip replacement	1180
Valve replacement for aortic stenosis	1140
Cholesterol testing and treatment	1480
Coronary artery bypass graft (patients with left main vessel disease, severe angina)	2090
Kidney transplantation	4710
Breast cancer screening	5780
Heart transplantation	7840
Cholesterol testing and treatment (incrementally) of all adults aged 25-39	14 150
Home haemodialysis	17 260
Coronary artery bypass graft (patients with one vessel disease, moderate angina)	18 830
Continuous ambulatory peritoneal dialysis	19 870
Hospital haemodialysis	21 970
Erythropoietin for anaemia in patients receiving dialysis (assuming 10% reduction in mortality)	54 380
Neurosurgical intervention for malignant intracranial tumours	107 780
Erythropoietin for anaemia in patients receiving dialysis (assuming no increase in survival)	126 290

From: Robinson, R., 'Cost Utility Analysis', *British Medical Journal*, 307, p. 861, *Table IV*

APPENDIX 1

Health and Social Services Secretaries and Ministers

Health Ministers 1919–1968

1919–21	Dr Christopher Addison	Liberal
1921–22	Sir Alfred Mond	Liberal
1922–23	Sir Arthur Griffith-Boscawen	Conservative
1923	Neville Chamberlain	Conservative
1923–24	Sir William Joynson-Hicks	Conservative
1924	John Wheatley	Labour
1924–29	Neville Chamberlain	Conservative
1929–31	Arthur Greenwood	Labour
1931	Neville Chamberlain	Conservative
1931–35	Sir E. Hilton-Young	Conservative
1935–38	Sir Kingsley Wood	National
1938–40	Walter Elliot	National
1940–41	Malcolm MacDonald	N. Labour
1941–43	Ernest Brown	L. National
1943–45	Henry Willink	Conservative
1945–51	Aneurin Bevan	Labour
1951	Hilary Marquand	Labour
1951–52	Harry Crookshank	Conservative
1952–55	Iain MacLeod	Conservative
1955–57	Robert Turton	Conservative
1957	Dennis Vosper	Conservative
1957–60	Derek Walker-Smith	Conservative
1960–63	Enoch Powell	Conservative
1963–64	Anthony Barber	Conservative
1964–68	Kenneth Robinson	Labour

Secretaries of State for Social Services

1968–70	Richard Crossman	Labour
	Minister of State:	
1968–70	David Ennals	
1969–70	Lady Serota	

1970–74	Sir Keith Joseph	Conservative
	Minister of State:	
1970–74	Lord Aberdare	
1974–76	Barbara Castle	Labour
	Minister of State:	
1974–76	David Owen	
1976–79	David Ennals	Labour
	Minister of State:	
1974–76	David Owen	
1976–79	Roland Moyle	
1979–81	Patrick Jenkin	Conservative
	Minister of State:	
1979–82	Gerard Vaughan	
1981–87	Norman Fowler	Conservative
	Minister of State:	
1979–82	Gerard Vaughan	
1982–85	Kenneth Clarke	
1985–86	Barney Hayhoe	
1987–88	Anthony Newton	
1987–88	John Moore	Conservative
	Minister of State:	
1986–88	Anthony Newton	

July 1988 The Department of Health and Social Security split

Secretary of State:

1988–90	Kenneth Clarke
1990–92	William Waldegrave
1992–to date	Virginia Bottomley
	Minister of State:
1988–89	David Mellor
1989	Lord Trafford
1989–92	Virginia Bottomley
1992–94	Brian Mawhinney
1994–to date	Gerald Malone

APPENDIX 2

List of reports and statutes 1858–1994

1858 Medical Act set up the General Medical Council.
1902 Midwives Act.
1911 National Insurance Act.
1918 Maternity and Child Welfare Act.
1919 Nurses Registration Act.
1920 The Ministry of Health. Consultative Council on Medical and Allied Services. Interim Report on the Future Provision of Medical Services and Allied Services (Dawson Report), HMSO.
1921 Ministry of Health Report on the Finance of Voluntary Hospitals (The Cave Committee), HMSO.
1926 Report on the Royal Commission on National Health Insurance, Cmnd 2596, HMSO.
1936 National Health Insurance Consolidating Act.
1937 PEP Report on the British Health Services. Political and Economic Planning.
1944 Ministry of Health. A National Health Service (Coalition government White Paper), Cmnd 6502, HMSO.
1946 National Health Service Act.
1956 Report of a Committee of Inquiry into the Cost of the National Health Service (Guillebaud Report), Cmnd 9663, HMSO.
1957 Royal Commission on Mental Illness and Mental Deficiency, HMSO.
1959 Report of the Committee on Maternity Services (Cranbrook Report), HMSO.
1959 Mental Health Act.
1960 Royal Commission Report on Doctor's and Dentist's Remuneration (Pilkington Report), Cmnd 939, HMSO.
1962 Ministry of Health. A Hospital Plan for England and Wales. Cmnd 1604, HMSO.
1962 Medical Services Review Committee. A Review of the Medical Services in Great Britain (Porritt Report), 1962.
1963 Ministry of Health. The Field of Work of the Family Doctor (Gillie Report), HMSO.
1966 Report of the Committee on Senior Nursing Staff Structure (Salmon Report), HMSO.

1968 Ministry of Health. The Administrative Structure of Medical and Related Services in England and Wales. 1st Green Paper, HMSO.

1968 Royal Commission on Medical Education (Todd Report), Cmnd 3569, HMSO.

1968 Department of Health and Social Security (DHSS) formed.

1969 DHSS. The Functions of the District General Hospital (Bonham-Carter Report), HMSO.

1970 Report of the Committee on Local Authority and Allied Personal Social Services (Seebohm Report), Cmnd 3703, HMSO.

1970 Social Services Act.

1970 DHSS. The Future Structure of the National Health Service. 2nd Green Paper, HMSO.

1971 DHSS. Better Services for the Mentally Handicapped, Cmnd 4683, HMSO.

1971 DHSS. The National Health Service Reorganisation: Consultative Document, HMSO.

1972 National Health Service Reorganisation: England. Cmnd 5055, HMSO.

1972 DHSS. Management Arrangements for the Reorganised National Health Service (The Grey Book), HMSO.

1972 Report of the Committee on Nursing (Briggs Report), Cmnd 5115, HMSO.

1973 The National Health Service Reorganisation Act.

1973 Report of the Committee on Hospital Complaints Procedure (Davies Report), HMSO.

1974 DHSS. Democracy in the National Health Service, HMSO.

1975 DHSS. Better Service for the Mentally Ill, Cmnd 6233, HMSO.

1975 Report of the Committee of Enquiry into the Regulation of the Medical Profession (Merrison Report), Cmnd 6018, HMSO.

1976 DHSS. Sharing Resources for Health in England: Report of the Resource Allocation Working Party, HMSO.

1976 DHSS. Report of the Committee on Child Health Services. Fit for the Future (Court Report), HMSO.

1976 DHSS. Priorities for Health and Social Services in England.

1976 DHSS. Prevention and Health: Everybody's Business: A Reassessment of Public and Personal Health, HMSO.

1977 DHSS. Priorities in the Health and Social Services: The Way Forward, HMSO.

1978 DHSS. A Happier Old Age. A Discussion Document on Elderly People in our Society, HMSO.

1979 Report of the Committee of Enquiry into Mental Handicap Nursing and Care (Chair: Peggy Jay), HMSO.

1979 Royal Commission on the National Health Service (Merrison Report), Cmnd 7615, HMSO.

1979 DHSS. Patients First. A Consultative Paper, HMSO.
1980 DHSS. Mental Handicap: Progress, Problems and Priorities, HMSO.
1980 DHSS. Report of a Working Group on Organisation and Management Problems of Mental Illness Hospitals.
1980 Health Service Act.
1980 DHSS. The Future Pattern of Hospital Provision in England – A Consultative Paper, HMSO.
1980 House of Commons Social Services Committee. Second Report, Perinatal and Neonatal Mortality. Session 1979/80, HMSO.
1980 House of Commons Social Services Committee. The Government's White Papers on Public Expenditure: the Social Services. Third Report, Session 1979/80. HC702, HMSO.
1981 DHSS. Care in the Community, a Consultative Document on Moving Resources for Care in England.
1981 DHSS. Growing Older, White Paper on the Elderly, 8173, HMSO.
1981 DHSS. Care in Action. A Handbook of Policies and Priorities for the Health and Personal Social Services in England, HMSO.
1981 DHSS. Report of a Study of Community Care.
1981 House of Commons Social Services Committee. Public Expenditure on the Social Services. Third Report, Session 1980/81, HC324, HMSO.
1981 DHSS. Health Services in England: Review of the NHS Planning System. A Consultative Document, HMSO.
1981 DHSS. Report on a Study Group on Community Care, HMSO.
1982 Health Advisory Service. The Rising Tide, Developing Services for Mental Illness in Old Age, NHS Advisory Service.
1983 DHSS. Health Care and its Costs. The Development of the National Health Service in England, HMSO. (See also Document 15 for reports on dependent groups.)
1985 DHSS Government Response to the Second Report from the Social Services Committee, 1984–85 Session: Community Care, Cmnd 9674, HMSO.
1986 Audit Commission. Making a Reality of Community Care, HMSO.
1987 National Audit Office. Community Care Developments, HMSO.
1987 DHSS. Promoting Better Health, HMSO.
1987 DHSS. Promoting Better Health: the Government Programme for Improving Primary Health Care, Cmnd, 259, HMSO.

1988 DHSS. Review of the Resource Allocation Working Party Formula: Final Report by the NHS Management Board, HMSO.

1988 DHSS. Community Care: Agenda for action (Griffiths Report), HMSO.

1989 Secretaries of State for Health. Working for Patients, Cmnd 555, HMSO.

1989 Secretaries of State for Health, Social Security Wales and Scotland. Caring for People, Community Care in the Next Decade and Beyond, HMSO.

1989 Department of Health. General Practice in the NHS: The 1990 Contract, Department of Health.

1990 Department of Health. Care in the Community: Making it Happen, HMSO.

1990 House of Commons Social Services Committee. Community Care: Carers. Fifth Report, Session 1989–90, HMSO.

1992 Audit Commission. The Community Revolution: Personal Social Services and Community Care, HMSO.

1992 Department of Health for England. The Patient's Charter, Department of Health.

1993 Department of Health. Managing the new NHS Department of Health, Department of Health.

1994 Department of Health. The NHS Complaints Review, Department of Health.

1994 Department of Health. Managing the new NHS, Functions and Responsibilities in the new NHS.

Select bibliography

Aaron, H. J. and Schwartz, W. B. (1984) *The Painful Prescription: Rationing Hospital Care*, Brookings Institution, Washington, DC.

Abel-Smith, B. (1964) The Hospitals 1800–1948, Heinemann, London.

Abel-Smith, B. (1960) *A History of the Nursing Profession*, Heinemann, London.

Alford, R. R. (1975) *Health Care Politics: Ideological and Interest Group Barriers to Reform*, University of Chicago Press, Chicago.

Allsop, J. and May, A. (1986) *The Emperor's New Clothes, Family Practitioner Committees in the 1980s*, King Edward's Hospital Fund for London, London.

Appleby, J. (1992), *Financing Healthcare in the 1990s*, Open University Press, Milton Keynes.

Audit Commission (1986) *Making a Reality of Community Care*, HMSO, London.

Audit Commission (1992) *Community Care: Managing the Cascade of Change*, HMSO, London.

Beck, E., Lonsdale, S., Newman, S. and Patterson, D. (1992) *In the Best of Health? The status and future of health care in the UK*, Chapman & Hall, London.

Blaxter, M. (1990) *Health and Lifestyles*, Tavistock/Routledge, London.

Bosanquet, N. and Leese, B. (1988) 'Family Doctors and Innovation in General Practice', *British Medical Journal*, 296, pp. 1576–80.

Butler, J. R. (1992) *Patients, Policies and Politics: before and after* working for patients, Open University Press, Milton Keynes.

Calnan, M. (1991) *Preventing Coronary Heart Disease: Prospects, policies and politics*, Routledge, London.

Cawson, A. (1982) *Corporatism and Welfare: Social Policy and State Intervention in Britain*. Heinemann Education Books, London.

Cochrane, A.L. (1971) *Effectiveness and Efficiency: Random Reflections on Health Services*, Nuffield Provincial Hospitals Trust, London.

Davey, B. and Popay, J. (1993) *Dilemmas in Health Care*, Open University Press, Milton Keynes.

Day, P. and Klein, R. E. (1987) *Accountabilities: five public services*, Tavistock, London.

Drucker, P. (1955) *The Practice of Management*, Pan Books, London.

Enthoven, A. C. (1985) Reflection on the management of the National Health Service, Occasional Paper 5, Nuffield Provincial Hospitals Trust, London.

Fisher, A. (1993) 'Fundholding', *British Medical Journal*, 303, 1003.

Freidson, E. (1970) *Profession of Medicine: a study of the sociology of applied knowledge*, Dodd Mead, New York.

Gabe, J., Calnan, M. and Bury, M. (eds) (1991) *The Sociology of the Health Service*, Routledge, London and New York.

Gabe, J., Kellcher, D. and Williams, G. (1994) *Challenging Medicine*, Routledge, London.

Glennerster, H., Matsaganis, M. and Owens, P. (1992) *A Foothold for Fundholding: a preliminary report on the introduction of GP fundholding*, King's Fund Institute, London.

Griffiths, R. (1992) Speech to the Audit Commission in 1991 published in full under the title 'Seven Years of Progress: General Management in the NHS', *Health Economics*, 1(1), pp. 61–70.

Ham, C. (1992) *Health and Policy in Britain, The politics and organisation of the NHS*, Macmillan, 3rd edn.

Harrison, S., Hunter, D. J. and Pollitt, C. (1990) *The Dynamics of British Health Policy*, Unwin & Hyman, London.

Harrison, S., Hunter, D. J., Marnock, G. and Pollitt, C. J. (1992) *Just Managing: Power and Culture in the National Health Service*, Macmillan, London.

Haywood, S. and Alaszewski, A. (1980) *Crisis in the Health Service*, Croom Helm, London.

Henwood, M. (1992) *Through a Glass Darkly: community care and elderly people*, Research Report No 14, King's Fund Institute, London.

Higgins, J. (1988) *The Business of Medicine: private health care in Britain*, Macmillan Education, London.

H.M. Treasury (1991) *Competing for Quality: Buying Better Public Services*, Cmnd 1730, HMSO, London.

Jacobson, B., Smith, A. and Whitehead, M. (eds) (1991) *The Nation's Health: a strategy for the 1990s*, King's Fund Institute, London.

Johnson, T. J. (1972) *Professions and Power*, Macmillan, London.

Kanter, R. M. (1990) *When Giants Learn to Dance: mastering the challenges of strategy, management and careers in the 1990s*, Unwin Hyman, London.

Klein, R. (1989) *The politics of the NHS*, 2nd edn, Longman, London.

Le Grand, J. (1982) *Strategies of Equality: redistribution and the social services*, Allen & Unwin, London.

Le Grand, J. and Bartlett, W. (1993) *Quasi-Markets and Social Policy*, Macmillan, London.

Leathard, A. (1990) *Health Care Provision: past, present and future*, Chapman & Hall, London.

Lipsky, M. (1980) *Street-level Bureaucracy*, Russell Sage Foundation, New York.

Lukes, S. (1974) *Power: a radical view*, Macmillan, London.

McKeown, T. (1979) *The Role of Medicine dream, mirage or nemesis?*, Blackwell, Oxford.

Mills, M. (ed.) (1993) *Prevention, Health and British Politics*, Avebury, Aldershot.

Navarro, V. (1978) *Class Struggle, the State and Medicine*, Robertson, Oxford.

O'Connor, J. (1973) *The Fiscal Crisis of the State*, St Martin's Press, New York.

Offe, C. (1984) *Contradictions of the Welfare State* (edited and translated by J. Keane) Hutchinson, London.

Parry, N. and Parry, J. (1976) *The Rise of the Medical Profession*, Croom Helm, London.

Pater, J.E. (1981) *The Making of the National Health Service*, King's Fund Historical Series I, King Edward's Hospital Fund for London.

Paton, C. (1992) *Competition and planning: the danger of unplanned markets*, Chapman & Hall, London.

Payer, L. (1988) *Medicine and Culture: varieties of treatment in the United States, England, West Germany and France*, Henry Holt & Co., New York.

Perrin, J. (1988) *Resource Management in the NHS*, Van Nostrand Reinhold, Wokingham.

Peters, T. J. and Waterman, R. H. (1982) *In Search of Excellence*, Harper & Row, New York.

Pollitt, C. J. (1993) *Managerialism and the Public Services: Cuts or cultural change*? 2nd edn, Blackwell, Oxford.

Pollitt, C. and Harrison, S. (1994) *Controlling Health Professionals*, Open University Press, Milton Keynes.

Ranade, W. (1994) *A Future for the NHS? Health care in the 1990s*, Longman, London.

Robinson, R. and Judge, K. (1987) *Public Expenditure and the NHS: trends and prospects*, King's Fund Institute, London.

Rodmell, S. and Watt, A. (eds) (1986) *The Politics of Health Education: raising the issues*, London: Routledge & Kegan Paul.

Saltman, R. B. and von Otter, C. (1992) *Planned Markets and Public Competition: Strategic reform in Northern European health systems*, Open University Press, Milton Keynes.

Stacey, M. (1991) *The Sociology of Health and Healing*, Routledge, London and New York.

Stanton Rogers, W. (1991) *Explaining Health and Illness: an exploration in diversity*, Harvester Wheatsheaf, London.

Stimson, G. and Webb, B. (1975) *Going to See Doctor: the consultation process in general practice*, Routledge & Kegan Paul, London.

Strong, P. and Robinson, J. (1990) *The NHS: under new management*, Open University Press, Milton Keynes.

Wadsworth, M. (1991) *The Imprint of Time*, Open University Press, Milton Keynes.

Watkin, B. (1978) *The National Health Service: the first phase – 1948 – 1974 and after*, Allen & Unwin, London.

Weale, A. (1988) *Cost and Choice in Health Care*, King's Fund Institute, London.

Webster, C. (1988) *The Health Services since the War*. Vol. 1, *Problems of Health Care: the national health service before 1957*, HMSO, London.

Whitehead, M. (1992) 'The Health Divide', 2nd edn, in *Inequalities in Health*, Penguin, London.

Wildavsky, A. (1980) *The Art and Craft of Policy Analysis*, Macmillan, London.

INDEX